# Health, Coping, and Well-Being

*Perspectives From Social Comparison Theory*

# Health, Coping, and Well-Being

## *Perspectives From Social Comparison Theory*

*Edited by*

Bram P. Buunk
*University of Groningen*

Frederick X. Gibbons
*Iowa State University*

Routledge
Taylor & Francis Group
NEW YORK AND LONDON

First Published by
Lawrence Erlbaum Associates, Inc., Publishers

This editions first published in 2009 by Psychology Press

Published 2016 by Routledge
711 Third Avenue, New York, NY 10017, USA
2 Park Square, Milton Park, Abingdon, Oxfordshire OX14 4RN

First issued in paperback 2016

*Routledge is an imprint of the Taylor and Francis Group, an informa business*



Cover design by Kathryn Houghtaling

**Library of Congress Cataloging-in-Publication Data**

Health, coping, and well-being : perspectives from social comparison theory / edited by Bram P. Buunk, Frderick X. Gibbons.
p. cm.
Includes bibliographical references and index.
ISBN 0-8058-1858-8 (alk. paper)
1. Clinical health psychology. 2. Social perception. 3. Self-perception. 4. Comparison (Psychology) 5. Health attitudes. 6. Health behavior. I. Buunk, Bram. II. Gibbons, Frederick X.
R726.7.H432 1997
362.1'042–dc21 96-54802
CIP

**Publisher's Note**
The publisher has gone to great lengths to ensure the quality of this reprint but points out that some imperfections in the original may be apparent.

ISBN 13: 978-1-138-97589-7 (pbk)
ISBN 13: 978-0-8058-1858-1 (hbk)

# Contents

# Preface

The idea for this book arose in 1993, during the meetings of the Society for Experimental Social Psychology, when we were having lunch on a pier in Santa Barbara. Both of us were involved in research in the boundary area of health and social psychology. Both of us were using social comparison theory as a theoretical framework in this research, and both of us had the clear impression that we were not alone. As many other researchers seemed to be heading in the same direction, we began to consider the idea of bringing together in a single volume the various perspectives and approaches that shared a common theme: applying social comparison theory to health-related issues.

Such a volume seemed timely for a variety of reasons. Social comparison theory has a long history in social psychology, and remains one of its most treasured theoretical constructions ("everybody's second favorite . . ."). It has considerable heuristic value. As much as any theory, it illustrates what is the central mission of our discipline—examining the influence of social factors on thinking, feeling, and behaving. Despite the central role that the theory plays in social psychology, however, its impact was not fully realized and appreciated until fairly recently. In the more than 40 years since Leon Festinger proposed the theory in an original paper, there have been only two volumes on social comparison theory, one edited by Jerry Suls and Rowland Miller in 1977, the other edited by Jerry Suls and Thomas Wills in 1991. Both books were very successful, sparking new interest in the theory, and were critical in its development. In many ways, the current volume is a direct result of the work prompted by each of these earlier volumes. The Suls and Wills book, in particular, stimulated a number of new ideas and new studies; hence the need now for a new collection. We hope this volume is as successful and useful as its predecessors.

About the time the Suls and Wills book appeared, the theory seemed to be heading in a slightly different direction. In particular, a significant number of researchers, including several contributors to that book, were becoming increasingly interested in health-related issues. That trend has clearly continued in the 1990s. In fact, literature searches with PsychLit indicate that mental and physical health, in a broad sense, is indeed one of the most popular focuses of empirical studies in the area of social comparison theory. The specific goal of this volume is to bring together some of the research that has been done on this topic in the past decade.

Despite their common focus on social comparison and health, the chapters of this book present many different perspectives within social comparison theory. Rather than a single narrowly defined statement, the theory constitutes a broad perspective on human behavior that has undergone a number of important developments, especially in the past decade, and that has become increasingly linked with recent work in social cognition. The present volume also illustrates the broad range of health-related issues to which social comparison theory is applied. Some of these issues and topics are health protective behaviors, such as condom use, and health impairing behaviors, such as smoking and drinking; perceptions of risk; coping with serious diseases, such as cancer and chronic pain disorders; preparation for surgery and postoperative recovery; stress coping during adolescence; seeking medical care; occupational stress and burnout; and depression and well-being.

Social comparison theory has both benefited from and contributed to the development of health psychology. On one hand, the research discussed in these chapters has furthered our understanding of the relation between health and behavior. On the other hand, health research in this applied context has made significant contributions to the development of the theory itself. As we hope the present volume testifies, the health area has become a fruitful arena for examining many theoretical issues and controversies that have long plagued and, at the same time, promoted social comparison theory. In fact, we would argue that many of the major theoretical developments in social comparison theory during the past two decades were achieved through examining comparison processes in the context of health and disease. Thus, we are hopeful that the present volume will contribute not only to the continued development of health psychology but to the evolution of social comparison theory as well.

We have tried to integrate the book as fully as possible by having all authors read and comment on the other chapters in the book most relevant to their own. We thank all contributors for helping us in this way and thereby sharing some of the editorial task. Of course, the final editorial responsibility is fully ours. We would also like to thank our departments for providing us with the necessary resources to complete this book. In addition, we thank Monica Reis-Bergan especially for all her help in the editing process. Finally, we would like to thank Jorie and Meg for their support all along the way.

*Bram P. Buunk*
*Frederick X. Gibbons*

# CHAPTER 1

# Social Comparison in Health and Illness: A Historical Overview

Bram P. Buunk
*University of Groningen*

Frederick X. Gibbons
Monica Reis-Bergan
*Iowa State University*

As the rapid growth of health psychology over the past few decades indicates, issues of health and disease have become major topics in contemprary psychological research (Adler & Matthews, 1994). Health psychology has been described as "devoted to understanding psychological influences on how people stay healthy, why they become ill, and how they respond when they do get ill" (Taylor, 1991, p. 6). According to some authors, health psychology is largely applied social psychology (Stroebe & Stroebe, 1995; cf. Salovey, Rothman, & Rodin, in press), or, more specifically, applied social cognition (Clark, 1994). Indeed, a number of social psychological theories have been applied productively to a wide range of health-related issues. Social-cognitive theories have been utilized to enhance our understanding of the coping process (see Clark, 1993); the theory of reasoned action has been used to understand behaviors aimed at weight loss and weight control (e.g., Sejwacz, Ajzen, & Fishbein, 1980); social learning theory has been invoked to understand the adoption of disease-prevention behaviors, such as exercise, cessation of cigarette smoking, and seat belt use (e.g., McAlister, 1987); behavioral decision theory has been applied to the perception of health risks (Slovic, Fischhoff, & Lichtenstein, 1987); self-identification theory has been used to illuminate the nature of stress (Schlenker, 1987); and attribution theory has been employed as a framework for understanding responses to victimization (e.g., Janoff-Bulman & Wortman, 1977).

It has become increasingly clear that among these many different social psychological approaches, social comparison theory is one of the most fruitful and most important for application to health-related cognitions and behaviors. As Clark (1994), among others, has "research on social comparison has shown a recent resurgence in the context of health psychology" (p. 242). Providing an overview of current research in this area, the present volume testifies to the significance of this resurgence. The research discussed in the book illustrates the myriad issues related to physical as well as mental health that, in one way or another, involve social comparison processes. In particular, there are studies that focus on smoking and AIDS risk behaviors; responses to one's own physical symptoms as related to the decision to seek medical help; adapting to serious diseases such as cancer; managing anxiety when facing surgery; coping with chronic pain disorders; and mental health and well-being, including depression and occupational burnout. This chapter offers a historical perspective of social comparison theory and outlines the theoretical and empirical developments that have stimulated and informed the research described in the book's subsequent chapters.

Within the general domain of social comparison, a number of theoretical traditions have had an especially strong impact on current research on health, coping, and well-being. Most noteworthy are four such traditions:

1. Early work on reference groups—much of it sociological—and, of course, Festinger's original theorizing and research.
2. Schachter's (1959) pioneering work on affiliation under stress, as well as his later work on emotional contagion (Schachter & Singer, 1962).
3. Downward comparison theory, including the early studies on downward comparison choices under threat (e.g., Hakmiller, 1966), as well as the very influential papers by Brickman and Bulman (1977) and Wills (1981), and the seminal work of Taylor, Wood, and Lichtman (1983) with cancer patients.
4. Work in social cognition, including research showing false consensus for undesirable attributes (e.g., Suls, Choi, & Sanders, 1988), and research on health risks, especially the research begun by Weinstein (1980) on unrealistic optimism.

In this chapter we outline these developments in social comparison theory briefly, and describe their relevance for the study of health-related issues. Throughout, we refer to research programs described in the book's other chapters so as to place them in some historical perspective.

## EARLY WORK ON REFERENCE GROUPS AND SOCIAL COMPARISON

### Reference Groups

Although it was Festinger (1954) who used the term *social comparison* for the first time, the notion that comparisons with others play an important role in evaluating and constructing reality goes back to Sherif (1936). In a series of classic experiments, Sherif demonstrated that two individuals who face the same unstable situation together develop, in a process of mutual social influence, a single characteristic reference point. Sherif showed that individuals faced with the autokinetic effect (a stable point of light in a dark room is perceived as moving) develop a unique reference point to which each successive experienced movement is compared. However, when an individual faces this situation together with another individual, they appear to develop a joint reference point that is peculiar to the dyad. Comparison processes were also highlighted in the sociological research on reference groups that was prompted by the work of Hyman (1942). In his classic paper, Hyman argued that the assessment of one's own status on such dimensions as financial position, intellectual capability, and physical attractiveness depends on the group with whom one compares oneself. In the same decade, the American Soldier studies (Stouffer, Suchman, DeVinney, Star, & Williams, 1949) provided evidence for what later was interpreted as the importance of social comparisons for satisfaction, or what we now would call subjective well-being. For example, African American soldiers in that study who were from northern states reported less satisfaction with their situations than did their counterparts from the south, supposedly because both compared themselves with Blacks outside the Army, a reference group that was, at the time, considerably worse off in the south. In subsequent work, particularly in sociology, the influence of reference groups on behavior continued to be an important issue (e.g., Singer, 1980).

In the current volume, the influence of this early work is most apparent in the chapter by Diener and Fujita on subjective well-being (chapter 11) and the chapter by Misovich, Fisher, and Fisher (chapter 4) on social comparison and AIDS preventive behavior. Misovich et al. make a strong case for the role of reference groups in influencing not only initial levels of AIDS awareness but attitudes and norms regarding AIDS risk perceptions and AIDS prevention. These investigators also show that interventions using social comparison, either in real life or on videotape, have a number of favorable effects. For example, because they enhance normative support for AIDS preventive behaviors, increase perceived vulnerability, and improve behavioral skills, they can be quite effective in reducing AIDS risk. On the other hand, Diener and Fujita find little evidence that social comparisons affect well-being directly. According to these authors, early empirical evidence of this impact was typically of a post hoc nature.

## Social Comparison Theory

Mettee and Smith (1977) provided one of the more useful definitions of social comparison theory; they suggest that it is a theory about "our quest to know ourselves, about the search for self-relevant information and how people gain self-knowledge and discover reality about themselves" (pp. 69–70). The theory states that individuals are driven by a desire for self-evaluation, a motivation to establish that their opinions are correct and to know precisely what they are capable of doing. According to Festinger (1954), individuals prefer objective information when evaluating their standing on a given attribute, but will, when such information is not available, turn to others for social information. In fact, the research described in this volume suggests that, if anything, Festinger may have underestimated both the strength of this motive to acquire social information and the impact such information can have on those who seek it.

Although Festinger (1954) did not relate social comparison to issues of health and disease, his theory would seem directly relevant to many health-related concerns because such concerns usually imply a strong need for self-evaluation. For instance, following Festinger's argument, one would expect that if people were interested in evaluating their chances of contracting a certain disease, they would compare themselves and their risk with other people they thought similar to themselves, that is, people of the same age and gender, and people with similar physical characteristics and risk behaviors. In a similiar vein, Suls, Martin, and Leventhal (see chapter 7) apply some of Festinger's original ideas to a discussion of how individuals may employ social comparison information when they are experiencing physical symptoms that are ambiguous or difficult to interpret, asking themselves such questions as, "Am I sick?" and "Should I go to a doctor?" According to Suls et al., the advice of social comparison others—the so-called lay referral network—can either inhibit or promote medical referral. This may account in part for the fact that many people visit their physicians when they are not ill, whereas others who are suffering from potentially serious symptoms fail to seek appropriate health care.

## STRESS, AFFILIATION, AND THE NEED FOR SOCIAL COMPARISON

The second theoretical tradition in social comparison theory that has relevance for health and coping was the pioneering work of Schachter (1959) on stress and affiliation. Indeed, despite the potential importance of the early work on social comparison and reference groups for health-related issues, the link between social comparison theory and health was not established explicitly until Schachter began investigating the ways in which social comparison is involved in the reaction to stress. Schachter's work stemmed from the convergence of two somewhat different research interests: first, the social comparison of opinions, and second, the dramatic effects of sensory deprivation. Schachter wondered whether social deprivation would have effects similar to those of sensory deprivation. He decided that the importance of social deprivation could best be studied by confronting an individual with a novel situation and then examining the strength of his or her desire for affiliation, that is his or her need to be with other people (Jones & Gerard, 1967). In his experiments with women students, Schachter showed that fear caused by the prospect of having to undergo an electric shock evoked in most people the desire to wait with someone else, and preferably someone anticipating the same event rather than someone in a different situation. As Schachter (1959) concluded: "Misery doesn't love just any kind of company, it loves only miserable company" (p. 24). Furthermore, Schachter argued and tried to demonstrate that social comparison was the main motive behind affiliation under stress, and in particular that this motive was more important than the desire for cognitive clarity about the nature of the threat. In line with the social comparison hypothesis, later studies have shown that fear of an electric shock leads to a desire for the company of others, especially when uncertainty about one's responses is induced experimentally, for instance by providing false feedback suggesting that one has quite unstable emotional reactions (Gerard, 1963), or by not providing any information about the responses of others (Gerard & Rabbie, 1961; see also Mills & Mintz, 1972).

### Health-Related Research

In retrospect, Schachter's work, which emphasized the threat of impending distress, has clear relevance for issues in health psychology, and, in fact this paradigm has certainly influenced a number of research traditions in the health area. That impact is readily apparent in this book. For example, in chapter 13, Ahrens and Alloy point out that depressed people experience a more or less chronically high level of distress, and are more interested in and more open to social comparison information than are nondepressed people. Buunk and his colleagues have examined affiliative desires in relation to coping with various types of stress, including marital and occupational stress. These researchers have shown that uncertainty over one's feelings and responses is associated with an enhanced desire for social comparison information and for affiliation with similar others (for a review, see Buunk, 1994; see also chapter 12, this volume). Furthermore, it must be noted that Schachter's (1959) original research led eventually to his classic 1962 experiment with Jerome Singer, which showed that when the cause of arousal is ambiguous, comparison with similar others can influence the way people interpret that arousal and the emotional label they place on it. Following on these experiments, a large number of studies have examined the role that attributions of arousal play in emotional experience (for a review, see Reisenzein, 1984). As Suls (1977) noted, however, it is ironic that Schachter and Singer's experiment is usually linked to attribution theory, when it really followed logically from Schachter's theorizing on social comparison. An important general implication of the work of Schachter and Singer is that especially when individuals are uncertain about their internal states, they may be very susceptible to the way others respond. Indeed, in this book's chapters by Suls et al. (chapter 7), and by Buunk and Ybema (chapter 12), the work of Schachter and Singer is related to situations in which individuals "adopt" the symptoms shown by others around them, such as occurs in the case of mass psychogenic illness.

The research program of Kulik and his colleagues on stress and affiliation in hospital settings (e.g., Kulik & Mahler, 1987a; Kulik, Mahler, & Earnest, 1994; see also chapter 8) appears to be the most directly influenced by Schachter's work. The research of these investigators focuses more on the informational value of affiliation, however, and as a result, they reach conclusions that differ from Schachter's. Employing an impressive variety of methods, including both laboratory studies and field research, Kulik and Mahler's research indicates that even though Schachter's research is still influential (after more than 35 years), some of his original ideas do not seem to apply well to real-life settings, and that the evidence for a number of widely cited conclusions from Schachter's research is scarce. For example, Schachter's conclusions that people prefer to affiliate with others under similar stress, and that the desire for cognitive clarity is a relatively unimportant element of this preference has been challenged. Various studies discussed by Kulik and Mahler (chapter 8) indicate that individuals who are anticipating some stressful event (such as surgery) actually prefer to affiliate with people who have the most information about the threat the subjects face. Not surprisingly, these are often people who have already experienced the stressor (e.g., postoperative patients) rather than similar others who are awaiting the same stressful event.

**The Support Group Phenomenon**

Schachter's work is directly relevant to the field of self-help and support groups. The proliferation of such groups over the last 15 to 20 years seems in itself clear evidence of the importance of affiliation with similar others for coping with stress. Surprisingly, however, the increase in lay interest in what is clearly a social-psychological phenomenon has not really been matched by an increase in empirical work by social psychologists. Indeed, the two major explanations proposed for why individuals facing some type of threat often decide to join support groups involve social comparison processes, and follow more or less directly from Schachter's (1959) work on fear and affiliation (cf. Medvene, 1992). The first explanation is that contact with others who are facing similar problems reduces anxiety by means of a shared stress type of process (cf. Coates & Winston, 1983). As noted above, a major implication of the work of Schachter is that individuals under stress often prefer contact with others in a broadly similar situation. Although this implication needs to be qualified, there is indeed evidence that people with similar problems are most effective at providing social support, and that is particularly true with regard to health problems. For example, evidence of this comes from research with quadriplegic psychotherapy clients (Rogers & Figone, 1978), and spinal cord-injured persons (Rohrer et al., 1980).

The second explanation of support group popularity is that participation in such groups reduces feelings of uniqueness or deviance (Medvene, 1992), but although a number of researchers have discussed this hypothesis few have actually examined it. In one notable exception, Barrett (1978) found that widows who had participated in support groups reported having fewer feelings of "unique experience" after their group disbanded. In another, Coates and Winston (1983) found that self-perceptions of deviance did decline among rape victims over the course of a support group. In discussing the topic, Coates and Winston suggested that people who have been victimized in some way suffer from a profound sense of uniqueness or deviance. One reason for this perception, according to Coates and Winston (1983), is that these people seldom have an opportunity to come in contact with others like themselves. Just seeing others around them who are experiencing some of the same difficulties allows them to feel less abnormal or deviant (Croyle, 1992).

Despite the impact of research using the stress–affiliation paradigm, we feel that its relevance for health psychology has not yet been fully appreciated. To begin with, except for the work of Kulik and his colleagues, very little attention has been focused on stress and affiliation in medical settings. Second, most of the numerous studies on social support have been concerned with the effects of support and not with the strength and nature of the desire for affiliation under stress. In fact, with a few exceptions (e.g., Buunk & Hoorens, 1992; Medvene, 1992; Stewart, 1989), social comparison theory has been notably absent in discussions of social support and of support group processes. One reason for this may be that social comparison theory, as noted by Taylor, Buunk, and Aspinwall (1990), suggests a much more active role of the person under stress than most social support research assumes. Third, although uncertainty is considered to be a characteristic aspect of stressful events (e.g., Lazarus & Folkman, 1984), and although Schachter suggested that it is especially uncertainty that generates social comparison needs, with the exception of the work by Buunk and his colleagues (Buunk, 1994), very few studies have examined the basic question of whether uncertainty about one's feelings, beliefs, and responses does in fact foster affiliation among individuals experiencing stress in real life. Finally, the influence of social comparison theory on the study of the development of physical symptoms has been quite limited; the important work of Pennebaker (1982) is a prime exception.

## DOWNWARD SOCIAL COMPARISON

The third research tradition that has significantly affected current thinking on social comparison as related to health and illness is downward comparison theory. Most of the research following on the work of Schachter (1959) emphasized the role of comparison with other people in a situation similar to that of the subject without paying much attention to whether these others were better or worse off than the subject. Festinger (1954) had emphasized that individuals compare in general *upward*. However, in a pioneering study, Hakmiller (1960) demonstrated that when individuals are threatened on a particular dimension they prefer to compare with others whom they believe are worse than they are on that dimension. The purpose of these downward comparisons, Hakmiller thought, was to allow individuals to feel better about themselves. This notion gained explicit attention when Thornton and Arrowood (1966) pointed out the potential conflict between the self-evaluation social comparison motive—finding out how well one is doing—and the self-enhancement motive—feeling good about how one is doing. These researchers conducted an experiment that showed that when a trait was pictured positively (e.g., as "social intelligence") many more persons wanted to see the score of someone who scored higher on this trait than when the trait was pictured negatively (e.g., as evidence of "neurotic conflicts"). Thornton and Arrowood suggested that in this last case, individuals avoided comparisons with others they thought were neurotic because this might provide some evidence of similarity to themselves. This important issue of perceived similarity to comparison targets—both upward and downward—appears in the research and theorizing of several contributors to this volume (Ahrens & Alloy; Aspinwall; Buunk & Ybema; Gibbons & Gerrard; Kulik & Mahler; Misovich et al.), and we discuss it later in this chapter.

A decade after these pioneering studies, Brickman and Bulman's (1977) chapter entitled "Pleasure and Pain in Social Comparison" elaborated the limitations of Festinger's basic assumption that comparison choice will typically be oriented toward superior others (i.e., upward comparison), because this type of comparison is most informative. Brickman and Bulman believed that comparison with others who are thought to be doing better, although potentially informative, can also be threatening. For this reason, such comparisons are often avoided, especially by persons who feel threatened in other ways. Instead, such people may seek comparisons with others who they think are worse off (see also Wilson & Benner, 1971).

## Coping

What eventually developed out of Hakmiller's work and Brickman and Bulman's chapter was a major modification of social comparison theory. This new direction was given further impetus by Wills' (1981) integrative paper on downward social comparison theory. Wills argued that in situations that produce a decrease in well-being, individuals will often compare with others who are they think are worse off in an effort to improve their well-being, particularly when they see no opportunity to take instrumental action. Wills' ideas had, and continue to have, direct relevance to research on coping.

***Downward Comparison and Coping.*** According to Lazarus and Folkman (1984), coping entails "constantly changing cognitive and behavioral efforts to manage specific external and/or internal demands that are appraised as taxing or exceeding the resources of the person" (p. 141). These writers suggest that there are two forms of coping: Problem-focused coping is aimed at managing or altering the problem that is causing the distress; emotion-focused coping is directed at regulating emotional responses to the problem. According to Wills, when problem-focused coping is not feasible (for whatever reason), individuals will engage in downward comparison as a means of improving negative mood. As Wills suggests in this book (chapter 6), this mood amelioration can act as an emotion-focused coping process. In so doing, it may facilitate the development of subsequent strategies that are actually more problem focused (see particularly chapter 9 by Tennen & Affleck, and chapter 14 by Leventhal, Hudson,& Robitaille for more discussion of definitions and theories of coping).

***Downward Comparison Among Cancer Patients.*** Although Wills' reasoning was provocative, at the time that his paper was published there was no direct evidence of downward comparisons in populations that were actively experiencing stress. Thus, a very important development in downward comparison theory was the research by Taylor and her colleagues, conducted among people who were experiencing a very real threat of decline and death from cancer. This work, which began with Taylor, Wood, and Lichtman's (1983) research with women breast cancer patients and their husbands (see also Wood, Taylor, & Lichtman, 1985), provided the first systematic investigation of downward comparison outside of the laboratory. Taylor et al. undertook their research to examine the psychological aspects of the strategies these people were using in coping with their disease. Although somewhat unexpected, evidence of downward, or favorable comparison (in which the self is better off than others) was quite apparent in this group. For example, when asked how well they were coping with their problems in comparison with other breast cancer victims, 80% of the women interviewed reported they were doing "somewhat" or "much" better than other women.

Perhaps more important, an analysis of the comments these women made *spontaneously* during the interview indicated that the vast majority of them had engaged in some kind of downward comparison with other cancer victims. No matter how serious these women's problems were, they believed that there were others who were worse off. If they did not know of a specific person who had been more seriously afflicted, they imagined others, or even fabricated a target. Although when the women's husbands were asked how well they were coping with their wife's illness, many admitted having a lot of difficulty, more than a quarter also claimed that they were not having nearly as much trouble as many other men they knew. One man said he was "much better off than those animals who leave their wives because of it." In fact, less than 4% of the marriages in the sample actually broke up as a consequence of the women's cancer. Thus, the stereotype of the poor coper with whom these men were comparing—or at least their estimates of the prevalence of bad copers—was apparently largely a figment of their imaginations. As a result, Taylor et al. referred to these fabricated downward comparison targets as "mythical men." The researchers concluded that comparison with these targets in particular and downward comparison in general somehow helped the women's husbands cope with their problems, perhaps, as Wills (1981) suggested, by allowing them to feel better about themselves and their own situation.

### Downward Versus Upward Comparisons

The conclusions from the pioneering research of Taylor and her colleagues that downward comparisons can facilitate coping efforts were supported by a number of subsequent field studies in populations facing different kinds of threat. Because several of the book's chapters describe these studies, we mention only a few examples here. For instance, research conducted in different types of support groups has indicated that participants with fairly serious behavioral problems (e.g., eating disorders—Gerrard, Gibbons, & Sharp, 1985; and smoking—Gibbons, Gerrard, Lando, & McGovern, 1991) prefer that their group include other members who have serious problems. Moreover, this downward preference declines over time, as perceived seriousness of the problem declines. Studies among victimized populations have shown that downward comparisons are, in fact, quite prevalent in such groups as mothers with medically fragile infants (Affleck, Tennen, Pfeiffer, Fifield, & Rowe, 1987), arthritis patients (DeVellis et al., 1991), and disabled individuals with a high degree of stress (Buunk & Ybema, 1995). One reason for this may be that the information that another individual is doing worse can help alleviate negative affect (e.g., Gibbons, 1986; for an overview, see Gibbons & Gerrard, 1991). In addition, Strack, Schwarz, Chassein, Kern, and Wagner (1990) found that subjects reported feeling better about their own situation when they were exposed to another person who had a serious health problem (i.e., a kidney disease, or being confined to a wheelchair). Similarly, Suls, Marco, and Tobin (1991) found that older persons' assessments of their health were more positive if they were presented with similar comparison targets who were in relatively poor health. As Aspinwall pointed out, however (see chapter 5), such positive reactions are more likely to occur among individuals who are experiencing threat.

Although these findings are quite strong and convincing, there is also a substantial amount of evidence suggesting that individuals who are experiencing stress may have a preference for upward comparisons. Again, we provide just a few examples. Ahrens and Alloy (chapter 13) note that depressed people often choose to compare upward rather than downward. This finding may be due to the dispositional tendency of depressed people to engage in negative thinking. Nevertheless, Wheeler and Miyake (1992) found that respondents reported that they were more likely to compare upward when they felt bad and downward when they felt good. Furthermore, Buunk, VanYperen, Taylor, and Collins (1991) showed that individuals with a high degree of marital stress preferred upward affiliation more than did individuals with a low degree of marital stress, whereas Ybema and Buunk (1993) found that individuals who had failed academically were more interested in upward comparison information than were those who had succeeded. There is also some evidence that the upward drive is particularly activated in situations in which there is some need or motivation to do better (cf. Nosanchuck & Erickson, 1985). Moreover, in a series of field experiments Ybema and Buunk (1995; Ybema, Buunk, & Heesink, 1996) found that disabled individuals and individuals facing a loss of their job experienced more positive mood after being confronted with an upward comparison rather than a downward comparison (see also chapter 12).

In an effort to reconcile such contradictory findings on the direction of social comparison under stress, Taylor and Lobel (1989) proposed a useful distinction between downward evaluations and upward affiliation. These investigators argued that individuals under stress will try to engage in both emotion-focused and problem-focused coping. On the one hand, affiliation with others coping well with their problems (or information about such others), can serve especially *problem-focused* coping. In particular, it may provide one with valuable clues to successful coping; it may also constitute a method for obtaining hope, motivation, and inspiration; and it may enhance the person's sense of self-efficacy. In short, it may serve as a means of improving one's current situation. This additional function of social comparison—*self-improvement*—was also addressed by Wood (1989), and was also identified earlier by Brickman and Bulman (1977), who emphasized that people seek social comparisons as one form of useful information that they can use to improve themselves. As they put it, "Comparison with superior others, although painful, is more valuable than comparison with inferior others, since more useful information may be acquired by observing superior others" (p. 179).

In line with Wills' original (1981) and current (chapter 6) reasoning, Taylor and Lobel (1989) suggested that individuals under stress often use social comparisons also as a means of *emotion-focused* coping, in order to alleviate the negative emotions that stress implies. For this goal, they will make self-enhancing downward evaluations by contrasting their situation with that of others they think are worse off, which, in turn, should make them feel better about themselves. According to Taylor and Lobel, these evaluations are not the result of actively seeking contact with worse-off others. Rather, they are based on unavoidable contacts with actual patients, or on the cognitive manufacturing of a comparison other who is doing worse. In other words, individuals may employ information about others they have met, but they may also cognitively construct hypothetical targets as well (Taylor et al., 1990). Thus, downward evaluations under stress seem primarily to reflect of a goal-directed, motivated, and dynamic process in which individuals aim to cognitively construct their situation as better than that of others. As Goethals, Messick, and Allison (1991) noted, "people wish to perceive themselves as superior to others, and they will in fact construct perceptions of themselves and social reality that support this wish to the maximum degree that physical and social reality permit" (p. 163). This notion of "constructive" social comparisons is apparent in many chapters of this book (e.g., Gibbons & Gerrard, chapter 3; Klein & Weinstein, chapter 2; Misovich et al., chapter 4).

Although the Taylor and Lobel approach does help in reconciling a number of contradictory findings on the direction of social comparison under stress and seems to incorporate Wills' model as well, Wood and VanderZee (chapter 10) argue that the Taylor and Lobel model still cannot account for a number of findings. First, Wood and VanderZee point out that the pattern of upward affiliation and downward evaluation is not only found under threat, but also among healthy, well-adjusted individuals. Second, Wood and VanderZee suggest that the major factor moderating the effects of social comparison information is whether one has the feeling that one can reach the target's level, which is in turn determined by the controllability of the dimension and the degree of contrast versus assimilation with the target.

***Similarity and Downward Comparison.*** Buunk and Ybema (chapter 12) come to similar conclusions in discussing the contradictory findings on the direction of social comparison under stress. In an effort to explain these findings, these researchers have proposed the identification–contrast model, which suggests that because people are motivated to feel superior to others, they will construe social comparison information as much as possible in this direction and will strongly resist acknowledging the superiority of others. Consequently, the more upward comparisons offer opportunity for identification with upward targets, the more people will prefer them, and the more opportunity downward comparisons they offer for contrast with downward targets the more people will favor them. Aspinwall (chapter 5) makes a similar point—as do Wood and VanderZee—but she focuses especially on the implications of social comparison for one's future standing on a dimension. For instance, Aspinwall argues that downward comparisons will evoke a negative response when they imply a possible downward shift in the future. As in various other models, a central dimension in the model proposed by Aspinwall is the amount of control that one has—or perceives one has—over one's situation. Finally, the theme that people often look for evidence of differences between themselves and a downward target and do so through a social comparison process is echoed in the work of Gibbons and his colleagues (Gibbons & Eggleston, 1996; Gibbons et al., 1991). These authors claim that people trying to overcome a health-relevant behavioral problem, such as smoking, engage in downward comparison with a prototype associated with the behavior (e.g., a "typical smoker") in an effort to distance themselves from that prototype and the group it represents. This form of downward comparison is thought to facilitate the quit attempt (see chapter 3, by Gibbons & Gerrard, for further discussion).

***The Meaning of Downward Comparisons.*** In line with a chapter by Wills (1987) that followed his classic downward comparison paper, most theoretical formulations have stated more or less explicitly that downward comparisons can and do function as a coping strategy in populations under stress. Two researchers who have investigated comparison processes among people with chronic illnesses, such as rheumatoid arthritis, are not entirely convinced of this, however. Tennen and Affleck argue in chapter 9 that if downward comparison is a coping strategy, it should behave like one; that is, it should be effortful, it should do more than just regulate mood, and it should bring about change in predictable ways over time in response to situational demands. Based on their review of the literature, Tennen and Affleck believe there is no convincing evidence that downward comparison does these things and thus conclude that it cannot be viewed as a coping strategy. In contrast, Wills (chapter 6), employing a number of data sets, comes to a very different conclusion: Because downward comparison items reliably load on the same factor as cognitive coping items, he holds, downward comparison should be seen as a form of cognitive coping. In part, the difference in opinion between Wills and Affleck and Tennen may be a matter of how one defines a coping strategy. It is not unlikely that many items of current coping inventories do not meet Tennen and Affleck's criteria for a coping strategy. For instance, many coping strategies as operationalized in these measures do not strike us as unequivocably effortful, nor do they necessarily seem to result in more than mood improvement. Indeed, as noted by Leventhal, Hudson, and Robitaille in their closing chapter (chapter 14), coping need not always be effortful. The debate on this issue should prove very productive for both coping and comparison researchers in the future.

***Comparative Ratings.*** Examining the impact of downward comparisons, many studies have assessed social comparisons by asking individuals to rate their situation in comparison to that of others. Tennen and Affleck (chapter 9) refer to such measures as *comparison conclusions*, Wood and VanderZee (chapter 10) use the term *comparative ratings*, whereas Buunk (1995) used the term *relative evaluations*. Diener and Fujita (chapter 11) and Wood and VanderZee (chapter 10) argue that such comparative ratings may not reflect the outcome of a comparison process at all, but—more so than other measures—something else, such as a positive mood. Although the meaning of comparative ratings may not be completely unambiguous, the evidence for positive associations between well-being and a feeling of being better off than most others is rather strong. To give just a few examples, Heidrich and Ryff (1993), Buunk (1995), and VanderZee, Buunk, and Sanderman (1995) all found that psychological well-being is affected directly by the perception of being better off than similar others, independent of physical health. Even more convincing, Affleck, Tennen, Pfeiffer, Fifield, and Rowe (1987) showed that persons with rheumatoid arthritis who thought their illness was less severe than that of other victims were rated by health care providers as more positively adjusted, even when data analysis controlled for the effects of disease activity, duration, and functional status of the patients. More generally, Tennen and Affleck point out (in chapter 9) that the conclusion that others are worse off is typically associated with positive adjustment. In a similar vein, Ahrens and Alloy (chapter 13) discuss the relation between depression and social comparison, and show that nondepressed people, in general, tend to see themselves as superior to others, whereas the self-perception of depressed individuals is more likely to include perceptions of inferiority. The influence of comparative evaluations on subjective well-being is discussed in detail in chapter 11 by Diener and Fujita.

We would suggest, that simply believing that there are others who are worse off is likely to benefit almost anyone who is experiencing problems. What this suggests is that a belief that one is relatively well off, which comes about through downward comparison, is an important step along the way to satisfactory adjustment. Although we cannot make a definitive statement at this point in time (and, indeed, the topic continues to generate a considerable amount of controversy and investigation), the research presented in this volume does shed considerable light on the issue of when downward comparisons will have favorable effects. In a nutshell, this research suggests that individuals are likely to receive some emotional benefit from such comparisons when they engage in some form of counterfactual thinking vis à vis the target, that is, when they believe there was, or is, some possibility that their own situation could have resembled that of the target but in fact will, or does, not. One implication of this is that individuals who believe their own situation will decline (such as those who are terminally ill or those who are depressed) are not likely to benefit from comparison with others who are more ill.

## SOCIAL COGNITION AND SOCIAL COMPARISON

Work on social cognition constitutes a fourth research tradition that has significantly influenced current health related work on social comparison. In the late 1980s and early 1990s, developments in social cognition research became linked to social comparison theory, particularly in the area of health, well-being, and illness. As will have become apparent, a recurrent theme in many of the chapters in this book is the idea that actual health status is strongly influenced by individuals' perceptions of how their status compares with that of others. Like other types of social information, people tend to have biased perceptions of others' health and health behavior that are often motivated, at a general level, by a desire to protect one's self-esteem, and at a more specific level, by an interest in creating favorable comparisons. These biased perceptions can affect all dimensions of health behavior and health cognitions, but they appear to be particularly influential in terms of behaviors that are either health-promoting or health-impairing.

### False Consensus

An oft-cited finding in the social cognition literature is that people tend to overestimate the extent to which their ideas and opinions are shared by others, a phenomenon known as the *false consensus effect* (Ross, Greene, & House, 1977). The same applies to perceptions of behavior. For example, people who align themselves with the Democratic party produce inflated estimates of the number of people who voted Democratic in the most recent election, just as people who smoke cigarettes or drink alcohol assume that those behaviors are more common than is actually the case (Marks, Graham, & Hansen, 1992; Sussman et al., 1988). One reason for this, at least with regard to health behaviors, is a belief that there is some safety in numbers. In other words, perceptions of prevalence and peril are negatively correlated. Research by Jemmott and Croyle and their colleagues (Jemmott, Croyle, & Ditto, 1986) offers experimental evidence in support of this interpretation of the false consensus effect. They have shown that when people are given bogus diagnoses suggesting they have some kind of ailment or susceptibility to an ailment, they tend to increase their estimates of the prevalence of that ailment in the population; then, the more prevalent they think the problem is, the less concerned they are about it.

The same basic process applies to health risk behavior. Overestimation of smoking prevalence by smokers, for example, is directly associated with an increase in smoking behavior—the more common the behavior is thought to be, the less dangerous it is thought to be, and the more likely one is to do it (Gibbons et al., 1995; Marks et al., 1992; Sherman, Presson, Chassin, Corty, & Olshavsksy, 1983). What this suggests is that when determining how safe their current health behavior is, people will use a form of comparison information—or, if necessary, create information—about what others are doing. The specific role that social comparison plays in this process is illustrated more clearly in the recent work on perceptions of risk by Weinstein and others.

### Illusion of Invulnerability

In an extensive program of research, Weinstein and his colleagues have documented a tendency for people to underestimate their vulnerability to negative events, ranging from tooth decay to terminal illness. A number of factors have been identified as contributing to this phenomenon, including false consensus of risk behaviors (for a review, see Weinstein, 1980). Certainly one of the more interesting factors has to do with how one's estimates of risk are influenced by comparison with others. Weinstein suggested that when people estimate their own risk for developing a disease, cancer for example, they are likely to compare their own vulnerability with that of other people. The target that is chosen, however, is usually not just another average person, like oneself; rather, it is someone whose behaviors and/or attributes make them especially likely to develop the disease. In other words, it is clearly a worse-off other, which is why Perloff (1987) suggested that the process is actually a form of downward comparison. Choosing to compare with a high-risk victim prototype is likely to leave the individual with a false sense of invulnerability–and this, in essence, is the basis of the illusion. Presumably, the less similar people believe they are to victim prototype, the safer they will feel and the less likely they are to take prophylactic actions (Janz & Becker, 1984). These issues are dealt with in depth by Klein and Weinstein in chapter 2. It is worth noting that this work of Weinstein and his colleagues, although not originating from social comparison theory, has moved more in the direction of examining issues relevant to the theory. In fact, their chapter deals with many classic issues in social comparison theory, such as determining which factors influence the choice of comparison others. A similar approach is taken by Misovich et al. (chapter 4), who argue that social comparisons, including target choice, have a significant impact on AIDS risk perceptions and risk behavior.

**Prototypes and Risk Behavior**

The notion that cognitive creations or images of social comparison targets can influence health behavior appears again in the research of Gibbons and Gerrard and their colleagues on adolescent health risk. This research indicates that risk images are prospectively related to health risk. For example, adolescents with a more positive image of the type of person who smokes or drives under the influence of alcohol are more likely to adopt or increase such behaviors than are people whose image is less favorable and less similar to themselves. On the other hand, for people who are trying to stop a risk behavior–adults who are trying to quit smoking, for example–those with a more negative image of the prototypical person who engages in the risk behavior (e.g., of the "typical smoker") are more likely to actually quit and maintain abstinence (Gibbons & Eggleston, 1996).

Gibbons and Gerrard's argument, which is outlined in chapter 3 (see also Gibbons, Helweg-Larsen, & Gerrard, 1995), is that these images influence behavior through a social comparison process. For example, although virtually all adolescents have an image of the typical teenage heavy drinker, whether that image actually affects an individual teenager's behavior depends on the extent to which she or he engages in social comparison. Those who are high in this tendency pay more attention to the images, and are more likely to compare themselves with it. Consequently, the nature of their images–how favorable they happen to be and how similar to the self (both are important)–is directly related to their decision to engage in the behavior.

## CONCLUSION

In a variety of ways, social comparison theory has augmented our knowledge about a number of important health outcomes, such as the determinants of health-impairing and health-protective behavior, and the ways in which people cope with stressful events. In fact, as this chapter has shown, social comparison theory is no longer a single, narrowly defined theory but rather is a broad perspective on human behavior that has undergone a number of important developments in the recent years and that has become increasingly linked to work in social cognition. As this volume aims to testify, social comparison theory has contributed significantly to the theoretical foundation of health psychology. At the same time, and at a more basic level, health, coping, and well-being currently constitute one of the major domains of social comparison research; moreover, research in this applied context has made significant contributions to the development of social comparison theory itself. Nevertheless, as noted by Leventhal et al. in their closing chapter, there still remain a number of fundamental theoretical issues to be resolved. For instance, an important question concerns to what extent social comparison actually deserves the independent role in health-related contexts that this volume attributes to it. According to Leventhal et al., people are not primarily social comparers, but rather problem solvers, who use social comparison as just one of many ways of dealing with the problems they are facing. Indeed, determining where social comparison processes "fit" in the taxonomy of coping and, more generally, health-related behaviors, will be important in conceptualizing a new generation of comparison studies. Nonetheless, although such issues remain to be considered in future research, this volume illustrates the various ways in which social comparison theory has already been applied productively to health-related issues, and also points out how these applications have contributed to our insight into the ways we all use social comparison information.

## REFERENCES

Adler, N., & Matthews, K. (1994). Health psychology: Why do some people get sick and some stay well? *Annual Review of Psychology, 45*, 229–259.

Affleck, G., Tennen, H., Pfeiffer, C., Fiflied, J., & Rowe, J. (1987). Downward comparison and coping with serious medical problems. *American Journal of Orthopsychiatry, 57*, 570–578.

Barrett, C. J. (1978). Effectiveness of widows' groups in facilitating change. *Journal of Consulting and Clinical Psychology, 46*, 20–31.

Brickman, P., & Bulman, R. J. (1977). Pleasure and pain in social comparison. In J. M. Suls

& R. L. Miller (Eds.), *Social comparison processes: Theoretical and empirical perspectives* (pp. 149–186). Washington, DC: Hemisphere.

Buunk, B. P. (1994). Social comparison processes under stress: Towards an integration of classic and recent perspectives. In W. Stroebe & M. Hewstone (Eds.), *European review of social psychology*: (Vol. 5, pp. 211–241). Chichester, UK: Wiley.

Buunk, B. P. (1995). Comparison direction and comparison dimension among disabled individuals: Towards a refined conceptualization of social comparison under stress. *Personality and Social Psychology Bulletin, 21,* 316–330.

Buunk, B. P., & Hoorens, V. (1992). Social support, social comparison and social exchange. *British Journal of Clinical Psychology, 31,* 445–457.

Buunk, B. P., Van Yperen, N. W., Taylor, S. E., & Collins, R. L. (1991). Social comparison and the drive upward revisited: Affiliation as a response to marital stress. *European Journal of Social Psychology, 21,* 529–546.

Buunk, B. P., & Ybema, J. F. (1995). Selective evaluation and downward comparison in coping with stress. *Journal of Applied Social Psychology, 25*(17), 1499–1517.

Clark, L. (1994). Social cognition and health psychology. In R. S. Wyer, Jr. & T. K. Srull (Eds.), *Handbook of social cognition: Vol. 2. Applications.* (pp. 239–288). Hillsdale, NJ: Lawrence Erlbaum Associates.

Coates, D., & Winston, T. (1983). Counteracting the deviance of depression: Peer support groups for victims. *Journal of Social Issues, 39,* 169–194.

Croyle, R. T. (1992). Appraisal of health threats: Cognition, motivation, and social comparison. *Cognitive Therapy and Research, 16,* 165–182.

Devellis, R. F., Blalock, S. J., Holt, K., Renner, B. R., Blanchard, L. W., & Klotz, M. L. (1991). Arthritis patients' reactions to unavoidable social comparisons. *Personality and Social Psychology Bulletin, 17,* 392–399.

Festinger, L. (1954). A theory of social comparison processes. *Human Relations, 7,* 117–140.

Gerard, H. B. (1963). Emotional uncertainty and social comparison. *Journal of Abnormal and Social Psychology, 66,* 586–592.

Gerard, H. B., & Rabbie, J. M. (1961). Fear and social comparison. *Journal of Abnormal and Social Psychology, 62,* 586–592.

Gerrard, M., Gibbons, F. X., & Sharp, J. (1985, August). *Social comparison in self help groups for bulimics.* Paper presented at the meeting of the American Psychological Association, Los Angeles, CA.

Gibbons, F. X. (1986). Social comparison and depression: Company's effect on misery. *Journal of Personality and Social Psychology, 51,* 140–148.

Gibbons, F. X., & Eggleston, T. J.(1996). Smoker networks and the "typical smoker": A prospective analysis of smoking cessation. *Health Psychology, 15,* 469–477.

Gibbons, F. X., & Gerrard, M. (1991). Downward comparison and coping with threat. In J. M. Suls & T. A. Wills (Eds.), *Social comparison: Contemporary theory and research* (pp. 317–345). Hillsdale, NJ: Lawrence Erlbaum Associates.

Gibbons, F. X., Gerrard, M., Lando, H. A., & McGovern, P. G. (1991). Social comparison and smoking cessation: The role of the "typical smoker." *Journal of Experimental Social Psychology, 27,* 239–258.

Gibbons, F. X., Helweg-Larsen, M., & Gerrard, M. (1995). Prevalence estimates and adolescent risk behavior: Cross-cultural differences in social influence. *Journal of Applied Psychology, 80,* 107–121.

Goethals, G. R., Messick, D. M., & Allison, S. T. (1991). The uniqueness bias: Studies of constructive social comparison. In J. M. Suls & T. A. Wills (Eds.), *Social comparison: Contemporary theory and research* (pp. 317–345). Hillsdale, NJ: Lawrence Erlbaum Associates.

Hakmiller, K. L. (1966). Threat as a determinant of downward comparison. *Journal of Experimental Social Psychology, (Supplement 1),* 32–39.

Heidrich, S. M., & Ryff, C. D. (1993). The role of social comparisons processes in the psychological adaptation of elderly adults. *Journal of Gerontology, 48,* 127–136.

Hyman, H. (1942). The psychology of subjective status. *Psychological Bulletin, 39,* 473–474.

Janoff-Bulman, R., & Wortman, C. B. (1977). Pleasure and pain in social comparison. In J. M. Suls & R. L. Miller (Eds.), *Social comparison processes: Theoretical and empirical perspectives* (pp. 149–186). Washington, DC: Hemisphere.

Janz, N. K., & Becker, M. H. (1984). The health belief model: A decade later. *Health Education Quarterly, 11,* 1–47.

Jemmott, J. B., Croyle, R. T., & Ditto, P. H. (1988). Commonsense epidemiology: Self-based judgements from laypersons and physicians. *Health Psychology, 7,* 55–73.

Jones, E. E., & Gerard, H. B. (1967). *Foundations of social psychology.* New York: Wiley.

Kulik, J. A., & Mahler, H. I. (1987a). Effects of preoperative roommate assignment on preoperative anxiety and recovery from coronary-bypass surgery. *Health Psychology, 6,* 525–543.

Kulik, J. A., & Mahler, H. I. (1987b). Health status, perceptions of risk, and prevention interest for health and nonhealth problems. *Health Psychology, 6,* 15–27.

Kulik, J. A., Mahler, H. I., & Earnest, A. (1994). Social comparison and affiliation under threat: Going beyond the affiliate-choice paradigm. *Journal of Personality and Social Psychology, 66,* 301–309.

Lazarus, R. S., & Folkman, S. (1984). *Stress, appraisal and coping.* New York: Springer-Verlag.

Marks, G., Graham, J., & Hansen, W. (1992). Social projection and social conformity in adolescent alcohol use: A longitudinal analysis. *Personality and Social Psychology Bulletin, 18,* 92–101.

McAlister, A. (1987). Social learning theory and preventive behavior. In N. D. Weinstein (Ed.), *Taking care: Understanding and encouraging self-protective behavior* (pp. 42–53). New York: Cambridge University Press.

Medvene, L. (1992). Self-help groups, peer helping, and social comparison. In S. Spacapan, & S. Oskamp (Eds.), *Helping and being helped: Naturalistic studies. The Claremont Symposium on applied psychology* (pp. 49–81). Newbury Park, CA: Sage.

Mettee, D. R., & Smith, G. (1977). Social comparison and interpersonal attraction: The case for dissimilarity. In J. M. Suls & R. L. Miller (Eds), *Social comparison processes: Theoretical and empirical perspectives* (pp. 69–102). Washington, DC: Hemisphere.

Mills, J., & Mintz, P. M. (1972). Effect of unexplained arousal on affiliation. *Journal of Personality and Social Psychology, 24,* 11–14.

Nosanchuck, T. A., & Erickson, B. H. (1985). How high is up? Calibrating social comparison in the real world. *Journal of Personality and Social Psychology, 48,* 624–634.

Pennebaker, J. W. (1982). Physical symptoms related to blood glucose insulin- dependent diabetics. *Psychophysiology, 19,* 201–210.

Perloff, R. (1987). Self-interest and personal responsibility redux. *American Psychologist, 42,* 3–11.

Reisenzein, R. (1984). Empiricism and analysis: Comments on Brandtstadter's "A priori elements in psychological research programs." *Zeitschrift fur Sozialpsycholgie, 15,* 74–80.

Rogers, J. C., & Figone, J. J. (1978). The avocational pursuits of rehabilitants with traumatic quadriplegia. *American Journal of Occupational Therapy, 32,* 571–576.

Rohrer, K., Adelman, B., Puckett, J., Toomey, B., Calver, G., & Johnson, E. W. (1980). Rehabilitation in spinal-cord injury: Use of patient–family group. *Archives of Physical Medicine and Rehabilitation, 61,* 255–229.

Ross, L., Greene, D., & House, P. (1977). The false consensus effect: An egocentric bias in social perception and attribution processes. *Journal of Experimental Social Psychology, 13,* 279–301.

Salovey, P., Rothman, A. J., & Rodin, J. (in press). Social psychology and health behavior.

In D. Gilbert, S. Fiske, & G. Lindzey (Eds.), *Handbook of social psychology*. New York: McGraw-Hill.

Schachter, S. (1959). *The psychology of affiliation*. Palo Alto, CA: Stanford University Press.

Schachter, S., & Singer, J. E. (1962). Cognitive, social, and physiological determinants of emotional state. *Psychological Review, 69*, 379-399.

Schlenker, B. R. (1987). Threats to identity: Self-identification and social stress. In C. R. Snyder & C. E. Ford (Eds.), *Coping with negative life events* (pp. 273-321). New York: Plenum.

Sejwacz, D., Ajzen, I., & Fishbein, M. (1980). Predicting and understanding weight loss. In I. Ajzen & M. Fishbein (Eds.), *Understanding attitudes and predicting social behavior* (pp. 101-112). Englewood Cliffs, NJ: Prentice-Hall.

Sherif, M. A. (1936). The psychology of social norms. New York: Harper.

Sherman, S. J., Presson, C. C., Chassin, L., Corty, E., & Olshavsky, R. (1983). The false consensus effect in estimates of smoking prevalence: Underlying mechanisms. *Personality and Social Psychology Bulletin, 9*, 197-207.

Singer, E. (1980). Reference groups and social evaluations. In M. Rosenberg & R. H. Turner (Eds.), *Social psychology: Sociological perspectives* (pp. 66-93). New York: Basic Books.

Slovic, P., Fischhoff, B., & Lichtenstein, S. (1987). Behavioral decision theory perspectives on protective behavior. In N. D. Weinstein (Ed.), *Taking care: Understanding and encouraging self-protective behavior* (pp. 14-41). New York: Cambridge University Press.

Stewart, M. J. (1989). Social support: Diverse theoretical perspectives. *Social Science and Medicine, 28*, 1275-1282.

Stouffer, S.A., Suchman, E.A., De Vinney, L.C., Star, S.A., & Williams, R.M., Jr. (1949). *The American soldier: Adjustment during army life* (Vol. 1). Princeton, NJ: Princeton University Press.

Strack, F., & Schwarz, N., Chassein, B., Kern, D., & Wagner, D. (1990). Salience of comparison standards and the activation of social norms. Consequences for judgements of happiness and their communication. *British Journal of Social Psychology, 29*, 749-754.

Stroebe, W., & Stroebe, M. S. (1995). *Social psychology and health*. Pacific Grove, CA: Brooks/Cole.

Suls, J. M. (1977). Social comparison theory and research. An overview from 1954. In J. M. Suls & R. L. Miller (Eds.), *Social comparison processes: Theoretical and empirical perspectives* (pp. 1-19). Washington, DC: Hemisphere.

Suls, J. M., Choi, K. W., & Sanders, G. S. (1988). False consensus and false uniqueness in estimating the prevalence of health protective behaviors. *Journal of Applied Social Psychology, 18*, 66-79.

Suls, J. M., Marco, C. A., & Tobin, S. (1991). The role of temporal comparison, social comparison, and direct appraisal in the elderly's self-evaluations of health. *Journal of Applied Social Psychology, 21*, 1125-1144.

Sussman, S., Dent, C. W., Mestel-Rauch, J., Johnson, C. A., Hansen, W. B., & Flay, B. R. (1988). Adolescent nonsmokers, triers, and regular smokers' estimates of cigarette smoking prevalence: When do overestimations occur and by whom? *Journal of Applied Social Psychology, 18*, 537-551.

Taylor, S. E. (1991). Asymmetrical effects of positive and negative events: The mobilization-minimization hypothesis. *Psychological Bulletin, 110*, 67–85.

Taylor, S. E., Buunk, B., & Aspinwall, L. (1990). Social comparison, stress and coping. *Personality and Social Psychology Bulletin, 16*(1), 74–89.

Taylor, S. E., & Lobel, M. (1989). Social comparison activity under threat: Downward evaluation and upward contacts. *Psychological Review, 96*, 569-575.

Taylor, S. E., Wood, J. V., & Lichtman, R. R. (1983). It could be worse: Selective evaluation as a response to victimization. *Journal of Social Issues, 39*, 19-40.

Thornton, D. A., & Arrowood, A. J. (1966). Self-evaluation, self-enhancement, and the locus of social comparison. *Journal of Experimental Social Psychology Supplement, 1,* 40–48.

VanderZee, K., Buunk, B. P., & Sanderman, R. (1995). Social comparison as a mediator between health problems and subjective health evaluations. *British Journal of Social Psychology, 34,* 53–65.

Weinstein, N. D. (1980). Unrealistic optimism about future events. *Journal of Personality and Social Psychology, 39,* 806–820.

Wheeler, L., & Miyake, K. (1992). Social comparison in everyday life. *Journal of Personality and Social Psychology, 62,* 760–773.

Wills, T. A. (1981). Downward comparison principles in social psychology. *Psychological Bulletin, 90,* 245–271.

Wills, T. A. (1987). Downward comparison as a coping mechanism. In C. R. Snyder & C. E. Ford (Eds.), *Coping with negative life events: Clinical and social psychological perspectives.* (pp. 243-268). New York: Plenum.

Wilson, S. R., & Benner, L. A. (1971). The effects of self-esteem and situation upon comparison choices during ability evaluation. *Sociometry, 34,* 381–397.

Wood, J. V. (1989). Theory and research concerning social comparisons of personal attributes. *Psychological Bulletin, 106,* 231–248.

Wood, J. V., Taylor, S. E., & Lichtman, R. R. (1985). Social comparison in adjustment to breast cancer. *Journal of Personality and Social Psychology, 49,* 1169–1183.

Ybema, J. F., & Buunk, B. P. (1993). Aiming at the top: Upward social comparison after failure. *European Journal of Social Psychology, 23,* 627–645.

Ybema, J. F., & Buunk, B. P. (1995). Affective responses to social comparison: A study among disabled individuals. *British Journal of Social Psychology, 34,* 279-292.

Ybema, J. F., Buunk, B. P., & Heesink, J. A. M. (1996). Affect and identification in social comparison after loss of work. *Basic and Applied Social Psychology, 18,* 151–169.

# CHAPTER 2

# Social Comparison and Unrealistic Optimism About Personal Risk

William M. Klein
*Colby College*

Neil D. Weinstein
*Rutgers, The State University of New Jersey*

> *So little are men [sic] governed by reason in their sentiments and opinions, that they always judge more of objects by comparison than from their intrinsic work and value . . . This no one can doubt of with regard to our passions and sensations.*
>
> —Hume (1739, p. 89)

> *We . . . are always trying to find out exactly what other people are doing in their lives in order to rate ourselves.—letter to the editor, Time magazine*
>
> —Worm (1994, p. 3)

The number of threats that people face is astonishing. Daily headlines and cocktail party conversations are filled with information about carcinogens, natural disasters, new viruses, chronic illnesses, AIDS, and numerous other health and safety concerns. Not surprisingly, the manner in which people appraise their chances of being victimized by these problems has captured the attention of psychologists in many fields. In this chapter, we explore the role that social comparison plays in judgments of personal risk.

We begin with the observation that personal judgments are made within a social milieu containing the feedback, scrutiny, and behavioral examples of others. People endeavor to make decisions whose outcomes will not lead to social embarrassment, and they look to others as sources of relevant information. As suggested by the quotations with which we opened this chapter, social comparison is one of the most important influences on our self-judgments (Festinger, 1954). Comparisons with others help us judge our abilities, opinions, emotions, and many other personal characteristics (Suls & Miller, 1977; Suls & Wills, 1991). Here we argue that judgments of our risk for health and safety problems are also shaped by social comparisons, and we consider the implications of this statement for the construction of successful health campaigns.

To demonstrate that social comparison plays an important role in how people respond to health and safety risks we need affirmative answers to several questions. First, when people judge their risk, are they sensitive to factors known to influence social comparisons? For example, if social comparison is important in determining whether Janice, a smoker, considers her risk of lung disease to be worrisome, we should be able to show that her observation of other women will strongly influence her judgment. In particular, according to social comparison theory and the research tradition that follows it, Janice should feel least vulnerable when faced with other smokers of similar sex, age, and socioeconomic status who smoke even more than she. And, as we show later, Janice should feel particularly invulnerable when her social comparison targets are vague or deindividuated and when they (rather than Janice herself) are used as the standard of comparison.

A stimulus to most of the research discussed in this chapter is the finding that, when judging personal risks, people not only engage in social comparison but enter into these comparisons with an ulterior motive of appearing better off than their comparison others (cf. Helgeson & Mickelson, 1995; Wood, 1989). With this in mind, we pose our second question: Do people attempt to maintain favorable beliefs about their comparative standing on risk dimensions when such beliefs are challenged? If so, what strategies do they employ in order to do so?

Third, we ask whether people engage in such social comparisons spontaneously when assessing personal risk. The thesis that risk assessment is partly a function of social comparison cannot be based solely on research in which people are asked to make explicit social comparisons, despite the fact that most relevant research has taken this approach. There is surprisingly little work on this issue, but we review the few studies that are relevant.

The demonstration that social comparison impacts risk judgments is academic if people's responses to health and safety threats are insensitive to these comparisons. Thus, a fourth question is whether social comparison information regarding personal risk influences people's affective, self-evaluative, and behavioral reactions to hazards. Consider John, a patient who learns that his blood cholesterol is 200 mg/dl, a level his physician says is perfectly acceptable. Upon discovering that his peers tend to have still lower levels of cholesterol, will John be upset and will he modify his diet and exercise regimen? If so, this would provide direct evidence that social comparisons about risk really make a difference.

In summary, we ask four questions: Do various elements of the social comparison process influence personal risk judgments? Do people attempt to preserve their favorable comparative standing on risk dimensions? Do social comparisons with others occur spontaneously when making judgments about personal risk in everyday life? Do people's social comparisons on risk dimensions predict their affective, self-evaluative, and behavioral responses? Our examination of these issues also allows us to address two related topics—how research on risk judgment may contribute to the development of social comparison theory, and how research linking social comparison with risk judgments may suggest ways of increasing desirable health behaviors and decreasing undesirable behaviors.

To answer these questions, we draw heavily from a body of research whose consistent message is that when people estimate their risk relative to that of others, they often are unrealistically optimistic. That is, they believe they are less at risk for experiencing negative life events than others are. In an early demonstration of this bias, students compared their likelihood of experiencing a variety of negative and positive life events to that of other students at the same institution (Weinstein, 1980). A large majority believed their likelihood of experiencing the negative events to be lower (and the positive events higher) than that of their peers. Because it is impossible for the majority of a sample to be below (or above) average (barring a skewed distribution), Weinstein (1980) was able to conclude that at least some of the sample was unrealistically optimistic. Because an individual's risk is so difficult to determine, such a conclusion would have been difficult to reach by contrasting participants' risk ratings with their actual chances of experiencing these events (although see Kreuter & Strecher, 1995; Shepperd, Ouellette, & Fernandez, 1996, for recent investigations that have measured the actual risk of individual participants).

We focus here on health and safety-related events, particularly negative events, because the little work that exists on beliefs about the likelihood of positive events suggests that the latter are conceptually distinct (e.g., Hoorens, 1996). We do not address the optimistic biases held by people coping with existing health problems such as breast cancer (Wood, Taylor, & Lichtman, 1985; Wood & Vander Zee, chapter 10, this volume) or AIDS (Taylor et al., 1992). These biases may have similar origins and goals, but they arise in quite different situations and may well be adaptive responses to victimization. We do not consider studies that only measure absolute personal risk, nor do we discuss dispositional optimism (Scheier & Carver, 1992), because this individual orientation does not necessarily involve either a social comparison or a risk judgment. We begin with a brief review of relevant literature on unrealistic optimism.

## UNREALISTIC OPTIMISM

There are two ways in which people can be unrealistically optimistic. First, people can underestimate their absolute or objective risk of having a problem, such as when a potential breast cancer victim believes her risk of getting breast cancer is below 20% when in fact her diet and family background cause her risk to be over 50%. We refer to this bias as *absolute unrealistic optimism.* Second, people can believe erroneously that their risk of having a health problem is lower than that of their peers. We refer to this bias as *comparative unrealistic optimism,* and because this latter type of optimism is more commonly investigated (and more prevalent; Rothman, Klein, & Weinstein, 1996) we sometimes just refer to it by the more general term *unrealistic optimism* (or optimistic bias).

Investigators have used three strategies to demonstrate comparative unrealistic optimism. A relative evaluation of these methods is currently impossible because very few studies employ more than one approach (however, see Otten & van der Pligt, 1996). The *direct* method has been mentioned earlier; participants rate their comparative risk for experiencing an event, and the sample mean is then compared to the midpoint of the scale (usually designated as "average"). The advantage of this method is that it is simple and straightforward; a weakness is that if an intervention is shown to decrease levels of unrealistic optimism the investigator is left unable to determine whether the intervention enhanced perceptions of own risk or reduced perceptions of average risk. A solution to this problem is to use the *indirect* method. In the within-group version of this method, participants rate their own absolute risk and then the average person's absolute risk on a separate but identical scale (e.g., Taylor & Gollwitzer, 1995). Absolute risk may be actuarial, or may appear on a scale ranging from, for example, "No chance" to "Extremely likely." If the sample mean of the self-ratings is less than the mean of the ratings for the average person, the sample is said to exhibit unrealistic optimism. In the between-group version, one group of people might rate their own risk, whereas a separate group rates the average person's risk. The difference between the two groups' ratings can then be examined to see if one mean is less than the other (e.g., Harris & Middleton, 1994). Indirect methods like these permit an investigator to determine whether a manipulation shown to increase or decrease unrealistic optimism affected self-ratings or other-ratings.

Using either the direct or indirect method, researchers have found unrealistic optimism about many health and safety problems (for reviews see Hoorens, 1993a; Perloff, 1987) including lung cancer, heart disease, alcohol and other drug addictions, gum disease, diabetes, AIDS and other sexually transmitted diseases (STD's), and pregnancy (e.g., Gerrard, Gibbons, & Warner, 1991; Harris & Middleton, 1994; Hoorens & Buunk, 1993; Perloff & Fetzer, 1986; Weinstein, 1980, 1982, 1983, 1984, 1987; Whitley & Hern, 1991). Unrealistic optimism tends not to be found for a few problems including ulcers, unspecified cancer, and high blood pressure (Weinstein, 1980, 1983, 1984). Biases emerge in all age groups (Quadrel, Fischhoff, & Davis, 1993; Weinstein, 1987), and it is unusual for any sample to be comparatively pessimistic (e.g., Dolinski, Gromski, & Zawisza, 1987) even if the sample is at high risk (e.g., van der Velde, van der Pligt, & Hooykaas, 1994). Thus, there is a great deal of evidence that, on average, people are unrealistically optimistic about their comparative risk,[1] although in only a few of these studies can we identify which members of the sample are biased. Moreover, unrealistic optimism appears in many different samples across a wide variety of demographics (e.g., Weinstein, 1987).

Despite the fact that all of these studies involve self-report, there is no evidence that the biases are artifacts of participants' self-presentational motives (Hoorens & Buunk, 1993), or that participants' answers are insensitive to the specific hazard they are asked to consider. For example, smokers are less optimistic about smoking-related hazards than about nonsmoking-related hazards (McKenna, Warburton, & Winwood, 1993); ill people feel more vulnerable to health problems than to nonhealth problems (Kulik & Mahler, 1987); and victims of natural disasters are less optimistic about their risk of those hazards than they are about other, unrelated hazards (Burger & Palmer, 1992; Dolinski et al., 1987).

Furthermore, when using the direct method, participants are attentive to the identity of the comparison target. For example, students rate the pregnancy risk of the average woman higher than that of the average woman at their university (e.g., Burger & Burns, 1988), and they see the risk of AIDS for the average same-age heterosexual college woman as lower than that of the average same-age heterosexual man, which in turn they see as lower than that of the average homosexual college man

[1]A bibliography containing more than 200 articles on unrealistic optimism is available from the second author. Furthermore, the Spring 1996 issue of the *Journal of Social and Clinical Psychology* is devoted to research on this bias.

(Mickler, 1991). This is important because if people use a high-risk reference group when making comparisons only because they disregard instructions, it becomes more difficult to argue that they are genuinely biased about their risk.

People also maintain self-serving biases about the specific behaviors associated with health problems. They tend to believe they consume less salt, butter, sweets, and alcohol; sunbathe and smoke less often; use birth control and seat belts more often; and have sex with fewer (and safer) partners than their peers (e.g., Harris & Middleton, 1994; Klein & Kunda, 1993, Perloff & Fetzer, 1986; Suls, Wan, & Sanders, 1988; Weinstein, 1984). These comparative judgments on specific risk factors are usually correlated with comparative judgments of overall risk (e.g., Gerrard et al., 1991; Weinstein, 1984, 1987).

Several consistent determinants of comparative unrealistic optimism have emerged. For example, people are more unrealistically optimistic both about events they believe they can control (DeJoy, 1989; Harris, 1996; Klein & Kunda, 1994), and about events they have not yet experienced (van der Pligt, Otten, Richard, & van der Velde, 1993; Weinstein, 1987, 1989). Some of these determinants are motivational in nature and others cognitive (for treatments of this distinction, see Hoorens, 1993a; van der Pligt et al., 1993). Moreover, many factors (such as control and experience) do not necessitate a social comparison, showing that unrealistic optimism derives in part from mechanisms unrelated to social comparison processes. Nevertheless, many antecedents of unrealistic optimism do invoke social comparison processes, and we focus on these in the sections that follow.

## SOCIAL COMPARISON AND UNREALISTIC OPTIMISM: THE FOUR QUESTIONS

### Question 1: Are People's Risk Judgments Sensitive to Factors Known to Influence Social Comparisons?

We now turn to the question of whether levels of comparative unrealistic optimism are influenced by social comparison. Research on social comparison processes offers several possible predictions. Although people tend to engage in upward comparison when choosing social contacts, they are more likely to engage in downward comparison (Wills, 1981, 1987, 1991) when undertaking self-evaluation, often leading to favorable self-assessments (e.g., Aspinwall & Taylor, 1993;

Reis, Gerrard, & Gibbons, 1993; Taylor & Lobel, 1989). Moreover, people are especially likely to engage in downward comparison under threat (e.g., DeVellis et al., 1990). Given that risk judgments are a form of self-evaluation and are made about potentially threatening negative life events, we might expect that people will exhibit downward comparison when judging their risk, and will consequently see their own risk as lower than that of their peers. Other interpretations of social comparison theory might lead to the prediction that people will choose similar others with whom to compare their risk levels (Wheeler, 1991), or to the prediction that they will construct hypothetical others as comparison targets (e.g., Gibbons & Gerrard, chapter 3, this volume; Goethals, Messick, & Allison, 1991; Wood, 1989; Wood et al., 1985).

To these possibilities we add three more variables that researchers have investigated in the context of unrealistic optimism and that are relevant to the comparison process: (a) the specificity, concreteness, and level of individuation of the comparison target; (b) the salience of own and others' standing on related dimensions; and (c) the standard of comparison used.

***Choice and Construction of Comparison Targets.*** Festinger's (1954) original theory predicts that people will choose targets who are slightly superior to them. Downward comparison theory (Wills, 1981, 1987, 1991), on the other hand, predicts that people will sometimes look to someone less well off as a target, particularly if self-esteem is threatened. From a functional perspective, it might be argued that people should compare with others less at risk, because doing so would help them learn how to reduce their own risk. Indeed, social comparison is often employed with the goal of self-improvement (e.g., Wood, 1989). However, people might find it threatening to be more at risk than their peers and thus might compare with those at higher risk (Affleck & Tennen, chapter 9, this volume; Wills, chapter 6, this volume). Indeed, one coping strategy that victims of health problems employ is to compare with others in still worse conditions (e.g., Wood et al., 1985). Support for downward comparison in risk judgments can be found in a study by Perloff and Fetzer (1986, Study 2), in which participants rated their own risk of experiencing several negative events and then provided similar ratings for the average student, their closest friend, or "one of your friends." In the last condition, participants were asked to choose a different friend for each negative event. Thus, participants in this last condition had a great deal of latitude in their comparison choices. As predicted, these participants were unrealistically optimistic; a majority chose friends who were especially vulnerable to the life events considered. (Optimistic biases were not obtained when participants did not have such latitude—that is, when they were asked to rate the risk of their best friend.) These findings suggest that people engage in downward comparison when judging health risk.

If people compare downwardly when assessing their risk, we should find that when participants are asked to compare themselves with the average person in a large reference group, they tend to focus their comparisons on a risky subgroup within the reference group. Indirect evidence for this prediction appears in a study by van der Velde et al. (1994). Four Dutch groups varying in their objective risk of contracting AIDS estimated their own risk of being infected in the next 2 years and then estimated the same risk for a random, same-sex, same-age individual from the general population. Listed from low to high risk, the samples consisted of Amsterdam citizens, heterosexuals with multiple private partners, gay men with many sexual partners, and visitors to an STD clinic who had recently engaged in sex with prostitutes. When rating their objective risk of getting AIDS, all groups seemed to be sensitive to their risk level: The high-risk group rated their risk the highest and the low-risk group rated theirs the lowest. However, the ratings of one's own risk were still lower than the ratings of the random citizen in all except the highest risk sample. These findings suggest that participants were using different reference groups, resulting in a significant downward comparison for three of the four samples.

People are especially likely to engage in downward social comparison when threatened (e.g., DeVellis et al., 1990; Wills, chapter 6, this volume). For example, when participants in the classic study by Hakmiller (1966) were led to believe that they were hostile toward their parents (a threatening assessment), they preferred to compare themselves with individuals perceived to be even more hostile. We might expect, then, that unrealistic optimism would be greater for negative life events that are particularly threatening. However, there is very little evidence for this; investigators rarely find that more threatening events elicit greater bias (e.g., DeJoy, 1989; Otten, 1995; Weinstein, 1980, 1982, 1987).

Finally, research has shown that people not only compare with actual individuals but also construct hypothetical targets, who often turn out to be inferior (e.g., Goethals et al., 1991; Wood, 1989). There is indirect evidence that this may occur in the risk domain as well. First, health problems for which people find it easy to picture typical victims elicit greater unrealistic optimism than those for which typical victims are hard to imagine (Moore & Rosenthal, 1991; Weinstein, 1980). Second, people distance themselves psychologically from such prototypes, just as smokers trying to quit do when thinking about how they compare with the "typical smoker" (Gibbons & Eggleston, 1996; Gibbons & Gerrard, chapter 3, this volume; Gibbons, Gerrard, Lando, & McGovern, 1991). Finally, when people are asked to compare themselves with the average person, they do not report having a specific individual in mind (Alicke, Klotz, Breitenbecher, Yurak, & Vredenburg, 1995), suggesting that they may be constructing a hypothetical target (or, alternatively, that they do not think significantly about the target).

If unrealistic optimism arises from downward comparison, what happens when people are forced to compare with fixed targets such as individuals similar to themselves? In the next two sections we consider how various manipulations of the comparison target may impact levels of unrealistic optimism.

***Effects of Target Similarity in Fixed Social Comparisons.*** When forced to compare their risk with similar others, are people less unrealistically optimistic? Perloff and Fetzer (1986, Study 2), found that participants exhibited less unrealistic optimism when comparing with a best friend (to whom they probably considered themselves most similar) than with "one of their friends," or with the average person (see also Whitley & Hern, 1991). Because ratings of personal risk were similar in this study's three conditions, these differences in unrealistic optimism levels were caused by differences in ratings of the comparison targets. Harris and Middleton (1994) had participants rate their own risk, the risk of an acquaintance ("someone you don't know very well but would like to know better"), or the risk of a friend's friend ("a friend of your best friend, someone you've heard about but never met"). The acquaintance was previously rated as more similar than the friend's friend. Participants estimating their own risk reported lower ratings than did participants rating either of the two comparison targets, yet the difference between self- and target ratings was greater when the target was a friend's friend than when the target was an acquaintance. Finally, Boney McCoy et al. (1992) reported that unrealistic optimism for smoking-related health problems was greatest among those smokers who considered themselves least similar to the typical smoker. These studies suggest that increasing similarity to a comparison target is associated with less comparative unrealistic optimism. Unfortunately, experimental manipulations of similarity in studies of unrealistic optimism are lacking, and they are often confounded with such factors as liking of, psychological closeness to, type of relationship with, and type of knowledge about the target.

If people prefer to engage in downward comparison when judging personal risk, then asking them to compare with similar targets could lead to compensatory strategies designed to maintain their risk perceptions vis-à-vis the target. One intriguing possibility is that people might reduce their perceptions of similarity to the target so as to preserve their optimistic beliefs. In a test of this hypothesis, students who learned that one of their peers was HIV-positive rated him as less similar to themselves than did students who learned the peer was HIV-negative, despite the fact that both groups received an identical behavioral profile for this peer (Gump & Kulik, 1995).

***Specificity, Concreteness, and Individuation of Fixed Comparison Targets.*** In addition to similarity, the specificity, concreteness, and individuation of a comparison target might be expected to affect the magnitude of unrealistic optimism observed. In early studies of unrealistic optimism, the comparison target was the average person of the participant's age and sex (e.g., Weinstein, 1980). Later researchers suggested that the "average person" might be a vague, deindividuated, and negatively evaluated target, and that comparisons with specific, concrete, and individuated targets might yield less unrealistic optimism. Most work in social comparison does not speak to this point because the convention is to use individuals (not groups or prototypes) as comparison targets.

The notion that comparisons with specific individuals will be less biased than comparisons with the average peer was first tested by Perloff and Fetzer (1986, Study 1). Participants compared their risk of experiencing several health and safety problems with that of the average same-sex college student, the average same-sex student at their particular university, their closest friend, the sibling closest in age to themselves, or a parent. Ratings of personal risk did not differ among these conditions. However, ratings of the comparison target differed in such a way that unrealistic optimism was found in both of the average-student conditions but in none of the single target conditions. Thus, unrealistic optimism was absent when the target was specific and concrete. In another study, when women participants were asked to compare their pregnancy risk with that of their best friend, the average student, or the average woman, unrealistic optimism was found only in the latter two conditions (Whitley & Hern, 1991).

Why did unrealistic optimism decrease when comparing with some of these targets? Later work has shown that even specific concrete comparison targets such as an "acquaintance" (Harris & Middleton, 1994), a "same-sex acquaintance" (Regan, Snyder, & Kassin, 1995), an "arbitrary random other" (Hoorens & Buunk, 1993), or an "arbitrary stranger" (Regan et al., 1995) elicit conventional levels of unrealistic optimism, suggesting that making the comparison target more specific and concrete is not itself a sufficient condition for reducing the bias significantly. Alicke et al. (1995) argued that individuation of the target is what reduces unrealistic optimism. Friends and family members are living, breathing individuals with unique traits, unlike the "average person." (Note that individuation may occur without an increase in perceived similarity.) In a series of studies, Alicke et al. (1995) increased individuation of the comparison target by having participants look at the person with whom they were comparing (on videotape or on a still image) or read a transcript of an interview with the target. In all cases, participants showed less unrealistic optimism than a control group that compared itself with the average person (although unrealistic optimism was not eliminated in any condition). The authors also found that unrealistic optimism was reduced even more when participants had personal contact with the comparison target. Ratings of personal risk did not differ among the various conditions, so these effects were due to changes in the comparison target.

Finally, it is plausible that greater amounts of unrealistic optimism are elicited when comparing with the average person than with an individuated target because people do not like to be average and therefore view the "average person" pejoratively. To test this idea, Alicke et al. (1995, Study 2) gave participants a series of 9-point rating scales for several bipolar trait dimensions (e.g., extremely dependable–extremely undependable), and asked them to estimate the percentage of undergraduates at their university who would fall into each of the nine categories. The distributions were used to calculate mean ratings. Another group merely provided point estimates of where the "average person" would fall on these scales. The mean response in the latter condition was actually more positive than that calculated from the distribution, suggesting that the average person was viewed more favorably than the mean of the distribution. These data argue against the notion that the average person is seen negatively.

In summary, studies show that unrealistic optimism is reduced (though not eliminated) by having people compare with an individuated target rather than the average person, and reduced still more when the participant has brief personal contact with the target. It is significant, however, that making the comparison target more specific and concrete does not suffice to reduce optimism; individuation and personal contact are required as well. The reduction in optimism for such targets does not appear to be due to pejorative associations with being "average." We note here that the effects described were not confounded with the amount of target information (which was equivalent in all conditions). This suggests that the reduced unrealistic optimism found in earlier studies for single targets such as friends and acquaintances was not necessarily due to the greater knowledge about these targets, though it could well be due to greater perceived similarity with them.

***Focusing Attention on One's Own or on Others' Relevant Behaviors.*** We have now reviewed evidence that one set of factors known to influence social comparisons—characteristics of the target—play a significant role in unrealistic optimism. Unrealistic optimism may also depend on the nature of the comparison, such as whether people focus their attention on themselves or on the comparison target. Although social comparison research does not generally consider such attentional variables, they may play a significant role in the outcome of a social comparison.

People's judgments are often egocentric in that they perceive their own behaviors and attributes more readily than those of others (e.g., Fenigstein, 1993; Krueger & Clement, 1994; Ross & Sicoly, 1979; Simon, 1993). Unrealistic optimism might occur, then, because people focus on their own risk-avoidant behavior rather than on the comparison target's behavior (suggesting a combination of egocentrism and selective focus on one's desirable attributes). Weinstein (1980) explored this idea by having some students list factors that increased or decreased their chances of experiencing several life events. In the actual experiment, one group reviewed the lists made by five of these students and then rated their own chances of experiencing these events. Relative to a control group, this group was less optimistic, presumably because reviewing information about others' risk factors reduced participants' egocentrism. However, unrealistic optimism was not eliminated. In a follow-up study, Weinstein (1983) was able to eliminate unrealistic optimism entirely by giving participants an explicit list of risk factors with the average student's standing on each factor. In another study, unrealistic optimism was attenuated even when people were merely asked to take the *perspective* of the comparison target (Weinstein & Lachendro, 1982). This last finding suggests that unrealistic optimism is generated at least in part by a failure to attend to the target, not necessarily by a lack of information about that target. Unfortunately, because all of these studies used the direct, comparative measure of risk, it is unclear whether participants reduced their perceptions of the average person's risk or enhanced perceptions of their own risk.

Of course, increasing attention to others will not decrease unrealistic optimism if people focus on others worse off than themselves. In the context of several unsuccessful attempts to reduce unrealistic optimism, Weinstein and Klein (1995) found that focusing on high-risk others may serve to increase the amount of bias. In one of their studies, participants were given a list of risk factors for weight problems and generated a vivid mental image of a person who was on the high-risk end of each factor. Participants later reported their own risk of having a weight problem relative to a same-age, same-sex peer. Unrealistic optimism in this condition was greater than in a no-image control group, even though participants were asked to compare themselves to an average peer and not to the person in the mental image. In this case, increasing the salience of (and presumably the focus on) a potential comparison target increased unrealistic optimism. Moreover, this greater optimism resulted from increased perceptions of the average peer's risk rather than reduced perceptions of the participants' own risk. In a related study, participants rated themselves as happier than a comparison target who had liver disease, but even more so when they were face-to-face with the target (Strack, Schwarz, Chassein, Kern, & Wagner, 1990).

The above studies address how information about others might influence unrealistic optimism. Additional work addresses the influence that information about the self might have. Given that unrealistic optimism is associated with egocentricity, we might expect that increasing attention toward the self will increase levels of unrealistic optimism. Indeed, when people are asked to report their standing on risk factors or to review their behavioral profile before estimating their risk, they sometimes end up being more unrealistically optimistic (Gerrard et al., 1991; Weinstein, 1983). This increase in optimism seems to result from reduced perceptions of personal vulnerability rather than increased perceptions of the average person's vulnerability (Gerrard et al., 1991). Similarly, in a study by Weinstein and Klein (1995, Study 4), participants who generated a list of personal attributes that decreased their risk of having a weight problem and then rated their comparative risk for this problem exhibited more unrealistic optimism than no-list controls. An opposite manipulation in which participants listed personal attributes that increased their risk did not reduce unrealistic optimism, suggesting that ego-enhancing processes may moderate the effects of self-focus on perceived risk.

It appears, then, that comparative risk judgments tend to be less optimistic when people are given information about (or take the perspective of) the comparison others, though when such comparison others are at especially high risk people may become even more convinced of their own invulnerability. The outcome of social comparisons about risk will also tend to be more optimistic when attention is turned inward, because people focus on what they do to decrease their risk (and even when they are asked to focus on what they do to increase their risk, their comparative risk judgments are unaffected).

***Standard of Comparison.*** To make a social comparison, people must start with one social object as the standard and then compare another social object to that standard. Comparative judgments of Objects A and B may differ depending on whether A or B serves as the comparison standard (cf. Wanke, Schwarz, & Noelle-Neumann, 1995). In most unrealistic optimism research, people are asked to compare themselves to the average person, making the average person the standard. How might people respond if the task were inverted and they were asked to use themselves as the standard of comparison? Past research has shown that people show a self–other asymmetry in similarity ratings such that others are considered more like the self than vice-versa (e.g., Codol, 1987; Holyoak & Gordon, 1983). This suggests that when the self is used as a standard, self–other differences in unrealistic optimism might decrease. Indeed, when Otten and van der Pligt (1996, Study 2) asked participants to compare the average person's risk to their own risk (thereby making self the standard of comparison) on a direct comparative scale, participants showed significantly lower levels of unrealistic optimism. Similar findings were reported by Hoorens (1995) for positive, but not negative, items. Thus, there is some preliminary evidence that unrealistic optimism is lower when people compare others to themselves.

These findings raise a more general question germane to most of the research in this chapter: When people compare their risk with that of others, do they begin this comparison with a well-articulated sense of the average person's risk and then use that information to assist them in judging their own risk (as classic social comparison research might suggest), or do they begin with a well-articulated view of their own risk and use that to construct an estimate of the average person's risk (as research on false uniqueness and false consensus effects might suggest)? In other words, what comparison standard do people normally use when judging their own risk? Because, as we discuss later, few data speak to people's everyday risk judgments, this is a difficult question to answer, although there is already evidence in other domains that people tend to use their own standing on various attributes to judge similar attributes in others (e.g., Dunning & Cohen, 1992; Fong & Markus, 1982). Given that self-judgments of risk can be modified by information about comparison others (Rothman et al., 1996), a likely model is that the self is used as a standard to judge others and that these judgments may be used in turn to modify beliefs about the self. This reflexive model awaits further research.

It is interesting that most research on unrealistic optimism has used the average person as the comparison standard (with the reference group to which this average person belongs varying widely among different studies). This approach has been appropriate because it is far easier in health campaigns to present information about others or "the average person" than about the numerous, separate individuals to whom the message is directed. However, if it turns out that the self is normally used as a standard for judging comparative risk, past research may have exaggerated the magnitude of optimistic biases by artificially changing the standard that people use (Hoorens, 1995).

***Summary.*** We set out in this section to show how several social comparison factors—direction of comparison; similarity, specificity, concreteness, and individuation of the target; attention toward own rather than others' behaviors; and standard of comparison—influence the degree to which people are unrealistically optimistic. We reviewed some evidence that, consistent with some elements of social comparison theory, people choose to compare their risk with that of real or hypothetical individuals whose risk is greater. People are less likely to believe that their risk is lower than that of a comparison target when they do not hold a stereotype of a typical victim, and when the target is individuated, physically present, and perceived to be similar to themselves. Furthermore, unrealistic optimism appears to be greater when people fail to take the perspective of others and when others are used as the standard of comparison. Because social comparison research rarely examines the individuality of the target, the salience of participants' own and others' behavior, or the standard of comparison, these findings are theoretically significant. It remains to be seen whether these findings may be generalized to other social comparison situations. For example, when receiving negative performance feedback, will people be more likely to engage in downward comparison when the comparison target is an abstract, deindividuated person?

These findings have a number of implications for health promotion campaigns. Given that attention to one's own behavior could exacerbate biases and that providing information about the risk of typical others is often ineffective, educational programs that rely on the dissemination of general risk information are unlikely to be successful. Instead, the use of similar, individuated, physically present others as comparison targets might lead people to exhibit less unrealistic optimism. Interventions that increase attention to these targets and that force the audience to compare these targets to themselves are also more likely to have an impact. We consider these recommendations in more detail in the final section of the chapter (see also Misovich, Fisher, & Fisher, chapter 4, this volume).

Clearly, there is much more to learn about the comparison targets people choose when judging their health risk. There is a particular need for experimental designs (e.g., Croyle & Ditto, 1990) in which risk feedback can be varied and target selection measured. Our understanding of unrealistic optimism would benefit greatly from such an approach, particularly given that social comparison studies using both target selection measures and comparative rating scales have sometimes yielded contradictory results (Wills, 1991; Wood & Taylor, 1991).

### Question 2: Do People Attempt to Maintain Favorable Risk Comparisons?

We have seen that a variety of social comparison variables directly affect the magnitude of unrealistic optimism. In this section, we go one step further. If people use social comparisons when judging risk, and prefer these social comparisons to be self-enhancing, they may be likely to engage in several compensatory strategies when their favorable social comparisons are challenged. That is, if people are given information that conflicts with their comparatively optimistic beliefs, they may attempt to restore these beliefs. How might unrealistically optimistic beliefs be challenged? Given that people tend to overestimate the risk of their peers (e.g., Whitley & Hern, 1991), accurate information about others may serve as negative feedback. When faced with such information, will people become less unrealistically optimistic?

Rothman and colleagues (1996, Study 2) addressed this issue by giving undergraduate women statistics about their peers' risk for several negative life events. The statistics were obtained from a variety of national health information sources. For example, the investigators told participants that the average risk for a college-educated individual to divorce sometime in her or his life was 38%. The researchers also included two additional conditions in which they manipulated the statistics given to participants. In the Deflated condition, the statistics were 50% of actual risk (e.g., participants in this group were told that the average risk of divorce was 19%). The Inflated group was given risk statistics inflated by 50% (e.g., participants in this group were told that the average risk of divorce was 57%). All participants then estimated their own absolute risk of experiencing these problems.

Because the researchers found in an earlier study that people tend to overestimate the average person's risk (Rothman et al., 1996, Study 1), they expected that the statistics offered in the Inflated condition of the current design would best match participants' own beliefs about the average person's risk and would therefore not be perceived as threatening. However, the risk statistics in the Actual and Deflated risk conditions were expected to challenge participants' overestimations of the average risk (and, in turn, their unrealistically optimistic beliefs). It was thus expected that participants in these two conditions would report lower personal risk than participants given inflated risk statistics. This is exactly what was found. Thus, participants appeared to be attempting to preserve a favorable difference between their own risk and others' risk.

***Changing Beliefs About One's Behavior.*** Another challenge to people's favorable risk comparisons may come in the form of information about the health behaviors of their peers. We might learn, for example, that most of our peers floss daily, avoid high cholesterol foods, and do not smoke. Because people tend to overestimate the frequency of others' undesirable behaviors (Goethals et al., 1991; Perloff & Fetzer, 1986), such information should challenge prior beliefs. Given that many of the effects reported in the first section of this chapter involve beliefs about behaviors (e.g., increased focus on one's own behaviors increases unrealistic optimism), one might expect that people would be motivated to sustain favorable beliefs about their relative standing on these behaviors.

Following this reasoning, Klein and Kunda (1993) hypothesized that people may lower their estimates of how often they engage in risk-increasing behaviors if they are given peer information that challenges their prior beliefs. The researchers placed participants in one of four conditions and asked them to report, on 7-point scales, how often they engaged in nine risk-increasing behaviors that generally elicit social comparison biases (i.e., people tend to believe that they engage in these behaviors less often than others). For example, participants indicated how many meals per week they ate red meat on a scale labeled *never*, *less than 1 meal*, *1–3 meals*, *4–7 meals*, *8–10 meals*, *11–13 meals*, and *more than 13 meals*. In three conditions, participants were told how often their peers engaged in these behaviors, designated by an "X" on each 7-point scale. One group was given actual frequencies (which had been obtained earlier from a pretest sample; see Table 2.1, first column), another was given frequencies that were *reduced* by one scale point, and the third was given frequencies that were *increased* by one scale point. A control condition received no peer information.

As Table 2.1 shows, participants in the Actual and Decrement (reduced frequency) conditions reported engaging in the behaviors *less often* than did participants in the Increment (increased frequency) and Control conditions. That is, when their beliefs about their comparative standing on these risk factors were challenged, participants seemed to modify their beliefs about how often they engaged in these behaviors in order to preserve their comparative superiority. Such modification was not necessary in the Increment condition, because the "average" frequencies provided closely approximated participants' expectations. Like

TABLE 2.1
Risk-Increasing Behaviors: Self-Reported Frequencies by Condition

| | Experimental Condition[b] | | | |
|---|---|---|---|---|
| *Behavior*[a] | *Control* | *Accurate* | *Increment* | *Decrement* |
| How often eat eggs (2.46) | 2.77 | 2.63 | 2.76 | 2.32 |
| How often lose one's temper (2.91) | 2.97 | 2.63 | 3.31 | 2.71 |
| How many alcoholic drinks consumed at one time (2.95) | 3.13 | 2.10 | 2.62 | 2.45 |
| How often eat red meat (3.23) | 3.39 | 2.87 | 3.28 | 2.77 |
| How often drink alcohol (3.28) | 3.68 | 2.70 | 2.79 | 2.71 |
| How often eat sweet baked goods (3.72) | 3.87 | 3.50 | 3.86 | 3.10 |
| How often eat candy (3.90) | 4.26 | 3.37 | 3.86 | 3.61 |
| How often get worried/anxious (4.22) | 4.61 | 4.03 | 5.38 | 4.32 |
| How often eat greasy food (5.02) | 5.39 | 4.77 | 4.97 | 4.42 |

*Note.* Responses ranged from 1 to 7; higher numbers indicate greater frequency. All numbers are group means. Multivariate tests revealed that means in the Control and Increment conditions, which did not themselves differ, were significantly greater than means in the Accurate and Decrement conditions, which did not themselves differ. Adapted from "Maintaining Self-Serving Social Comparisons: Biased Reconstruction of One's Past Behaviors," by W. M. Klein and Z. Kunda (1993), *Personality and Social Psychology Bulletin.*

[a]Mean self-reported frequency in pretest appears in parentheses.

[b]Subjects in the four conditions received no information (Control), accurate information about normative means (Accurate), ostensibly normative means that were inflated by one scale point (Increment), or ostensibly normative means that were reduced by one scale point (Decrement).

the Rothman et al. (1996) study, this investigation shows that people may revise beliefs about themselves in order to preserve their comparative superiority.

It could be argued, of course, that people have neither well-articulated beliefs about their precise numerical risk nor a good sense of how often they engage in risky behaviors. According to this argument, people's beliefs are inherently comparative: they believe only that their risk is lower and their risky behaviors fewer than those of their peers, and when given an anchor, they simply generate self-estimates that are consistent with their prior social comparisons. However, an anchoring explanation cannot fully account for the range of findings reported here. For example, when participants received inflated peer frequencies, they did not increase reports of their own self-frequencies. Also, whether we accept the former or latter argument, both lead to interpretations of the data that acknowledge an important role for social comparison in judging risk. Indeed, the latter argument posits that judgments of risk and risk behaviors are based entirely on social comparison. In the next section, we present further evidence that lowering reports of personal risk behaviors is a strategy for preserving one's own perceived superiority.

Of course, such changes must be made within the limits imposed by reality (Kunda, 1990). Indeed, although participants in Klein and Kunda's (1993) Decrement condition gave the lowest estimates of frequency of risky behaviors, these estimates were still higher than the peer means that participants were given—in other words, participants stated that they engaged in these behaviors *more* often than what they thought the average was. Relative to the standards they were given, then, these participants actually rated their own behavior as inferior. When people are no longer able to distort beliefs about their own or others' behavior in a way that preserves their superiority, what do they do?

***Changing Beliefs About Risk Factors.*** One strategy people may follow when they hear that others engage in risk-increasing behaviors less than they do is to alter their evaluation of these behaviors. For example, if we learn that other people consume less salt than we do and we are unable to revise estimates of how often we use salt, we may become less convinced of the relationship between salt and hypertension, thereby preserving our unrealistic optimism about this health problem. As an alternative, we might devalue the personal importance we ascribe to avoiding this behavior. These two strategies are not the same—we can believe a behavior is risky for others and still not consider it important for us to avoid, a distinction that may be critical in whether or not we adopt a precaution (cf. Weinstein, 1988). The personal importance people ascribe to a behavior may depend partly on its perceived relevance to health, but importance may also reflect such factors as peer pressure, religious practice, and the enjoyment the behavior provides.

In a study assessing both of these strategies (Klein, 1996, Study 1), participants reported how often they engaged in each of nine risk-increasing behaviors, and did so again 1 month later. At Time 2, the investigators gave the experimental group the mean responses collected at Time 1. A control group did not receive such information. At both times, participants rated how *relevant* they believed each of these behaviors was to the general risk of having health problems and how *personally important* they considered it to avoid these behaviors. At Time 2, participants also recalled the ratings they had provided at Time 1.

Upon receiving the peer information at Time 2, the experimental group responded in the same way as those in the Klein and Kunda (1993) study, that is, by reducing their estimates of how often they engaged in these behaviors. However, experimental participants at Time 2 also exhibited two other strategies: they rated these behaviors both as less relevant to health and as less personally important to avoid than did the control group. Interestingly, participants did not tend to engage in all of these strategies at once: Those who reduced their self-frequencies were significantly less likely to alter their beliefs about the health relevance and personal importance of the items (changes in the latter two beliefs were highly correlated). Thus, changing self-frequency beliefs and changing relevance–importance beliefs seem to be at least partially substitutable strategies. Furthermore, analyses of participants' memory for their Time 1 ratings showed that they had distorted their memory of all three types of beliefs (self-frequencies, health relevance, and personal importance) in the direction of their Time 2 beliefs, suggesting that they were not aware that they had engaged in these comparison-preserving strategies.

In a second study by Klein (1996, Study 2), participants were told their peers engaged in nine risk-increasing behaviors (related to heart disease or alcoholism) very infrequently and then immediately reported their own behavior frequencies. The distorted peer information made it difficult for participants to see their own behavior as better than average. (Indeed, when participants reported their own frequencies of engaging in these behaviors, they lowered their self-frequencies but were unable to bring them below the extremely low peer frequencies they had been given.) Participants also rated the health relevance and personal importance of each of these behaviors—they did this before or after providing their frequency estimates—and also reported their comparative risk for heart disease and alcoholism. The relevance and importance ratings were completed on 11-point scales ranging from 1 (*not at all*) to 11 (*extremely*).

Klein predicted that participants would compensate for their inability to preserve their favorable standing on these behaviors by coming to see the behaviors as less relevant to health and less personally important to avoid. Indeed, when participants made their health relevance and personal importance ratings after rather than before reporting their self-frequencies, they availed themselves of this opportunity to compensate for their inferior standing by modifying their ratings on these other dimensions. In particular, they rated the behaviors as significantly less relevant to health and as less personally important than did participants in a control condition who had rated relevance and importance before reporting their self-frequencies (see Table 2.2). Remarkably, the comparative risk judgments in both conditions remained unrealistically optimistic despite participants' acknowledgment that they engaged in the risky behaviors far more than their peers, according to the peer

TABLE 2.2
Health Relevance and Personal Importance Rating Means

| | *Condition* | |
|---|---|---|
| | *Control* | *Experimental* |
| Heart disease risk factors | | |
| Health relevance | 7.07 | 6.77† |
| Personal importance | 6.19 | 5.75* |
| Alcoholism risk factors | | |
| Health relevance | 7.38 | 6.60*** |
| Personal importance | 6.83 | 5.88*** |

*Note.* Numbers in table are group means. Significance levels refer to difference between the two conditions. The higher the number the more relevant to their health subjects judged risky behaviors to be and the more personally important they felt it was to avoid them. Adapted from "Maintaining Self-Serving Social Comparisons: Attenuating the Perceived Significance of Risk-Increasing Behaviors," by W. M. Klein (1996), *Journal of Social and Clinical Psychology*. Reprinted by permission of Sage Publications © 1996 by Sage.

†$p < .10$. *$p < .05$. **$p < .01$. ***$p < .001$.

means they were given. This finding is a testament to the resistance of people's optimistic risk comparisons to correction.

These findings are consistent with Tesser's (1991) self-evaluation maintenance (SEM) model, which predicts that when people are outperformed on a dimension important to their self-definition, they respond by decreasing their view of the importance of this dimension. The current findings also fit into a growing literature showing that people may even modify the importance to their self-definition of highly consequential attributes. For example, in a study by Gibbons, Benbow, and Gerrard (1994), gifted children came to see academic achievement as less important when their own performance was inferior to that of other children. Moreover, Gerrard, Gibbons, Benthin, and Hessling (1996) reported that adolescents came to see risk-increasing behaviors as less problematic the more they engaged in these behaviors. Taken all together, these findings warn health researchers and professionals that information about others' performance of desirable health behaviors could lead people to be less rather than more convinced of the relevance and importance of those behaviors.

The successful use of strategies such as modifying beliefs about one's behavior or about the relevance of risk factors to a health problem is likely to produce contentment with one's current behavioral patterns and a disinterest in taking precautions. Indeed, it is conceivable that these strategies might lead individuals to become even more convinced of their invulnerability, thereby making them even less likely to modify their behavior. As an example, a smoker who has relapsed after an attempt at quitting may come to devalue the danger of smoking and thus make no further attempts to quit (cf. Festinger, 1957; Gibbons, Eggleston, & Benthin, 1997). Clearly, additional research is needed to determine the consequences of each of the strategies just listed for subsequent precautionary behavior.

***Summary.*** People maintain unrealistic optimism by distorting beliefs about others, about themselves, and about related behaviors. We also saw earlier that people may preserve beliefs about their favorable risk status by reducing their perceived similarity to a target who is said to be at high risk (Gump & Kulik, 1995). These strategies do not exhaust the possibilities. People might give more credit to other health-related behaviors (e.g., on hearing that their diets are only average, people might increase the perceived importance of exercise), or might invent new behaviors of questionable relevance (e.g., people might convince themselves that showering after intercourse reduces the risk of AIDS transmission; Bauman & Siegel, 1987). People could also choose to highlight the presumed health benefits of risky behaviors (e.g., the iron in red meat). Other work shows that people employ a variety of strategies to buffer themselves against the pain of negative feedback (e.g., Taylor & Brown, 1988; Taylor, Collins, Skokan, & Aspinwall, 1989). We need further research to identify these strategies, to specify when each is most likely to be used, and to find ways to counteract them. It is likely that people will use the strategies that are most economical (cf. Abelson, 1968). The strategies that have already been demonstrated, however, provide strong support for the claim that social comparison—and self-enhancing social comparison in particular—is an important component of risk judgment.

### Question 3: Do People Use Social Comparison in Everyday Risk Judgments?

We have now argued that social comparison factors influence the magnitude of unrealistic optimism and that people engage in a variety of strategies to maintain their unrealistic optimism. This work provides convergent evidence that social comparison plays a significant role in the way people respond to risk. The experiments so far described establish that people respond to comparison information when the investigators provide it. Information about others is surely available in everyday life, but do people make use of such information on their own without being prompted by eager experimenters? Although this might seem to be the most important question of those we have addressed, there are surprisingly few relevant studies available.

In one study (Suls, Marco, & Tobin, 1991), 54% of an elderly sample mentioned individual or group social comparisons when asked what types of information they used when they evaluated their overall health. Of course, these participants were rating health status, not risk. In a study by Wheeler and Miyake (1992), undergraduates kept a record of their social comparisons over a 2-week period and noted in each case the dimension on which they were comparing. Approximately 55% of the comparisons were on academic, personality, and physical appearance dimensions. The next most mentioned dimension was "lifestyle" (12%), which, of the dimensions listed, is probably the closest to judgments about one's health. Finally, Helweg-Larsen (1996) asked participants to explain their ratings on a series of comparative risk scales. Surprisingly, despite the comparative nature of these scales, paticipants generally referred only to their own behavior (and not to others' behavior) when attempting to account for their ratings. Although it is certainly possible that they were unaware of the role of social comparison in their judgments (cf. Nisbett & Wilson, 1977) or did not think to mention their comparison targets, Helweg-Larsen's data do not support the notion that unrealistically optimistic judgments arise from social comparison.

In sum, the evidence from naturalistic studies for the role of social comparison in everyday risk judgment is scant and mixed. Further research employing methodologies such as those used by Wheeler and Miyake (1992) in which participants carried beepers and reported their social comparisons when beeped might help us understand the extent to which people rely on social comparison spontaneously in personal risk assessment. Naturalistic studies will also be useful to determine the effects of comparative risk judgments on subsequent behavior, a topic that we address in the next section. If people's risk comparisons in everyday life affect their risk-related behavior, it will be easier to argue that social comparison is important in beliefs about personal risk. One plausible outcome of such research is that people use social comparison more for some health problems (particularly those that are threatening, ambiguous, and caused by controllable risk factors) than for others.

### Question 4: Are Reactions to Hazards Sensitive to Risk Comparisons?

Health is one domain in which objective information, such as the significance of family history, medical tests, and a risky lifestyle, is readily available. With access to abundant information and with apparently objective criteria—health and life versus illness and death—people might not consider social comparison information particularly important when judging their own risk. Thus, we now turn to our fourth and final question: Are people's affective, self-evaluative, and behavioral reactions to risk sensitive to social comparisons on risk status?

To assess the consequences of social comparisons, it is useful to contrast their impact with that of the knowledge people have about their *absolute (or actuarial) risk* of experiencing an event. At least at the aggregate level, estimates of absolute personal risk turn out to be fairly accurate (e.g., Rothman et al., 1996). And, as noted previously, objective information about health risk is often widely available. According to social comparison theory (Festinger, 1954), objective standards are the first source of information used in self-evaluation, and social comparison is initiated only when objective standards are not available. Thus, social comparison theory predicts that judgments of risk will be more dependent on absolute than on comparative standing. The notion that objective information is considered first has rarely been tested in social comparison research, however, because most of the dimensions studied (e.g., intelligence, attractiveness, and coping) do not possess objective standards. Not surprisingly, people are sensitive to comparison information when such attributes are involved. Indeed, people are more motivated to engage in an activity in which they perform better than others than in an activity in which their performance is objectively superior but no better than others (Tesser & Campbell, 1980). For example,a student who scores more highly on a math task than on a literature task may still prefer to engage in the literature task if his or her performance is better than that of a peer on the literature task but is equivalent to that of the peer on the math task. Will this greater sensitivity to comparative standing also hold for beliefs about risk, such as one's objective chances of having heart disease?

Note that although comparative risk ratings and absolute risk ratings are positively correlated, they are not redundant. In one study correlations between the two were sometimes as low as .22 (Weinstein, 1984). When participants believe their risk for an event is objectively high, it does not necessarily mean that they consider their risk to be above average (nor should they).

***Social Comparison and Affective Reactions to Risk.*** If comparisons with others are important in judgments of personal risk, we should find that such comparisons have a significant impact on emotional responses to risk. For example, if a gay man with a risky behavioral profile learns that his risk of getting AIDS is below the average of other gay men, he should exhibit a more positive emotional response than if his level of risk is said to be above this average (even if his risk is high in absolute terms). Klein (in press) tested this idea by asking participants to imagine that they had tested positive on a salivary litmus test of a genetic marker for pancreatic disease and that their risk of having this disease was either above average by 20% or below average by 20% (constituting *relative* risk). Moreover, in order to determine whether participants would be sensitive to their objective risk level, Klein asked some participants to imagine that their own risk was 30% and others that it was 60% (constituting *absolute* risk). This resulted in four conditions, with each absolute risk group being told that their risk was either above or below average (e.g., participants in the 30% conditions were told that the average person's risk was 10% in the above-average condition and 50% in the below-average condition). Participants then estimated how disturbed they would be with their test results.

Participants' absolute level of risk had no effect on how disturbed they believed they would be; participants who were said to have a 60% chance of having this disease did not believe they would be any more disturbed than participants who were said to have a 30% chance of having the disease. This finding is inconsistent with past research showing that people are less worried about a health risk the more prevalent it is said to be (Jemmott, Ditto, & Croyle, 1986); in this case, prevalence was not influential. However, there was a strong main effect of comparative standing: participants believed they would be more disturbed by a worse-than-average than by a better-than-average test. Indeed, participants whose risk of 30% was said to be above average expected to be more disturbed than participants whose risk of 60% was said to be below average. These findings suggest that affective responses to personal risk information are sensitive to social comparison, and, at least in some situations, even more so than to objective risk information.

***Social Comparison and Self-Evaluative Reactions to Risk.*** Although people's comparisons with others may influence affective reactions to personal risk, such comparisons may not necessarily influence their self-evaluations, which are more constrained than emotional responses by factual information and prior knowledge (Kunda, 1990). In our AIDS example, gay men may be comforted by the fact that their risk is below average yet they may still believe that their objective behavior is dangerous. In an attempt to assess the effect of social comparison on self-evaluation, Klein (in press) asked participants to imagine that, because of their driving habits, they had either a 30% or a 60% chance of causing an automobile accident. As before, half imagined that the average person's risk was 20% higher than this figure and half imagined that it was 20% lower. The self-evaluation measure employed was participants' judgments of how safe they would consider their driving to be upon hearing this information. Once again, absolute risk had no effect on participants' safety judgments. However, analyses revealed a main effect of comparative risk such that participants thought they were safer drivers when their risk was said to be below average than when it was said to be above average. Participants in the 60% risk/below-average group believed they were safer drivers than those in the 30% risk/above-average group. These findings suggest that social comparison influences not only affective responses to personal risk levels but self-assessments as well.

***Social Comparison and Behavioral Reactions to Risk.*** The question of most interest to health researchers and public health workers is whether behavior is influenced by social comparison. Continuing with the AIDS example, would a high-risk gay man who learned that his AIDS risk was below the average of other gay men be less interested in precautionary behaviors despite the fact that he faces a substantial, life-threatening hazard? (See also Misovich, Fisher, & Fisher, chapter 4, this volume.) Although people's affective and self-evaluative responses to risk information may depend more on relative than on absolute risk, the often immediate consequences of risky behaviors may lead behavioral responses to reflect a more realistic understanding of the correlation between one's objective risk standing and the consequences of one's behavior (and thus encourage less attention to relative information). In Klein's (in press) next problem, participants again imagined that they had a 30% or 60% absolute risk of causing an automobile accident, and that their risk was 20% above or below the average. Participants then indicated the extent to which they might change several different driving behaviors. The same pattern found earlier for judgments of driving safety was observed for participants' behavioral intentions. Participants whose risk was said to be above average (rather than below average) indicated that they would be more likely to drive slower on the highway, use seat belts more often, and take public transportation more frequently. There were no effects of absolute risk on behavioral intentions.

Of course, it is difficult to draw strong conclusions from studies involving scenarios that are hypothetical and that do not measure actual behavior. Are people responsive to comparative risk when making a decision with a real outcome? In the next study, Klein (in press) informed participants that they correctly answered 8 or 12 out of 20 items on a judgment task. Half were told that the average score was 50% higher (and half 50% lower) than the participant's score. Participants could then engage in one of two games with the chance of winning a prize. The first game was to complete 20 more items on the same judgment task; participants would win if they answered 10 or more correctly. The other option was a chance game in which participants would spin a roulette wheel 20 times and win if the ball landed on red 10 times or more. Task choice was the primary measure. Note that among participants who had scored an 8 on the first judgment task, the only reason they should choose to perform this task again instead of the chance task was if they believed they could improve their score to 10 or higher on a second try.

The data showed that participants were sensitive to their absolute score—participants scoring 12 were more likely than those scoring 8 to choose the judgment task again. However, participants also exhibited attention to the comparison information: significantly more "above-average" participants than "below-average" participants chose the judgment task again. Thus, when thinking about their risk of succeeding at the second judgment task, participants were influenced by their comparative standing. A follow-up study (Klein, in press) that contrasted these two conditions with a no-information control group showed that the above-average group was somewhat more likely and the below-average group somewhat less likely to choose the judgment task, suggesting that the effects of comparative risk in the first study were unrelated to the desirability of the information. Mediational analyses showed that relative standing affected task choice by modifying beliefs about the self. Returning once more to the AIDS example, this study suggests that a high risk gay man who hears that his risk of AIDS is below that of others may come to see his behavior in an even more favorable light, and, in turn, neglect to make important behavioral changes.

***Correlational Studies Linking Risk to Behavior.*** The issue of whether social comparison influences behavioral reactions to risk may also be addressed by consulting the extensive literature correlating risk perceptions with health behaviors. Given our interest in contrasting the influence of relative risk estimates on subsequent behavior with that of absolute risk estimates, the studies of most relevance are those that measure both types of risk perceptions. Many investigators assess just one of these risk variables (e.g., Kulik & Mahler, 1987) and others measure both but combine them into a single variable when analyzing their data (e.g., Aspinwall, Kemeny, Taylor, Schneider, & Dudley, 1991). Among the few studies that analyze the variables separately, findings are mixed. Some report that behavior correlates more highly with absolute risk than with comparative risk (e.g., Gladis, Michela, Walter, & Vaughan, 1992; Hoorens & Buunk, 1993), whereas others report the opposite (van der Velde et al., 1994). This inconsistency could reflect variations in the timing of behaviors. Cross-sectional correlations between risk and behavior usually indicate the accuracy of risk perceptions, whereas prospective correlations between risk perceptions and future behavior pertain to the effects of risk perceptions on behavior (Gerrard, Gibbons, & Bushman, 1996; Weinstein & Nicolich, 1993; Weinstein, Rothman, & Nicolich, in press). Several of the prospective studies find that future behavior is predicted better by comparative risk than by absolute risk (e.g., Blalock, DeVellis, & Afifi, 1990; van der Velde, van der Pligt, & Hooykaas, 1992; although see Weinstein, Sandman, & Roberts, 1990). We encourage researchers to use both risk variables in order to determine which best predicts precaution adoption.

***Summary.*** The studies reviewed show that people are sensitive to the comparison between their risk and the risk of their peers. In fact, some reactions seem more sensitive to comparative than to absolute risk status, arguing against the assumption in social comparison theory that objective information is used first. In other ways these findings provide strong support for social comparison theory because they show that social comparison may be even more ubiquitous than the theory predicts.

In addition to highlighting the importance of social comparison in the way people feel about risk, these studies suggest that any interventions focusing solely on one's personal, actuarial risk may not be successful in changing behavior. Campaigns that provide personal risk information may be more effective if they add information about a person's relative risk. Of course, this adjustment may sometimes backfire, because if people learn that their risk is below the average for their reference group they may become even less interested in behavioral change. We consider this possibility further in the next section.

## DILEMMAS OF THE HEALTH PROFESSIONAL

For anyone hoping to change people's health habits, the findings reviewed here might appear quite discouraging. People not only hold optimistically biased beliefs about their health, but vigorously attempt to maintain these beliefs when challenged. However, knowledge about the importance of social comparison in risk judgments suggests a number of approaches for designing more effective interventions. In our first section, we found that comparative unrealistic optimism is attenuated under a variety of conditions: when people compare with similar, individuated, or physically present others; when people pay attention to what others are doing to decrease their risk; and when people compare others to themselves (rather than vice-versa). In our last section, we discussed research that showed that people's affective, self-evaluative, and behavioral reactions to risk information are sensitive to comparisons with others. These two bodies of work suggest that people will feel particularly concerned about their own risk if they are forced to compare with a similar, highly individuated peer who has a healthier lifestyle (and thus a relatively lower risk) than they do. Alternatively, people may become strongly concerned about their risk by comparing themselves to another who is at high risk but similar on all other dimensions. Indeed, this assumption is at the heart of work by Misovich, Fisher, and Fisher (chapter 4, this volume): these researchers showed that films of seemingly normal undergraduates who also happen to be HIV-positive have a great impact on viewers' beliefs about (and behavioral reactions to) their own HIV risk. Of course, it is essential to reduce biases about risk without creating feelings of hopelessness and helplessness (cf. Janoff-Bulman, 1989). With this caveat in mind, researchers should determine which comparison targets elicit the most behavior change.

The picture becomes more complicated when we recognize that people harness several strategies to maintain biased beliefs about their comparative risk and their comparative standing on relevant risk factors. Interventions that merely include the use of comparison targets without taking these strategies into account are probably doomed to fail and may even exacerbate biases (Weinstein & Klein, 1995). For example, presenting a comparison target that is a prototype of the type of person who contracts a particular disease may not only be ineffective but may make people believe they are even less at risk than they thought before. One promising implication of the Klein (1996) studies is that if people report their risky behaviors and health beliefs before rather than after an intervention they may be prevented from reducing estimates of how often they engage in these behaviors or from changing their beliefs about the significance of these behaviors to their health. According to this argument, having people report their beliefs prior to a social comparison intervention will make them feel a greater need to justify any changes they make in these beliefs after the intervention. Further research will determine the kinds of interventions that work best, but one thing is clear: the effect of educational interventions will in all likelihood be enhanced by the inclusion of carefully chosen social comparisons and further enhanced if these comparisons block people's bias maintenance strategies.

## CONCLUSIONS AND REFLECTIONS

Our inquiry into the role of social comparison in biased comparative assessments of personal risk addressed four questions. On balance, the available research suggests that social comparison may play an important role in risk appraisal. We found that several aspects of the social comparison process influence the magnitude of unrealistic optimism, that people try to maintain favorable comparisons with others on risk dimensions, and that in their affective, self-evaluative, and behavioral reactions to risk people are sensitive to social comparison information. We also reported very preliminary and mixed research on the role social comparison plays in everyday risk perceptions.

Several interesting questions remain. First, does the importance of social comparison in judging personal risk match the importance of social comparison in other life domains? Although research on social indicators has provided some sense of the value of social comparison in judging different life dimensions (e.g., Diener & Fujita, chapter 11, this volume; Emmons & Diener, 1985; Fox & Kahneman, 1992), health is rarely among the dimensions examined. This question awaits further research.

Could it be that the processes reported here are present in other self-enhancement biases, such as false consensus (e.g., Marks & Miller, 1987), false uniqueness (e.g., Goethals et al., 1991), and positivity biases in judgments of personality (Brown, 1986) and ability (Larwood & Whittaker, 1977)? Given that processes of self-assessment are generally related (e.g., Hoorens, 1993b; Tesser & Cornell, 1991), we think the answer is yes. Indeed, Klein and Goethals (1997) have recently shown that people's attempts to maintain favorable comparisons in the face of challenging information may increase uniqueness biases.

Moreover, it is likely that social comparison is relevant to other risk-specific issues such as the decision to see a medical professional or submit to a risky medical procedure. In general, an integration of these research findings will be helpful in constructing a theoretical understanding of self-enhancing social comparison and its effects on everyday functioning (see also Suls, Martin, & Leventhal, chapter 7, this volume).

Another interesting question is whether cultural factors determine the role of social comparison in risk perception. Optimistic biases have been found among individuals in Singapore (Lek & Bishop, 1995), Denmark (Helweg-Larsen, 1994), and the Netherlands (van der Pligt et al., 1993), as well as among American Indians (Lightdale, Oken,Klein, Welty, & Landrigan, in press). It remains to be seen whether social comparison influences risk judgment equally in these and other cultures. For example, in cultures where one is taught not to stand out from others, seeking favorable social comparisons may be avoided (cf. Markus & Kitayama, 1991); in this context, optimistic biases would presumably have their roots in some phenomenon other than social comparison. In some cases, cultural tendencies may even prevent unrealistic optimism from appearing at all (e.g., Heine & Lehman, 1995). The role of cultural and other individual differences such as SES and personality deserves further attention.

It is important to emphasize that when social comparison is used to judge risk, self-enhancement is only one possible goal (cf. Helgeson & Mickelson, 1995). People may be genuinely interested in risk information about similar others, especially when new health problems such as AIDS and skin cancer arise or receive additional public attention. Individuals will also be interested to know that members of their in-group are especially susceptible to a health problem, as are Jews to Tay-Sachs disease and African Americans to sickle-cell anemia. Learning that others in one's ethnic group have been victimized by a problem is likely to increase personal risk perceptions. People may also use low-risk targets as models (upward comparison) in order to ascertain how to lead healthier lifestyles.

Still, social comparison in risk judgment often appears more focused on self-enhancement. Although this makes reducing comparison biases a major challenge, the search for successful interventions is under way. As we discover what works, we will undoubtedly learn more about the many ways that social comparison and risk judgment are intertwined.

## ACKNOWLEDGMENTS

The writing of this chapter was supported by a sabbatical extension grant and Social Science grants 01-2230 and 01-2242 from Colby College and was completed while the first author was a visiting researcher at Rutgers University. We thank Bram Buunk, Meg Gerrard, Rick Gibbons, Marie Helweg-Larsen, Steve Misovich, and Elise Phillips for their helpful suggestions on earlier versions of the chapter.

## REFERENCES

Abelson, R. P. (1968). Psychological implication. In R. P. Abelson, E. Aronson, W. J. McGuire, T. M. Newcomb, M. J. Rosenberg, & P. H. Tannenbaum (Eds.) *Theories of cognitive consistency: A sourcebook* (pp. 112–139). Chicago: Rand McNally.

Alicke, M. D., Klotz, M. L., Breitenbecher, D. L., Yurak, T. J., & Vredenburg, D. S. (1995). Personal contact, individuation, and the better-than-average effect. *Journal of Personality and Social Psychology, 68,* 804–825.

Aspinwall, L. G., Kemeny, M. E., Taylor, S. E., Schneider, S. G., & Dudley, J. P. (1991). Psychosocial predictors of gay men's AIDS risk-reduction behavior. *Health Psychology, 10,* 432–444.

Aspinwall, L. G., & Taylor, S. E. (1993). Effects of social comparison direction, threat, and self-esteem on affect, self-evaluation, and expected success. *Journal of Personality and Social Psychology, 64*, 708–722.

Bauman, L. J., & Siegel, K. (1987). Misperception among gay men of the risk for AIDS associated with their sexual behavior. *Journal of Applied Social Psychology, 17*, 329–350.

Blalock, S. J., DeVellis, B. M., Afifi, R. A., & Sandler, R. S. (1990). Risk perceptions and participation in colorectal cancer screening. *Health Psychology, 9*, 792–806.

Boney McCoy, S., Gibbons, F. X., Reis, T. J., Gerrard, M., Luus, C. A. E., & Sufka, A. V. W. (1992). Perceptions of smoking risk as a function of smoking status. *Journal of Behavioral Medicine, 15*, 469–488.

Brown, J. D. (1986). Evaluations of self and others: Self-enhancement biases in social judgments. *Social Cognition, 4*, 353–376.

Burger, J. M., & Burns, L. (1988). The illusion of unique invulnerability and the use of effective contraception. *Personality and Social Psychology Bulletin, 14*, 264–270.

Burger, J. M., & Palmer, M. L. (1992). Changes in and generalization of unrealistic optimism following experiences with stressful events: Reactions to the 1989 California earthquake. *Personality and Social Psychology Bulletin, 18*, 39–43.

Codol, J. P. (1987). Comparability and incomparability between oneself and others: Means of differentiation and comparison reference points. *European Journal of Cognitive Psychology, 7*, 87–105.

Croyle, R. T., & Ditto, P. H. (1990). Illness cognition and behavior: An experimental approach. *Journal of Behavioral Medicine, 13*, 31–52.

DeJoy, D. M. (1989). The optimism bias and traffic accident risk perception. *Accident Analysis and Prevention, 21*, 333–340.

DeVellis, R. F., Holt, K., Renner, B. R., Blalock, S. J., Blanchard, L. W., Cook, H. L., Klotz, M. L., Mikow, V., & Harring, K. (1990). The relationship of social comparison to rheumatoid arthritis symptoms and affect. *Basic and Applied Social Psychology, 11*, 1–18.

Dolinski, D., Gromski, W., & Zawisza, E. (1987). Unrealistic pessimism. *Journal of Social Psychology, 127*, 511–516.

Dunning, D., & Cohen, G. L. (1992). Egocentric definitions of traits and abilities in social judgment. *Journal of Personality and Social Psychology, 63*, 341–355.

Emmons, R. A., & Diener, E. (1985). Factors predicting satisfaction judgments: A comparative examination. *Social Indicators Research, 16*, 157–167.

Fenigstein, A. (1993). Self-attention and the egocentric assumption of shared perspectives. *Journal of Experimental Social Psychology, 29*, 287–303.

Festinger, L. (1954). A theory of social comparison processes. *Human Relations, 7*, 117–140.

Festinger, L. (1957). *A theory of cognitive dissonance.* Evanston, IL: Row, Peterson.

Fong, G. T., & Markus, H. (1982). Self-schemas and judgments about others. *Social Cognition, 1*, 191–205.

Fox, C. R., & Kahneman, D. (1992). Correlations, causes, and heuristics in surveys of life satisfaction. *Social Indicators Research, 27*, 221–234.

Gerrard, M., Gibbons, F. X., Benthin, A. C., & Hessling, R. M. (1996). The reciprocal nature of risk behaviors and cognitions: What you think shapes what you do, and vice versa. *Health Psychology, 15*, 344–354.

Gerrard, M., Gibbons, F. X., & Bushman, B. J. (1996). The relation between perceived vulnerability to HIV and precautionary sexual behavior. *Psychological Bulletin, 119*, 390–409.

Gerrard, M., Gibbons, F. X., & Warner, T. (1991). Effects of reviewing risk-relevant behavior on perceived vulnerability among women marines. *Health Psychology, 10*, 173–179.

Gibbons, F. X., Benbow, C. P., & Gerrard M. (1994). From top dog to bottom half: Social comparison strategies in response to poor performance. *Journal of Personality and Social*

*Psychology, 67,* 638–652.

Gibbons, F. X., & Eggleston, T. J. (1996). Smoker networks and the "typical smoker": A prospective analysis of smoking cessation. *Health Psychology, 15,* 469–477.

Gibbons, F. X., Eggleston, T. J., & Benthin, A. C. (1997). Cognitive reactions to smoking relapse: The reciprocal relation of dissonance and self-esteem. *Journal of Personality and Social Psychology, 72,* 184–195.

Gibbons, F. X., Gerrard, M., Lando, H. A., & McGovern, P. G. (1991). Social comparison and smoking cessation: The role of the "typical smoker." *Journal of Experimental Social Psychology, 27,* 239–258.

Gladis, M. M., Michela, J. L., Walter, H. J., & Vaughan, R. D. (1992). High school students' perceptions of AIDS risk: Realistic appraisal or motivated denial? *Health Psychology, 11,* 307–316.

Goethals, G. R., Messick, D. M., & Allison, S. T. (1991). The uniqueness bias: Studies of constructive social comparison. In J. Suls & T. A. Wills (Eds.), *Social comparison research: Contemporary theory and research* (pp. 149–176). Hilsdale, NJ: Lawrence Erlbaum Associates.

Gump, B. B., & Kulik, J. A. (1995). The effect of a model's HIV status on self-perceptions: A self-protective similarity bias. *Personality and Social Psychology Bulletin, 21,* 827–833.

Hakmiller, K. L. (1966). Threat as a determinant of downward comparison. *Journal of Experimental Social Psychology* (Suppl. 1), 32–39.

Harris, P. (1996). Sufficient grounds for optimism? The relationship between perceived controllability and optimistic bias. *Journal of Social and Clinical Psychology, 15,* 9–52.

Harris, P., & Middleton, W. (1994). The illusion of control and optimism about health: On being less at risk but no more in control than others. *British Journal of Social Psychology, 33,* 369–386.

Heine, S. J., & Lehman, D. R. (1995). Cultural variation in unrealistic optimism: Does the West feel more invulnerable than the East? *Journal of Personality and Social Psychology, 68,* 595–607.

Helgeson, V. S., & Mickelson, K. D. (1995). Motives for social comparison. *Personality and Social Psychology Bulletin, 21,* 1200–1209.

Helweg-Larsen, M. (1994). *Why it won't happen to me: A cross-cultural investigation of social comparison as a cause of the optimistic bias.* Unpublished doctoral dissertation, University of California, Los Angeles.

Holyoak, K. J., & Gordon, P. C. (1983). Social reference points. *Journal of Personality and Social Psychology, 44,* 881–887.

Hoorens, V. (1993a). Unrealistic optimism in social comparison of health and safety risks. In L. D. Rutter & L. Quine (Eds.), *The social psychology of health and safety: European perspectives.* Aldershot, UK: Avebury.

Hoorens, V. (1993b). Self-enhancement and superiority biases in social comparison. In W. Stroebe & M. Hewstone (Eds.), *European Review of Social Psychology* (pp. 113–139). New York: Wiley.

Hoorens, V. (1995). Self-favoring biases, self-presentation and the self-other asymmetry in social comparison. *Journal of Personality, 63,* 793–817.

Hoorens, V. (1996). Self-favoring biases for positive and negative characteristics: Independent phenomena? *Journal of Social and Clinical Psychology, 15,* 53–67.

Hoorens, V., & Buunk, B. P. (1993). Social comparison of health risks: Locus of control, the person–positivity bias, and unrealistic optimism. *Journal of Applied Social Psychology, 23,* 291–302.

Hume, D. (1911). Treatise of human nature. In E. Rhys (Ed.), *Everyman's library. (p. 89). New York: Dutton. (Original work published in 1739)*

Janoff-Bulman, R. (1989). The benefits of illusions, the threat of disillusionment, and the limitations of inaccuracy. *Journal of Social and Clinical Psychology, 8,* 158–175.

Jemmott, J. B. III, Ditto, P. H., & Croyle, R. T. (1986). Judging health status: Effects of perceived prevalence and personal relevance. *Journal of Personality and Social Psychology, 50,* 899–905.
Klein, W. M. (in press). Objective standards are not enough: Affective, self-evaluative, and behavioral responses to social comparison information. *Journal of Personality and Social Psychology.*
Klein, W. M. (1996). Maintaining self-serving social comparisons: Attenuating the perceived significance of risk-increasing behaviors. *Journal of Social and Clinical Psychology, 15,* 120–142.
Klein, W. M., & Goethals, G. R. (1997). *Social reality and self-construction.* Manuscript submitted for publication.
Klein, W. M., & Kunda, Z. (1993). Maintaining self-serving social comparisons: Biased reconstruction of one's past behaviors. *Personality and Social Psychology Bulletin, 19,* 732–739.
Klein, W. M., & Kunda, Z. (1994). Exaggerated self-assessments and the preference for controllable risks. *Organizational Behavior and Human Decision Processes, 59,* 410–427.
Kreuter, M. W., & Strecher, V. J. (1995). Changing inaccurate perceptions of health risk: Results from a randomized trial. *Health Psychology, 14,* 56–63.
Krueger, J., & Clement, R. W. (1994). The truly false consensus effect: An ineradicable and egocentric bias in social perception. *Journal of Personality and Social Psychology, 67,* 596–610.
Kulik, J. A., & Mahler, H. I. M. (1987). Health status, perceptions of risk, and prevention interest for health and non-health problems. *Health Psychology, 6,* 15–27.
Kunda, Z. (1990). The case for motivated reasoning. *Psychological Bulletin, 108,* 480–498.
Larwood, L., & Whittaker, W. (1977). Managerial myopia: Self-serving biases in organizational planning. *Journal of Applied Psychology, 62,* 194–198.
Lek, Y. Y., & Bishop, G. D. (1995). Perceived vulnerability to illness threats: The role of disease type, risk factor perception and attributions. *Psychology and Health, 10,* 205–217.
Lightdale, J. R., Oken, E., Klein, W. M., Welty, T. K., & Landrigan, P. J. (in press). Psychosocial barriers to health promotion in an American Indian population. *Journal of the National Center for American Indian and Alaska Native Mental Health Research.*
Markus, H., & Kitayama, S. (1991). Culture and the self: Implications for cognition, emotion, and motivation. *Psychological Review, 98,* 224–252.
Marks, G., & Miller, N. (1987). Ten years of research on the false-consensus effect: An empirical and theoretical review. *Psychological Bulletin, 102,* 72–90.
McKenna, F. P., Warburton, D. M., & Winwood, M. (1993). Exploring the limits of optimism: The case of smokers' decision making. *British Journal of Psychology, 84,* 389–394.
Mickler, S. E. (1991, April). *Perceptions of vulnerability: Impact on AIDS-preventive behavior among college adolescents.* Paper presented at the annual meeting of the Eastern Psychological Association, New York.
Moore, S., & Rosenthal, D. (1991). Adolescent invulnerability and perceptions of AIDS risk. *Journal of Adolescent Research, 6,* 164–180.
Nisbett, R. E., & Wilson, T. D. (1977). Telling more than we can know: Verbal reports on mental processes. *Psychological Review, 84,* 231–259.
Otten, W. (1995). *Optimism.* Unpublished doctoral dissertation, University of Amsterdam, Amsterdam, The Netherlands.
Otten, W., & van der Pligt, J. (1996). Context effects in the measurement of comparative optimism in probability judgments. *Journal of Social and Clinical Psychology, 15,* 80–101.
Perloff, L. S. (1987). Social comparison and illusions of vulnerability to negative life events. In C. R. Snyder & C. E. Ford (Eds.), *Coping with negative life events* (pp. 217–242). New York: Plenum.

Perloff, L. S., & Fetzer, B. K. (1986). Self-other judgments and perceived vulnerability to victimization. *Journal of Personality and Social Psychology, 50,* 502–510.

Quadrel, M. J., Fischhoff, B., & Davis, W. (1993). Adolescent (in)vulnerability. *American Psychologist, 48,* 102–117.

Regan, P. C., Snyder, M., & Kassin, S. M. (1995). Unrealistic optimism: Self-enhancement or person positivity? *Personality and Social Psychology Bulletin, 10,* 1073–1082.

Reis, T. J., Gerrard, M., & Gibbons, F. X. (1993). Social comparison and the pill: Reactions to upward and downward social comparison of contraceptive behavior. *Personality and Social Psychology Bulletin, 19,* 13–20.

Ross, M., & Sicoly, F. (1979). Egocentric biases in availability and attribution. *Journal of Personality and Social Psychology, 37,* 322–337.

Rothman, A. J., Klein, W. M., & Weinstein, N. D. (1996). Absolute and relative biases in estimations of personal risk. *Journal of Applied Social Psychology, 26,* 1213–1236.

Scheier, M. F., & Carver, C. S. (1992). Effects of optimism on psychological and physical well-being: Theoretical overview and empirical update. *Cognitive Therapy and Research, 16,* 201–228.

Shepperd, J. A., Ouellette, J. A., & Fernandez, J. K. (1996). Abandoning unrealistic optimism: Performance estimates and the temporal proximity of self-relevant feedback. *Journal of Personality and Social Psychology, 70,* 844–855.

Simon, B. (1993). On the asymmetry in the cognitive construal of ingroup and outgroup: A model of egocentric social categorization. *European Journal of Social Psychology, 23,* 131–147.

Strack, F., Schwarz, N., Chassein, B., Kern, D., & Wagner, D. (1990). Salience of comparison standards and activation of social norms: Consequences for judgments of happiness and their communication. *British Journal of Social Psychology, 29,* 303–313.

Suls, J., Marco, C. A., & Tobin, S. (1991). The role of temporal comparison, social comparison, and direct appraisal in the elderly's self-evaluations of health. *Journal of Applied Social Psychology, 21,* 1125–1144.

Suls, J., & Miller, R. L. (Eds.). (1977). *Social comparison processes: Theoretical and empirical perspectives.* Washington, DC: Hemisphere.

Suls, J., Wan, C. K., & Sanders, G. S. (1988). False consensus and false uniqueness in estimating the prevalence of health-protective behaviors. *Journal of Applied Social Psychology, 18,* 66–79.

Suls, J., & Wills, T. A. (Eds.) (1991). *Social comparison: Contemporary theory and research.* Hillsdale, NJ: Lawrence Erlbaum Associates.

Taylor, S. E., & Brown, J. D. (1988). Illusion and well-being: A social psychological perspective on mental health. *Psychological Bulletin, 103,* 193–210.

Taylor, S. E., Collins, R. L., Skokan, L. A., & Aspinwall, L. G. (1989). Maintaining positive illusions in the face of negative information: Getting the facts without letting them get to you. *Journal of Social and Clinical Psychology, 8,* 114–129.

Taylor, S. E., & Gollwitzer, P. M. (1995). Effects of mindset on positive illusions. *Journal of Personality and Social Psychology, 69,* 213–226.

Taylor, S. E., Kemeny, M., Aspinwall, L. G., Schneider, S. C., Rodriguez, R., & Herbert, M. (1992). Optimism, coping, psychological distress, and high-risk sexual behavior among men at risk for AIDS. *Journal of Personality and Social Psychology, 63,* 460–473.

Taylor, S. E., & Lobel, M. (1989). Social comparison activity under threat: Downward evaluation and upward contacts. *Psychological Review, 96,* 569–575.

Tesser, A. (1991). Emotion in social comparison and reflection processes. In J. Suls & T. A. Wills (Eds.), *Social comparison: Contemporary theory and research* (pp. 115–145). Hillsdale, NJ: Lawrence Erlbaum Associates.

Tesser, A., & Campbell, J. (1980). Self-definition: The impact of the relative performance and similarity of others. *Social Psychology Quarterly, 43,* 341–347.

Tesser, A., & Cornell, D. P. (1991). On the confluence of self processes. *Journal of Experimental Social Psychology, 27,* 501–526.
van der Pligt, J., Otten, W., Richard, R., & van der Velde, F. (1993). Perceived risk of AIDS: Unrealistic optimism and self-protective action. In J. B. Pryor & G. D. Reeder (Eds.), *The social psychology of HIV infection* (pp. 39–58). Hillsdale, NJ: Lawrence Erlbaum Associates.
van der Velde, F. W., van der Pligt, J., & Hooykaas, C. (1992). Risk perception and behavior: Pessimism, realism, and optimism about AIDS-related behavior. *Psychology and Health, 6,* 23–28.
van der Velde, F. W., van der Pligt, J., & Hooykaas, C. (1994). Perceiving AIDS-related risk: Accuracy as a function of differences in actual risk. *Health Psychology, 13,* 25–33.
Wanke, M., Schwarz, N., & Noelle-Neumann, E. (1995). Asking comparative questions: The impact of the direction of comparison. *Public Opinion Quarterly, 59,* 347–372.
Weinstein, N. D. (1980). Unrealistic optimism about future life events. *Journal of Personality and Social Psychology, 39,* 806–820.
Weinstein, N. D. (1982). Unrealistic optimism about susceptibility to health problems. *Journal of Behavioral Medicine, 5,* 441–460.
Weinstein, N. D. (1983). Reducing unrealistic optimism about illness susceptibility. *Health Psychology, 2,* 11–20.
Weinstein, N. D. (1984). Why it won't happen to me: Perceptions of risk factors and susceptibility. *Health Psychology, 3,* 431–457.
Weinstein, N. D. (1987). Unrealistic optimism about susceptibility to health problems: Conclusions from a community-wide sample. *Journal of Behavioral Medicine, 10,* 481–500.
Weinstein, N. D. (1988). The precaution adoption process. *Health Psychology, 7,* 355–386.
Weinstein, N. D. (1989). Effects of personal experience on self-protective behavior. *Psychological Bulletin, 105,* 31–50.
Weinstein, N. D., & Klein, W. M. (1995). Resistance of personal risk perceptions to debiasing interventions. *Health Psychology, 14,* 132–140.
Weinstein, N. D., & Lachendro, E. (1982). Egocentrism as a source of unrealistic optimism. *Personality and Social Psychology Bulletin, 8,* 195–200.
Weinstein, N. D., & Nicolich, M. (1993). Correct and incorrect interpretations of correlations between risk perceptions and risk behaviors. *Health Psychology, 12,* 235–245.
Weinstein, N. D., Rothman, A. J., & Nicolich, M. (in press). Use of correlational data to examine the effects of risk perceptions on precautionary behavior. *Psychology and Health.*
Weinstein, N. D., Sandman, P. M., & Roberts, N. E. (1990). Determinants of self-protective behavior: Home radon testing. *Journal of Applied Social Psychology, 20,* 783–801.
Wheeler, L. (1991). A brief history of social comparison theory. In J. Suls & T. A. Wills (Eds.), *Social comparison: Contemporary theory and research* (pp. 3–21). Hillsdale, NJ: Lawrence Erlbaum Associates.
Wheeler, L., & Miyake, K. (1992). Social comparison in everyday life. *Journal of Personality and Social Psychology, 62,* 760–773.
Whitley, B. E., & Hern, A. L. (1991). Perceptions of vulnerability to pregnancy and the use of effective contraception. *Personality and Social Psychology Bulletin, 17,* 104–110.
Wills, T. A. (1981). Downward comparison principles in social psychology. *Psychological Bulletin, 90,* 245–271.
Wills, T. A. (1987). Downward comparison as a coping mechanism. In C. R. Snyder & C. Ford (Eds.), *Coping with negative life events: Clinical and social-psychological perspectives* (pp. 243–268). New York: Plenum.
Wills, T. A. (1991). Similarity and self-esteem in downward comparison. In J. Suls & T. A. Wills (Eds.), *Social comparison: Contemporary research and beyond* (pp. 51–78). Hillsdale,

NJ: Lawrence Erlbaum Associates.
Wood, J. V. (1989). Theory and research concerning social comparisons of personal attributes. *Psychological Bulletin, 106,* 231–248.
Wood, J. V., & Taylor, K. L. (1991). Serving self-relevant goals through social comparison. In J. Suls & T. A. Wills (Eds.), *Social comparison: Contemporary theory and research* (pp. 23–49). Hillsdale, NJ: Lawrence Erlbaum Associates.
Wood, J. V., Taylor, S. E., & Lichtman, R. R. (1985). Social comparison in adjustment to breast cancer. *Journal of Personality and Social Psychology, 49,* 1169–1183.
Worm, T. (1994). [Letter to the editor]. *Time, 144,* p. 3.

# CHAPTER 3

# Health Images and Their Effects on Health Behavior

Frederick X. Gibbons
Meg Gerrard
*Iowa State University*

Imagine the prototypical "couch potato." If you think for a minute about this common image, more than likely you will generate a description that includes one or more of the following adjectives: sedentary, boring, slovenly, lazy. A quick survey of the graduate and undergraduate assistants in our laboratory one afternoon revealed a great deal of consensus about what couch potatoes are like and how they typically behave. Our assistants' images were both very rich and very detailed. In fact, most people maintain a wealth of images of typical members of many categories—movie actresses, professional athletes, joggers, to name just a few. Moreover, a growing body of literature demonstrates, convincingly, that these *images* or *prototypes* (we use both words interchangeably in this chapter) can have a significant impact on behavior. This chapter concerns one group of images that appears to be particularly influential, that associated with health and health behaviors.

Behaviors that are relevant to health and health risk and the people who engage in them are often quite visible or salient. For example, most of us have a pretty clear image of the type of person who smokes or the type of college student who likes to go on drinking binges. Like other images, health images can be favorable or unfavorable, and they can have positive as well as negative effects on behavior. Sometimes they facilitate healthy behavior; often, however, they seem to interfere with a healthy lifestyle. Like other images, health images are more influential for some people than they are for others.

Our aim in this chapter is to present and discuss research that examines health images and the impact that they have on health behavior. We also present a model of how images influence behavior. A fundamental assumption of the model (and a focus of the chapter) is our belief that images influence behavior through a process of social comparison. Our own research, as well as most of that conducted by others, has focused on adolescents and young adults, and so most of our discussion deals with these age groups. We believe that the processes remain essentially the same as people age, however, even though preliminary analyses of our data suggest that the impact of images probably diminishes later in life (Gibbons & Buunk, 1997). Finally, we present some thoughts on types of interventions, suggested by our own work and that of others, that might help alter risk-taking behavior among adolescents and young adults.

## PROTOTYPES

When we form an impression of someone we have an almost automatic tendency to try to assign that individual to a particular category or group with which we are already familiar (Cantor & Mischel, 1979). These categories may be defined by one or more of a wide variety of traits. Grandparents would be one such group, politicians would be another group, juvenile delinquents yet another, and so forth. Each of these categories has a typical member or representative associated with it, an image or prototype that embodies many of the characteristics that are thought to covary with the central trait, and that as a result are attributed, in varying degrees, to all members of the category. The central or defining features may be physical (e.g., weight); demographic (e.g., age or ethnic group), or they could be behavioral, something that members of the group do (e.g., snowboarding). Thus, people can just as easily generate a list of behaviors associated with a specific prototype (e.g., grandparents spoil their grandchildren), as they can generate a list of characteristics associated with a prototype that is defined by a particular behavior (rock climbers are intense, chefs are creative).

The categories themselves are often loosely constructed (i.e., "fuzzy sets;" see Rosch, 1978); thus a particular individual need not necessarily match the prototype perfectly in order to be assigned to the category that the prototype represents. Instead, a general similarity or "family resemblance" may be sufficient for inclusion (Mervis & Rosch, 1981). As long as the central or defining feature is identified or approximated, variability is tolerated. At the same time, the group must be distinctive in some manner. Categories that are very large (e.g., men) and groups that are very obscure (e.g., pinot noir drinkers) are not likely to have a clearly defined image. On the other hand, some groups are readily defined by virtue of their visibility and assumed homogeneity, even though their actual size is quite small (e.g., TV talk show hosts). Another contributor to prototype clarity or definition is the extremity of the behavior in question. In particular, negative or unusual behaviors are more salient and tend to carry more weight in the impression formation process (Birnbaum, 1972; Skowronski & Carlston, 1989; Taylor, 1991), just as they are more likely to be associated with clearly defined prototypes. For example, most people could easily identify and describe their prototypes of professional soccer players or of men who beat their wives. By the same token (and more pertinent to the current discussion), adolescents who smoke, take drugs, or drive recklessly also comprise recognizable categories with prototypes that other adolescents can readily define and to which they can relate.

## Prototypes and the Self

Although prototypes are frequently based in reality and experience, they are nevertheless cognitive constructions. As such, their formation is subject to idiosyncrasies and biases that often reflect an underlying motive. Frequently that motive involves protection of self-esteem. As Dunning et al. (1991) suggested, "if people wish to achieve positive self-images, there is no more convenient avenue than defining relevant social categories on the unique proficiencies and strengths that they themselves possess" (p. 967). Thus, one individual's perception of the prototypical "smart" person is likely to include a number of attributes that that individual believes characterize herself or himself (e.g., takes chances, accepts social norms), apparently whether or not those attributes are actually related to intelligence. By assuming similarity with a specific favorable prototype (e.g., handsome young men; see the discussion by Sherman, Presson, & Chassin, 1984, of the "similarity principle"), an individual can align himself or herself with a particular desirable image or group.

***Images as Goal States.*** Early work on the relation between prototypes and behavior suggested that the image itself, perhaps even more than membership in the group, may become a goal for young people (Leventhal & Cleary, 1980). Citing prior research indicating that children may have fairly distinct images of smokers well before they start smoking (e.g., Bland, Bewley, & Day, 1975; Bynner, 1970; McKennel & Bynner, 1969), Leventhal and Cleary claimed that many young people become interested in smoking not so much because of its physiological effects but because they wish to possess some of the characteristics they associate with their image of the smoker. These young people, it was thought, believe that if they start smoking, others will be more likely to view them as having some of these valued characteristics (e.g., toughness, precocity). Although there is some disagreement as to exactly how this process occurs, most theorists believe that the impact of images is mediated by a comparison of the image with the self. In other words, in order for the images that most of us maintain to affect our behavior, we must in some way compare the prototype and its attributes with ourselves.

The idea of a self-prototype comparison was first addressed by Cantor and her colleagues. In one of their earlier studies, Niedenthal, Cantor, and Kihlstrom (1985) asked students first to describe, with various adjectives, the type of person who would be "happy and comfortable" living in each of seven different types of university residences and then to rate themselves on the same adjectives. As expected, the closer the match between self-perception and prototype-perception, the greater the interest in becoming a member of the group. In a similar study, Moss and Frieze (1993) asked participants to describe themselves, using a series of adjectives, and then to describe the typical person working in certain types of jobs. Self-prototype difference scores (on each adjective) were smallest for the careers in which the subject had previously expressed the greatest interest (cf. Burke & Reitzes, 1981). Given the level of commitment represented by these choices (e.g., selecting a career or a residence hall), one would expect that membership in the group most likely was a goal state for these young people. Because the prototypes are representatives of those goal states, then, it is not hard to understand why an individual might want to become as much like the representative as possible. Whether health images represent goal states, however, is a different issue, to which we return later.

***Individual Differences in the Impact of Prototypes on Behavior.*** As is the case with many social psychological phenomena, it is informative to ask whether there are meaningful individual differences in the extent to which the prototype construct influences behavior, and if so, what these differences say about the processes involved. Two studies by Cantor and her colleagues indicate that the answer to the first question is yes. First, the Niedenthal et al. (1985) study cited above provided evidence of an important individual difference in image influence. Participants who described themselves as having many different personality characteristics and as being able to adapt to different situations ("low" in "distinctiveness") were less likely to demonstrate a high correspondence between self-prototype match and housing preference. In the second of these studies, Cantor, Mackie, and Lord (1984) had participants choose a partner to work with them on an art project. These investigators found that people preferred a partner who resembled their prototype for artists or for artistic ability. Cantor et al. also reported that this preference was especially pronounced among individuals who felt that they (themselves) could not easily adapt to social situations and, presumably, would be more likely to rely on others for social "guidance." In short, these two studies suggest that prototypes are more influential for individuals who report being more socially dependent. This finding is consistent with our belief that the process of image influence involves social comparison. Because such differences are informative, we return to this idea later in the chapter.

*Negative Images and the Self.* Hazel Markus has argued that people maintain images of what they might be like in the future, what she calls "possible selves," that can have a significant impact on their behavior (Markus & Nurius, 1986). Markus's influential work in this area provides an intrapersonal analog to the prototype matching research we discussed earlier. For example, some young people maintain a positive possible self that includes the attributes they associate with drinkers (e.g., sophisticated, friendly). Markus has pointed out, however, that there are two sides to the possible-self coin, and in many respects the other side is more interesting; that is, people also maintain images of the future self that are negative and unwanted. One such negative possible self that comes readily to mind for most is being overweight or out of shape. Markus suggests that negative selves of this nature are important because of their motivating qualities: the desire to avoid becoming the negative possible self motivates certain types of behaviors.

The idea that people will use negative images of the self, or of others similar to the self, to motivate behavior has some precedence in psychology. Lewin, for example, used the term "negative chauvinism" to describe a tendency he had observed among small groups of Jews in Europe in the 1930s to openly criticize and reject other Jews, mostly out of a desire to dissociate themselves publicly from a group at risk. More recently, Marques and his colleagues (Marques, Robalo, & Rocho, 1992; Marques, Yzerbyt, & Leyens, 1988) have demonstrated that disliked ingroup members—what they called "black sheep"—tend to be rejected more than outgroup members with the same negative attributes. It is not hard to imagine why people with negative characteristics who happen to be similar to the self might be particularly threatening. A primary reason is the implication that the self may share some of these negative characteristics or may become like this distasteful image. It is for essentially the same reason that social comparison with others who are thought to be similar to the self tends to have more impact than comparison with dissimilar others (Goethals & Darley, 1977).

## Distancing

A similar type of dissociative process can be seen in our earlier research involving stigmatized groups. In one study we asked higher level mentally handicapped persons to describe themselves and the typical person with mental retardation, and then to compare the two (Gibbons, 1985). The participants in this study had very clear images of the prototype, and these images were both negative (similar to the stereotype that nonhandicapped persons might maintain) and quite distinct from the self; for example, participants saw the typical person with mental retardation as less intelligent, less friendly, and less socially skilled than nondisabled people. In discussing these results, we suggested that the mentally handicapped persons were using the images—which they had created—as downward comparison targets. By comparing with, and looking for evidence of distinction from the image, they might convince others and themselves that they are different. Thus, the downward comparison process was part of an effort on their part to distance themselves from a category to which they did not want to belong. (Buunk & Ybema describe a similar process in their discussion of "contrasting" from downward comparison targets; see chapter 12, this volume).

Similar motives, albeit at a different level, are apparent in the responses of subjects in a study by Niedenthal and Mordkoff (1991). This study concerned prototype matching, but with a different twist. The researchers forced participants to choose which of several stigmatized groups they must join. In particular, they were asked to imagine they had a "pressing personal problem," and then they were asked which type of therapist (e.g., psychiatrist, social worker) they would prefer to see to treat this "problem." The authors hypothesized that because seeing a therapist has a negative connotationfor many people, participants would be motivated to minimize their identification with the prototypical patient of their chosen therapist. Results supported the hypothesis: participants chose therapists whose typical patients (they thought) were different from themselves. The investigators suggest that because of the nature of the category, the pattern of responses was opposite to that evidenced in most matching studies. When membership in the group is desirable (e.g., joining a fraternity or becoming an attorney), a close match with the prototype should be self-enhancing. When membership is undesirable or stigmatizing, however, self-image distinction should be self-enhancing. As we discuss in the next major section of this chapter, our own research suggests that this distinction is very important when trying to understand and predict health behavior.

### Summary

Prototypes are based on reality and experience, but they are nonetheless cognitive creations, and their construction often reflects a self-serving bias. People tend to form images of desirable groups that are similar to the self, whereas those of undesirable groups or categories are formulated in such a way as to highlight self-other distinction. Once constructed, the images serve as social comparison targets, and this comparison influences behavior in a variety of ways. Moreover, this process is dynamic: images change over time as a function of experience with the behaviors or groups they represent. For example, one's image of a smoker is likely to become more favorable after one starts smoking, more negative after one quits. Because they are mutable, prototypes have a certain utility that real comparison targets or exemplars do not have (cf. Misovich, Fisher, & Fisher, chapter 4, this volume). This flexibility and mutability are primary reasons why prototypes have a significant effect on behavior, especially in the domain of health.

## PROTOTYPES AND HEALTH

In reviewing the research on prototypes and health, we have found it most helpful to use a taxonomy that is based on two more or less distinct dimensions. The first has to do with the nature of the behavior the image fosters—does it promote health or facilitate coping, or does it interfere? On the one hand, it is clear that images of the type of person who engages in risky behavior exist, the typical smoker or alcoholic being prime examples. On the other hand, one might assume that there are countervailing images, such as that of the type of person who engages in health-promoting behavior, or avoids risk (e.g., the typical nondrinker). As we will see, however, it is not clear that such positive images do exist. The second dimension has to do with the nature of the image itself—how favorable or acceptable is it? Some images are influential because of their negative qualities; they represent groups or categories that most people are motivated to avoid, and so they are similar to Markus's negative possible selves. Other images are more positive, closer to actual goal states. Although we will discuss the dimensions in dichotomous terms, we acknowledge that both are actually continua. For example, our own research suggests that many images have both favorable and unfavorable elements, which means that the same image can promote risky behavior for some, reduce it for others, and have no impact at all on still others.

**Health Promotion and Coping: Favorable Images**

Anyone who has spent time in an exercise club knows that such establishments are full of possible selves. These images do have a significant effect on behavior (exercise) and are probably one of the primary reasons why club members are there in the first place. In this regard, a survey conducted by Cross and Markus (1991) suggested that physical possible selves may be the most common and most influential of all self-images. These researchers asked a group of 173 adults between the ages of 18 and 86 to list as many possible selves as they could think of. For all age groups, health images were the most common type of imagined future self, although this finding was stronger for negative images (e.g., the self as sick or obese) than it was for positive images. A follow-up study by Hooker (1992) suggested that the importance of these images increases with age: Of her sample of older adults, 75% mentioned health-relevant possible selves as their most important hoped-for or most dreaded self (cf. Hooker & Kaus, 1994). Moreover, these positive health self-images were related to self-reports of health behavior: The more importance adults assigned to their positive health-relevant selves, the more likely they were to report engaging in health-maintaining behaviors (e.g., medical check-ups, stress management program) and not engaging in health-impairing behaviors (e.g., smoking; Hooker & Kaus, 1992).

Surprisingly, however, very little research has looked at how positive health images influence behavior. At this point, it is not clear whether this is an oversight or a reflection of reality. It does appear that negative health images, or feared selves, have more motivational power. Hooker and Kaus (1994) found that feared health selves are more common and more salient than hoped-for health selves, and suggested "it is unfortunate that conceptualizations of self in the future tend to be focused on negative and feared health images" (p. 130). Perhaps the people in the exercise club are driven more by a desire to avoid old age than to retain or regain youth. At any rate, the image of the fit and healthy athlete (e.g., the svelte stair-stepper in the health club) is certainly one that most would recognize and could describe in some detail, and it would seem likely that positive images of this nature would have some motivating capability. If we exclude the elements of this image that are attributable solely to physical attractiveness, however, there aren't many other positive health images that come readily to mind. Moreover, even the physically attractive or healthy self-image has not received much empirical attention. In contrast, the impact of negative images on behavior has received considerable attention. One reason for this is that most of the research on health images has concerned health risk, and these images usually are fairly negative.

### Health Promotion and Coping: Unfavorable Images

Another variation on the negative self-image (or "black sheep"; Marques et al., 1988) theme can be seen in Taylor's original research with cancer patients and their spouses (see chapter 10, by Wood & VanderZee, for further discussion of this work). Taylor, Wood, and Lichtman (1983) asked the husbands of the women who had breast cancer how they were coping with their wives' illness. Many men indicated that they were having trouble, but as one suggested, at least he wasn't like "all those other animals," referring to what he assumed was a significant proportion of men in this situation who leave their wives because of the illness. The fact that the evidence does not support this man's assumption (only 4% of the marriages in Taylor's sample dissolved as a result of the illness) led Taylor and her colleagues to label these fabricated downward comparison targets "mythical men." Nevertheless, the husbands in Taylor's study evidently profited from believing that there were others who were doing worse than they were and who were clearly different from them. These men appeared to be engaging in a form of what Wills (1981) has called "active downward comparison" (i.e., derogation of a target in order to facilitate or set up a downward comparison; see Wills, chapter 6, this volume), in order to help them cope with the problem they faced. The reasoning appears quite similar to that displayed by the mentally handicapped persons in our research (Gibbons, 1985, discussed earlier), who also derogated images of a category or group with which they did not want to be associated.

The possibility that the men in the Taylor et al. study and the people with mental retardation in our study were actually using "mythical" images as a means of facilitating coping with their situations led us to formulate a new hypothesis involving coping with a health problem. In particular, there were two related aspects of the mythical man image that were especially interesting and relevant to us. One is the fact that the image was clearly a fabrication. The other is that it was constructed, more or less independent of reality, in such a way that it was both worse off and different from the self—the two primary characteristics of an "ideal" downward comparison target. As the Taylor et al. study suggests, individuals in this situation are not constrained by reality. They can create images that are imbued with characteristics that highlight the images' inferiority and their distinction from the self. Social comparison with these images, in turn, is likely to focus on both the distinction and the inferiority. Our hypothesis in this first study (Gibbons, Gerrard, Lando, & McGovern, 1991), then, was that individuals who are trying to overcome a particular behavioral problem will use the prototype associated with that behavior as a downward comparison target in order to facilitate coping with (i.e., resolving) the problem.

The behavioral problem that we chose was smoking, although any behavior that has a recognizable image associated with it (e.g., heavy drinker, drug user, spouse abuser) should work just as well. We asked adult smokers who had joined smoking cessation clinics about their smoking habits and their images of the typical smoker. (Both open-ended items and adjective descriptors produced similar results; only the latter are reported here.) We also asked them to tell us what kind of person they would like to have in their group in terms of the individual's ability to quit smoking, both in absolute terms and relative to the self. What we were looking for in this latter item was evidence of downward comparison target preferences, and change in those preferences over time.

As expected, initial images for most of these smokers were relatively favorable (although more negative than the same images formed by smokers who had not decided to quit) and then became more negative over time and more dissimilar to the self, as the participants tried to quit smoking. This pattern was significant for all smokers, but it was much stronger among those who quit and then maintained abstinence. A recent replication and extension of this study (Gibbons & Eggleston, 1996) has indicated that the image maintained by smokers at the time they enter the cessation clinics is a significant predictor of eventual outcome: the more negative the original image the more likely eventual abstinence. This suggests two things. First, a negative image may have been partly responsible for the decision to join the clinic; in fact, our data indicate that smokers who have made a decision to quit and have joined a cessation clinic do have more negative images, even though they tend to smoke more, than those who have not made that decision. Second, the desire to distance from the image may have contributed to the success of both the cessation attempt and the maintenance of abstinence. One additional finding from this study is worth noting. We assessed smokers' perceptions of a positive image—the "typical former smoker"—to see if it was related to outcome. It was not. Once again, this suggests that positive images (or goals) may have less motivating capability, in terms of health behavior, than negative images.

We believe that the smokers in the clinics were engaging in a form of motivated downward comparison with these fabricated targets, as they looked for evidence of superiority and especially distinction from the self. Of course, that evidence wasn't hard to find. The images had been created by the smokers in the first place and they were dynamic, evolving, presumably, in ways that fit the smokers' interests (cf. Dunning et al., 1991). Moreover, as the image of the typical smoker changed over time, so did smokers' preferences with regard to other clinic participants. The correlation between downward comparison target preference and perceived seriousness was significant at Time 1—the more serious participants' smoking problems, the more interested they were in having someone in the group with them who was having a lot of difficulty quitting. Perhaps more important, these two measures also covaried over time ($r = -.44$). In other words, as people's perceptions of their smoking problems declined and their coping improved, their comparison target preferences gradually shifted upward. Finally, a more recent study (Gibbons, Blanton, Gerrard, & Eggleston, 1997) indicated that smokers' Time 1 affiliation–comparison preferences predicted outcome: those who initially preferred to have others in their group who were having a lot of difficulty quitting were more likely to fail at their own attempt to quit.

Comparison with someone who is having more difficulty in dealing with their problem is not likely to provide much useful information about coping strategies (Brickman & Bulman, 1977; Buunk, 1994; Gibbons et al., 1997; Taylor & Lobel, 1989; Wills, 1987). On the other hand, downward comparison theory and research both suggest that this type of comparison should result in a favorable affective response (Gibbons, 1986; Gibbons & Boney-McCoy, 1991; Wills, 1981, 1991). The gradual shift away from downward comparison preference may be a reflection of smokers' increased confidence in their ability to quit smoking, which, in turn, is accompanied by a declining interest in mood regulation and increasing interest in more active coping strategies. This issue of downward comparison and coping is discussed in more detail by Tennen and Affleck in this volume (chapter 9), as well as by Buunk and Ybema (chapter 12), Wills (chapter 6), and Wood and VanderZee (chapter 10).

### Health-Impairing Behaviors: Unfavorable Images

Of course, not all of the research examining images and health risk has focused on their role in health promotion or in coping with illness. An even larger body of research suggests that health images can have the opposite effect: They can facilitate health risk behavior. Once again, social comparison appears to be an integral part of the process.

***Perceptions of Vulnerability.*** The hypothesis that perceptions of vulnerability motivate precautionary behavior is a central component of most current theories of health behavior. More central to the current discussion, however, is the fact that the converse also appears to be true—perceptions of invulnerability reduce precautionary behavior. Support for this relation has been provided by a substantial number of studies, and by three major reviews of the literature (Becker, 1974; Harrison, Mullen, & Green, 1992; Janz & Becker, 1984). A closely related body of literature documents the tendency for individuals to believe that they are less vulnerable to negative events than are others. This optimistic bias, as it has been called, definitely includes illness. People see themselves as less likely than others to develop a variety of health problems, ranging from poison ivy and tooth decay to cancer and heart attacks (Weinstein, 1980, 1987).

The role of social comparison in optimistic bias, which is discussed by Klein and Weinstein in chapter 2 of this volume, was initially investigated by Perloff and Fetzer (1986). In one of their studies, subjects were asked to consider their own risk for health problems, such as heart attack or cancer, as well as the risk of an average student, a friend, or their closest friend. Results indicated that when the comparison target was not specified (e.g., imagine "any friend"), subjects tended to choose an individual who was particularly susceptible to the event. For example, when considering cancer risk, two thirds of the subjects reported that they chose a friend who was particularly vulnerable to the disease. As Perloff and Fetzer suggested, "Because the [comparison target] . . . has been selected to match the typical victim, subjects are likely to see themselves as less vulnerable in relation..." (p. 508; cf. Weinstein, 1980). A more recent study by Weinstein and Klein (1995) found that focusing on high risk (downward comparison) targets led to an increase in perceptions of the risk of others (peers). In short, social comparison with these (negative) prototypes of the typical victim promotes a sense of invulnerability that may decrease motivation to engage in preventive or precautionary behavior or even facilitate risk behavior. (Klein & Weinstein make a persuasive argument in chapter 2 of this book that social comparison is an integral part of risk perceptions even when comparison is not explicitly elicited.)

***Symptoms and Illness Representations.*** Leventhal was the first to suggest that people have illness images that motivate health behavior (Leventhal 1970, 1975; see also chapters 7 and 14 in this volume).

According to his "common sense model of illness," people interpret and elaborate on their experience of a specific illness and their knowledge of its characteristics to form images of that illness (cf. Pennebaker, 1982). Bishop and his colleagues have expanded the construct of illness representations into what they call a "prototype model of symptom interpretation" (Bishop, 1991; Bishop, Briede, Cavazos, Grotzinger, & McMahon, 1987; Bishop & Converse, 1986). This model suggests that people form representations of particular diseases, or disease prototypes, based on commonly shared information, prior experience, and cultural factors. According to both Leventhal's common sense model and Bishop's prototype model, when individuals experience illness symptoms, they test the match of their symptoms against these mental representations of specific illnesses in an effort to assess whether they are in fact ill. This procedure may involve temporal (intrapersonal) comparison: Are my current symptoms similar to those I have experienced in the past? Or it may involve social comparison: Are any close associates suffering from the same symptoms? Did any of last night's dinner companions awaken feeling the same way? (See discussions of this process in chapter 7 by Suls, Martin, & Leventhal, and in chapter 14 by Leventhal, Hudson, & Robitaille, in this volume).

Research on these negative illness images has suggested that they can have important negative consequences. For example, Meyer, Leventhal, and Gutmann (1985) reported that hypertensives have mental representations of the symptoms of hypertension (even though, in reality, hypertension is asymptomatic until its later stages), which they believe are closely related to their blood pressure, and which guide their behavior. Moreover, Meyer et al.'s data suggest that hypertension patients' misguided confidence in their ability to control their blood pressure predicts noncompliance with physicians' recommendations. In other words, when patients' images of an illness are inconsistent with either the medical facts or physicians' recommendations, they are more likely to avoid medical treatment, to self-treat, or to ignore the prescribed regimen altogether. Finally, Bishop et al. (1987) also demonstrated that symptoms that are thought to be inconsistent with the prototype are less often remembered and reported, and are less likely to affect health behavior.

### Health-Impairing Behaviors: Favorable Images

When we ask participants in our own research to describe a health-risk prototype (e.g., the typical smoker) they are initially reluctant to do so—after all, prototype sounds a lot like stereotype and that implies some prejudice. With some encouragement, however, most eventually respond, and what they have to say tends to be fairly negative. Years of listening to health education messages warning of the dangers of substance use and unprotected sex have taken their toll. They see the behaviors as risky, and those who do them as foolish or reckless, with only a sprinkling of positive traits (e.g., "independent"). That has not always been the case, however; in fact, some research suggests that the opposite used to be true. As was noted earlier, Leventhal and Cleary (1980) suggested that one reason adolescents start smoking is because they believe it will help them acquire some of the traits they associate with smoking, traits that they view as desirable.

Once again, there is less information available about the process than about its outcome. There is, however, considerable evidence of the impact that images have on adolescents' health risk behavior, especially smoking. In an extensive series of studies, Laurie Chassin and her colleagues have shown that smoker images are related to interest in smoking behavior. In the first of these studies, Chassin et al. (1981) found that non-smoking adolescents whose self-images matched the smoker stereotype (derived by combining all participants' smoker stereotypes) were more likely to report that they intended to smoke sometime in the future. Similarly, adolescents who have more rather than less favorable smoker images also report greater interest in the behavior (cf. Burton et al., 1989). The same appears to be true with alcohol. Adolescents who drink have self-concepts, as well as ideal and "admired" self-concepts (i.e., beliefs about what friends would admire), that are similar to their drinker images (Chassin, Tetzloff, & Hershey, 1985), and they have more favorable drinker images than those who do not drink (Snortum et al., 1987). Comparable results have also been reported for smokeless tobacco (Chassin et al., 1985).

Although the smoker prototype does comprise some desirable qualities, the image is certainly not uniformly positive, not even among those who are interested in the behavior. As we noted earlier, the first smoker image studies, conducted more than 25 years ago (Bynner, 1970; McKennell & Bynner, 1969), reported that adolescent boys, the group most favorably disposed to the smoker image, indicated they were ambivalent about it. Moreover, the tremendous amount of negative media attention that has been focused on smoking and smokers over the last 10 to 15 years has exacerbated the negative aspects of that image (e.g., Cooper & Kohn, 1989; Goldstein, 1991). The same is true for alcohol images, even though they have not been reviled to nearly the extent that smoker images and smokers have. Snortum et al. (1987) found that even among adolescents who drank, their drinker images were more negative than their self-images. For this reason, they concluded that adolescent drinking does not reflect an attempt at (positive) image acquisition. We agree. But, of course, this raises a basic question of how and why the images are influential.

Social influence plays a prominent role in almost all models of substance use, and, indeed, a number of researchers believe it is the primary precipitating factor among adolescents (Graham et al., 1991; Kandel, 1980). One reason for this has to do with the social orientation of adolescents. As Erikson (1950, 1968) has suggested, the primary "task" of this stage of life is establishing an identity, and adolescents often look to their peers for guidance in this process (Sebald, 1989). More generally, adolescence is a time during which reliance on others for such things as information, social resources, and advice is peaking (Coleman, 1978), and that reliance, of course, involves social comparison. One important element of this other-directedness is an enhanced concern about one's social image (e.g., heightened self-consciousness; see Simmons, Rosenberg, & Simmons, 1973). According to Elkind (1985), it is during adolescence that we are most likely to believe that others are preoccupied with our behavior and our appearance (cf. Adams & Jones, 1981; Goosens, 1984). Thus, there is good reason to expect that social images will be most influential at this stage of life. And, given that health risk behaviors are particularly salient because of their unusual nature and visibility, image influence should be especially strong for this type of behavior.

## A MODEL OF ADOLESCENT HEALTH RISK BEHAVIOR

Our own research has included health images as part of an effort to predict onset and change in health risk behavior among adolescents and young adults. Toward this end, we have collected data from two samples and are now beginning a third. The first sample comprises 500 adolescents (mean age of 14 at Time 1) whom we interviewed in their homes (along with their families) at 12-month intervals. We completed the sixth and most recent wave of these interviews in early 1997. The second sample was composed of 680 college students whom we interviewed first at the time they entered the university, and whom we have continued to survey annually or semi-annually since that time. In both samples we have assessed participants' health risk behaviors (drinking, reckless driving, smoking, and unprotected sex), as well as the prototypes they associate with these behaviors (e.g., the "typical teenager who drinks frequently"), in terms of both favorability and similarity to the self. We assess favorability by means of a list of adjective descriptors (e.g., *smart, friendly, careless*), and similarity to the self by a single item ("How similar are you to the typical person your age who . . ."). For comparison purposes, we have also asked subjects to evaluate themselves and their ideal selves using the same adjectives. In addition, because our model shares some assumptions about the antecedents of risk behavior with the Theory of Reasoned Action and its update, the Theory of Planned Behavior, we also assessed constructs suggested by these models (e.g., behavioral intentions, norm perceptions, attitudes toward the behavior; see Ajzen, 1991; Ajzen & Fishbein, 1980; Fishbein & Ajzen, 1975). These two theories contain the models of decision making that have been most often and most successfully used in efforts to predict health behavior.

### Theoretical Assumptions

***Risk Prototypes.*** We began this research with several basic assumptions that were eventually supported by our data. First, we assumed that health risk behaviors for adolescents are primarily social events. Unlike adults, who often drink alone, smoke whenever they want to, and tend to drive more carefully when others are with them, adolescents and young adults perform much of their risk behavior in front of, and often for the benefit of, their friends and peers. This assumption received considerable support in the data. The vast majority of our participants indicated they did these behaviors most or all of the time with friends. Second, because these behaviors are both very salient and very social, we assumed they would have clear and identifiable images associated with them. Again, the support was strong and unambiguous, as the majority of adolescents answered our open-ended questions describing the various prototypes and did so in some detail. Similarly, the adjective checklists that we have used to evaluate prototypes have proven to be both valid and reliable. A third and final assumption is that prototypes influence behavior by means of social comparison, that is, comparison of the self with the image. The first two assumptions together led to the primary hypothesis of our initial analysis, which was that social (risk) images would predict changes in risk behavior. More specifically, the more favorable and similar to the self the image happens to be, the more likely the adolescent will be to start or increase the behavior.

***Preliminary Analyses.*** Our first set of analyses, which was preliminary, was conducted on just the adolescent sample. We ran a series of hierarchical regression analyses in which we entered Time 1 behavior, intention, and then the prototype into the equations to predict Time 2 risk behavior. Results indicated that the prototypes predicted change in all four behaviors (i.e., prototype favorability was positively linked with Time 2 behavior, taking into account Time 1 behavior), and did so in each case after the other variables had been entered into the equation.

We also ran analyses comparing prototype perceptions with self-perceptions on several dimensions. These analyses indicated, first of all, that prototype perception was considerably more negative than was self-perception. Even among those who were engaging in the behavior, all of the prototypes were evaluated more negatively than the self on every one of the 12 adjectives (all $p < .001$). Second, we replaced the prototype evaluation index with the mean of the 12 (self–prototype) difference scores to construct a matching index, as in previous prototype studies (e.g., Niedenthal et al., 1985). Because the prototype evaluations were all more negative than the self-evaluations, however, this new matching index added nothing to the prototype mean other than a measure of self-evaluation or self-esteem. In fact, the match score did not predict as well as did the straight prototype mean score. We'll discuss this point again later. Now we turn to an additional and important element of our model.

## Willingness

Like most models of attitude–behavior consistency, the Theories of Reasoned Action and Planned Behavior are based on a fundamental assumption that all human social activities are, essentially, rational. Consequently, according to these theories the best predictor of behavior, whether health-relevant or not, is intention to engage in that behavior. We believe, however, that adolescent risk behaviors are not always intended. Rather, they are reactions to risk-conducive circumstances; that is, situations that facilitate (but don't demand) experimentation with and involvement in these behaviors. These are frequently situations that adolescents have not planned to be in (e.g., a party where their peers are smoking marijuana) but have not actively avoided, either. The question then becomes what they are willing to do under these specific circumstances. Thus, we have proposed a distinction between, on the one hand, *intention* (planning to engage in the behavior) and the closely related *expectation* (acknowledgment that one will probably engage in the behavior; Warshaw & Davis, 1985), and, on the other hand, *willingness* (recognition that one would be willing to engage in the behavior under some circumstances).

An important component of the distinction between willingness and the two types of intentions is the locus of responsibility. When one states an intention there is an explicit element of planning and therefore an assumption of responsibility for one's own behavior. Expressing a willingness, however, is only an acknowledgment that certain circumstances (or social influences) could lead one to engage in the behavior; thus some (perhaps even all) of the responsibility for acting is deflected outward.[1] Certainly the adolescent's ability to control the behavior and to (just) say no is relevant here. And, in fact, recent tests of Ajzen's Theory of Planned Behavior (Ajzen, 1991), which includes perceived control over the behavior–typically translated as "refusal efficacy" when examining risk behavior–have shown this to be a useful predictor (see Ellickson & Hays, 1991; van den Putte, 1993; Wills, Baker, & Botvin, 1989). For a number of adolescents, however, saying no is not the issue. Some can, but when the opportunity presents itself, decide they don't want to. Others may very well find it difficult to resist peer pressure but may also be somewhat interested in or at least ambivalent about engaging in the behavior. In both cases, the adolescents in these categories have reasonable ability to "control" the behavior: They can refuse, but, for whatever reason, they decide not to.

To assess willingness, we present participants with a series of hypothetical situations that are common for people of this age (e.g., they have had several drinks and need to get home). We then ask them how willing they would be to do each of several things (e.g., go ahead and drive home; ask a friend to give them a ride). Separate constructs can then be defined that assess willingness to engage in each of a variety of different risk behaviors. These constructs, along with intention and the associated prototypes, are used to predict a variety of different risk behaviors, such as unprotected sex or heavy drinking.[2]

## Social Comparison

Our initial study with the adolescent sample did not include a social comparison measure. We did have one item that assessed general comparison tendencies, however, which was "How often do you compare how well things are going for you in general (socially, personally, etc.) with other people?" This allowed us to look at the relation between comparison tendencies and several measures of prototype consideration. These correlations indicated that those adolescents who reported frequently engaging in social comparison were also

---

[1]Evidence that willingness does not denote acceptance of responsibility is the fact that although both willingness and intention predict changes in risk behavior independently, only intention is related to perceptions of vulnerability. For example, intention and willingness to smoke both predict adolescent smoking behavior. However, whereas intention is accompanied by an increase in perceptions of smoking-related health risk, increased willingness is not accompanied by an increase in perceived vulnerability (Gibbons, Gerrard, Ouellete, & Burzette, in press).

[2]Our attempts to compare the predictive power of refusal efficacy with willingness to proceed with a given behavior have suggested that, at least for these behaviors in this age group, the latter is more closely linked with eventual behavior.

more likely to report that they had thought about the four prototypes (smoking, drinking, reckless driving, and unprotected sex), and had socially compared with them (all $p < .001$). Prompted in part by this finding, we attempted to construct a social comparison scale that would allow us to further investigate the role that comparison plays in the image influence process. We began this task with our college sample, but we have continued to develop the scale since that time (Gibbons & Buunk, 1997). In its initial form the scale included a subset of three items that appeared to provide a reasonable measure of "social-behavior comparison" (e.g., "How often do you compare with others in terms of social behavior [social skills, popularity, etc.]?"; alpha = .74). In both the adolescent and college samples, this scale correlated with all our measures of prototype consideration (e.g., "How often have you thought about this typical person?" and "How often have you compared yourself with this type of person?").[3] In addition, the overall means on these prototype items indicated that virtually all of the subjects had spent some time considering the prototypes.

***Predicting Behavior.*** We then attempted to replicate with the college sample the regression analyses that we had performed originally with the adolescent sample (Gibbons & Gerrard, 1995). Our first attempt at this met with mixed success: prototype favorability predicted increases in one of the risk behaviors (unprotected sex; $p < .002$), and came close on a second (reckless driving; $p < .08$). We then tested our primary hypothesis, which was that the prototype would be maximally predictive for those subjects who were more inclined to socially compare. We did this by entering a Prototype × Social Comparison interaction term. We also entered a three-way interaction, Prototype × Social Comparison × Gender, to determine if there were any gender differences in image influence. These results supported our hypothesis: The two-way and/or the three-way interactions were significant on all four risk behaviors. The two-way interactions indicated that the images were much more impactful for high social-comparison people. The pattern of the three-way interactions, which occurred on the smoking and drinking measures, was such that the prototype (i.e., prototype favorability and similarity to self) was most predictive of behavior change for men who were high in social-comparison tendencies. We had not anticipated this gender difference (although there is some precedence in the literature for the idea that males may be more influenced by social images; Brown, Classen, & Eicher, 1986), but we have now found

[3]All $p < .001$, except comparison with the smoker prototype ($p < .04$), which we think reflects the very low prevalence rate of smoking in this sample (i.e., < 6%).

evidence of it in several different analyses. We will explore it further in future research.

Once again, the prototype evaluations were much more negative than the self-evaluations, and the self-prototype match index was not as effective at predicting the behaviors as was the prototype by itself. In addition, we included a measure of ideal self, consisting of self-ratings on each of the 12 adjectives, which enabled us to calculate an ideal-self-prototype match score. The assumption here was that the match score would be a better indication of the extent to which the prototype represented a goal for these subjects. As we had expected, however, the gap between ideal-self and the prototype was even greater than that between self and prototype, and, once again, the mean-difference score did not predict as well as did the prototype alone (self and ideal-self did not predict at all). In short, there was no evidence in any of our data that these adolescents were trying to acquire characteristics that they associated with the prototypes or that they aspired to be like the members of the different categories the prototypes represented.

***A Reciprocal Relation.*** One final point to be mentioned is that in addition to looking at the prospective effect of the prototypes on behavior, we also looked at the reverse relation—the impact that behavior change had on prototype perceptions. As in the "typical smoker" research (Gibbons et al., 1991), prototype favorability and similarity both declined over time among those who reduced their risk behavior. The opposite occurred among those who increased their risk behavior, what we have termed an "assimilation effect" (subsequent analyses indicated that perception of the prototype changes noticeably whereas self-perception on these dimensions changes only slightly). What this suggests is that the relation between image and behavior is nonrecursive; each one influences and is influenced by the other (cf. Gerrard, Gibbons, Benthin, & Hessling, 1996). Thus, the child who has developed a favorable image of a heavy drinker is predisposed to drink. Then, when he does start drinking and spending more time with friends who drink, his image gradually becomes more favorable, which in turn, facilitates or promotes more drinking, and so on. On the other hand, the child who decreases his drinking, and engages in distancing from the group develops a more negative image, which, in turn, reduces the likelihood of future use. This reciprocal relation has implications for interventions, which we discuss later.

## The Model: An Overview

We have continued to develop our model of health risk over the last 4 years as we have collected more data and conducted more analyses of existing data from the two longitudinal samples. Currently, our assessment of the role of prototypes and willingness in risk behavior is as follows: Adolescents develop a sense of what the typical "perpetrator" is like for a given risky behavior from a variety of sources, including TV, advertising, and most important, their friends (Blanton, Gibbons, Gerrard, Conger, & Smith, in press). Owing to the nature of these behaviors, these images are quite salient and remain that way for most people. Moreover, because the images are widely recognized and identifiable, and because the behaviors they are associated with are typically visible and social, young people realize that by engaging in the behaviors even a few times they will come to assume the images themselves. Over time, they will, in essence, become the typical smoker or the typical drinker—whether they want to or not. That awareness has a significant impact on their decision to engage in or refrain from engaging in the risk behavior.

In general, the adolescents in our studies have risk images that are much more negative than their self-images. We suspect that is largely a result of the warnings that they have heard many times in school and elsewhere. At any rate, it does raise the question of why they would adopt behaviors associated with images that are fairly negative. First, it would appear that most young people (today) do not engage in these behaviors in order to acquire the images or aspects of them; few would want to acquire an image that was more negative than the one they currently think they have. Second, there is evidence of "pluralistic ignorance" in our data (cf. Prentice & Miller, 1993); i.e., young people often mistakenly assume that others hold a much more favorable impression of the behaviors, and those who engage in them, than they themselves do. In other words, their personal image of the typical smoker may not be that positive, but they think their peers' images are. Thus, a positive image isn't likely, nor is it necessary. The question, then, is not so much do I want to acquire this image but rather, how acceptable is it to me, especially given that (I assume) many of my peers admire it? The more acceptable it is, the more willing the adolescent is to engage in the behavior should the opportunity present itself (Gibbons, Gerrard, & Boney McCoy, 1995). For many adolescents, that will happen sooner or later.

## The Role of Social Comparison

The specific manner in which the prototype influences behavior involves social comparison as both a moderator and a mediator. First, some minimum level of comparison activity is necessary for the image even to be considered. Those who tend not to compare are not going to pay much attention to the image. They are likely to have an idea of what the typical perpetrator is like, perhaps a very good idea, and that image may even be moderately favorable, but it won't make much difference for their own behavior. In fact, when we split our college sample at the median in terms of social-comparison tendencies, we found that there were just as many low-comparison students as high-comparison students who had favorable risk images (i.e., comparison tendencies were not correlated with prototype favorability). Those images were not at all related to risk behaviors for the former group, however.

Those who are inclined to compare will do so with the images they maintain. If they find the behavior appealing and have some interest in doing it (some inclination, pro or con, is necessary before the adolescent will pay much attention to the image), then the comparison will be biased toward finding evidence of similarity. The combination of a relatively favorable or acceptable image with perceived similarity to the self is likely to translate into willingness to do the behavior and, eventually, into the behavior itself. By the same token, having a negative image (especially if it is dissimilar to the self) is likely to lead to comparisons that are biased toward discovery of differences, in other words, toward downward comparison and distancing. This, in turn, translates into both less willingness and less behavior.

### Testing the Model

***College Students.*** In a recent paper (Gibbons, Gerrard, Blanton, & Russell, in press), we used structural equation modeling to test the overall fit of our complete model. The results of one of those analyses, presented in Fig. 3.1, provide some illustration of how the prototype affects behavior. The model was run with the college sample, predicting change in their unprotected sexual behavior, as assessed by two measures of sex without birth control. As can be seen in the right-hand side of the figure, the model proposes two distinct pathways to risk behavior. One path involves constructs suggested by the Theory of Reasoned Action, including attitudes toward the behavior and perceived norms. This, the *intentional* path, explains that part of risk behavior that is reasoned or premeditated (although not necessarily *rational*). The other path includes the prototype and proceeds through *willingness*; we have labeled this the *social reaction* path. Each pathway explains a significant percentage of the variance in risky sexual behavior; most important, the social reaction pathway does add significantly to the rational pathway, as we had predicted. In addition, we split the sample into top and bottom thirds, based on scores on the social-comparison index, and analyzed these relations among the two groups separately. The results of these analyses indicated that, as expected, the

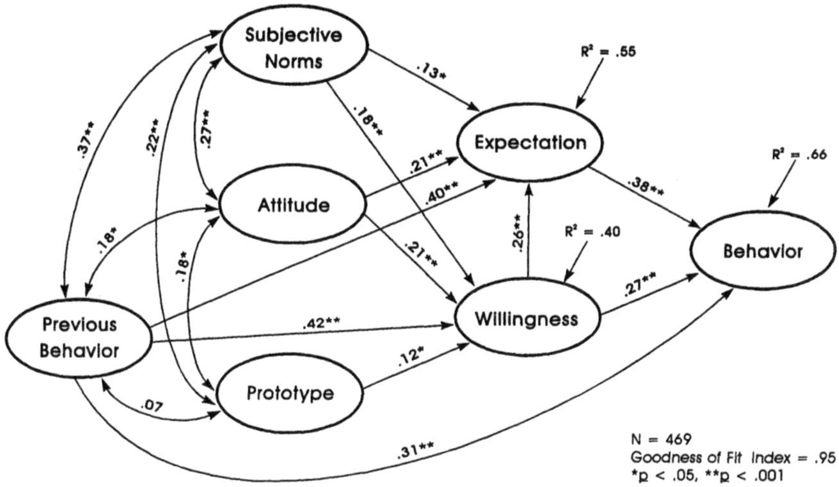


FIG. 3.1. Predicting change in college students' risky sexual behavior (from Gibbons et al., in press).

pathways from prototype to willingness and willingness to behavior (see Fig. 3.1) were both significantly stronger for those who were high in social comparison tendencies ($\beta$s > .23, *ps* ≤ .005), than they were for those low in such tendencies ($\beta$s < .14, *ps* > .15).

***Adolescents.*** We conducted similar analyses with our adolescent sample and found no differences between groups high and low in social comparison tendencies in terms of the magnitude of the willingness pathways. Our interpretation of this lack of effect is that social comparison tendencies are so common among adolescents (Bixenstine, DeCorte, & Bixenstine, 1976) that it does not discriminate within this age group. In other words, for most adolescents, images affect their health and health-risk behaviors by way of a social comparison process. Later in life, however, these images lose impact for some people, apparently because interest in the images and in social comparison itself has declined for those individuals (Buunk & Gibbons, 1997).

## Other Moderators of Prototype Influence

An obvious limitation of our model and our research is that almost all of it has involved young people in Iowa, a state that is almost exclusively white and has a very high education level. It is quite possible that adolescents from other backgrounds (e.g., youths from inner cities) or other parts of the country have more positive or sympathetic images of the typical smoker or drinker (cf. Mosbach & Leventhal, 1988; Sussman et al., 1990). A main effect of ethnicity or geographical location on prototype favorability, as this would suggest, should not influence the predictive power of our model. On the other hand, it does raise an interesting alternative possibility regarding which types of images are influential and why.

***Unconventionality.*** A number of theorists, Jessor perhaps being the most well-known (e.g., Jessor & Jessor, 1977), have argued that some young people reject the idea of using conventional means to achieve success, and actually maintain a negative image of those who don't drink or use drugs and who do the right thing (i.e., a "goody two-shoes" sort of prototype). It is possible that such "deviant" young people may actually try to distance themselves from this straight or conventional image, and that their health risk behavior, in turn, is a reflection of this effort (Wills, Duhamel, & Vaccaro, 1995; cf. Sussman et al., 1990). We find this possibility to be both intriguing and ironic—the process is the antithesis of what we believe happens with many smokers trying to quit, and of course, it has the exact opposite result. We will be exploring this question in a new study using a third sample, begun in early 1997, consisting of lower socioeconomic status Black youngsters in rural communities.

***Age.*** We would argue that health behavior decisions are often the result of a comparison between the self and negative health images, and that that process occurs throughout the life span. The consequences of that comparison often vary considerably as a function of age, however. Among adolescents, health risk behavior frequently results from comparisons with a risk image (e.g., the typical smoker), whereas the same image may be used by adults to help them stop such behavior. In fact, adolescents' negative health images are often very similar to those of adults. The difference is that adolescents' versions of the images are more socially oriented and, perhaps more important, represent an earlier stage in the possible development of a behavior and its consequences. Instead of the typical lung cancer patient, for example, it's a kid with a cigarette in his mouth; instead of the unemployed alcoholic, it's the young party-goer. Even these images are not that favorable, however, and few young people aspire to acquire them. For both adults and adolescents, the question, once again, becomes how willing am I to adopt the unfavorable image that comes with this behavior (e.g., smoking) or lack of behavior (e.g., exercise)? In short, social images are certainly not the only factors that affect whether people, even adolescents, engage in risky behaviors; there are numerous other dispositional, physiological, and social influences that must be considered. Still, the role played by these cognitive factors appears to be both quantifiable and important.

**Prototype Favorability: A Summary**

Our review of the relevant literature turned up very few examples of studies of positive health images. The lack of research surprised us, and we think it is a deficit that should certainly be addressed. It is possible, however, that one reason the topic has been largely overlooked is that positive images actually have less impact on behavior than negative images. There are three reasons why we think this might be the case.

First, positive or healthy images are usually much less vivid than risky images (e.g., safe driver vs. reckless driver), just as inaction is much less salient than is action (e.g., nonsmoker vs. smoker), a variation of the "feature positive" effect (Fazio, Sherman, & Herr, 1982). If the images are not well-defined, they are not likely to have much effect on behavior. More generally, research has indicated that negative events elicit more reaction from individuals than positive events (Stokols, Ohlig, & Resnick, 1978). Similarly, research in the area of impression formation has indicated that information about others' negative or unusual behaviors elicits more reaction from observers (cognitive response, attributions, physiological response: Birnbaum, 1972; Dreben, Fiske, & Hastie, 1979) and, as a consequence, is likely to have more impact on impressions (see Taylor, 1991, for a review). That being the case, it seems likely that this type of information may also have more impact on behavior.

Second, negative images can serve as downward comparison targets and, as such, are more reinforcing. One can feel better about one's risk behavior, or lack of healthy behavior, by comparing with others who are thought to be in worse shape (Gibbons, 1986; Wills, 1981). This is consistent with a general tendency, found in the perceived-risk literature, for people to focus on their own risk-reducing behavior and on the risk-increasing behavior of others more than on their own risk-increasing behavior (Gerrard, Gibbons, & Warner, 1991; Weinstein, 1980).

Third, healthy images are less relevant to most people. Among adolescents, for example, it is not even clear that healthy images are widely recognized. Almost all adolescents think they are healthy and, of course, most of them are. The closest relevant image that comes to mind for young people would be that of the jock or athlete. Positive health images do become more important later in life (Hooker & Kaus, 1992), but even then they appear to be less influential than negative images.

With age comes wisdom (usually) and often the realization that the lifeguard body is just not going to happen, whereas the seven essential food groups are likely to be replaced, from time to time, with a Big Mac or a scotch and soda. In short, images of unhealthy lifestyles are both very real and realistic.

## IMPLICATIONS

### Intervention

The research and theory presented here have some implications for interventions that are intended to reduce health risk among young people. First is the fact that adolescents are especially concerned with social images; these images are very influential. Second, results from both our adolescent and young adult samples indicate that risk images are dynamic. They tend to change as the behavior changes, which means they are also malleable. Thus, there is reason to believe that efforts to alter them stand a good chance of success; that alteration should, in turn, translate into a change in behavior. Third, the fact that images not only affect risk behavior but are also affected by it—becoming more positive, for example, as behavior increases (Gibbons & Gerrard, 1995)— suggests that interventions should be initiated at an early age (cf. Leventhal & Cleary, 1980). Ideally, this should occur before the adolescent has experimented with the risk behaviors or had much exposure to peers who engage in them, as both of these experiences are likely to influence the image.

Fourth, our data and that of others, suggest that few adolescents have a good sense of their peers' risk images. They tend to overestimate the favorability of others' images, much as they tend to overestimate how much risk behavior their peers are engaging in (Graham et al., 1991; Sherman, Presson, Chassin, Corty, & Olshavsky, 1983), and for apparently the same reasons. Prentice and Miller (1993) believe this prevalence overestimation is the result of pluralistic ignorance: Those who don't engage in the behaviors tend not to talk about them; those who are engaging in them do talk, perhaps even exaggerating somewhat. The result is that most assume that the behaviors are more common and the images more favorable than they actually are. Consistent with this analysis, Hansen and Graham (1991) demonstrated that a substance use intervention that includes information about other adolescents' use of and attitudes toward substances can be successful at disabusing adolescents of their misperceptions and reducing their substance use.

Finally, along the same lines, even the adolescents who are engaging in the risk behaviors recognize that the prototypes have negative components. If future research can further identify those negative components, and in so doing, determine in what ways the images are actually "vulnerable," efforts could then be directed at emphasizing the negative elements, thereby further reducing the likelihood that young people will experiment with the behaviors.

**Future Research**

In addition to the need for research aimed at identifying negative elements of the images, we believe more research should be focused, in general, on their composition. For example, are there certain characteristics (e.g., maturity, selfishness, pessimism) that are more closely linked to the behaviors? Similarly, in order to more fully understand how health images work and how they can be modified, research examining the development of these images should prove fruitful. Toward this end, our current research is following up on data we collected earlier from adolescents pertaining to the antecedents of their images. The sources that they have suggested to us include (in descending order of frequency and impact): friends, TV and other media, family, and other adults. As mentioned earlier, this impending study will include samples of African-American pre-adolescents of lower socioeconomic status, in Georgia and Iowa, as well as their early teen siblings, and their parents.

This new study will also provide information about another important issue, that is, whether individual differences in temperament moderate the development and/or the influence of prototypes. For example, recent research linking impulsivity and hyperactivity to adolescent risk behavior (Cloninger, Sigvardsson, & Bohman, 1988; Wills et al., 1995) suggests the possibility that children with these characteristics may have more favorable prototypes of the typical smoker, the reckless driver, and so on and may feel more similar to those prototypes well before they experiment with risky behavior themselves. Once again, we would argue that the model still holds for these young people in that their images, though different, are still very influential, and that influence is mediated by willingness. Nonetheless, the issue of image etiology is clearly an important one with many implications, and it is worthy of additional attention.

We are also attempting to determine to what extent positive health images exist among adolescents as well as adults. Is there, for example, a recognizable image of the young person who doesn't drink or drive recklessly? of a young adult who engages in safe sex? If so, how influential are these positive images? What effect do healthy images have on adults' day-to-day behaviors, other than visits to the health club? Finally, research to date appears to have established the importance of health images in influencing behavior; but we have really only begun to investigate the process whereby this influence occurs. More work is needed in this area, including additional examination of the role that social comparison plays, specifically as a mediator, in the link between images and health behavior.

## REFERENCES

Adams, G. R., & Jones, R. M. (1981). Imaginary audience behavior: A validation study. *Journal of Early Adolescence, 1,* 1–10.

Ajzen, I. (1991). The theory of planned behavior. *Organizational Behavior and Human Decision Processes, 50,* 179–211.

Ajzen, I., & Fishbein, M. (1980). *Understanding attitudes and predicting social behavior.* Englewood Cliffs, NJ: Prentice Hall.

Becker, M. H. (Ed.). (1974). The health belief model and personal health behavior. *Health Education Monographs, 2*(4).

Birnbaum, M. H. (1972). Morality judgments: Tests of an averaging model. *Journal of Experimental Social Psychology, 93,* 35–42.

Bishop, G. D. (1991). Lay disease representations and responses to the victims of disease. *Basic and Applied Social Psychology, 12,* 115–132.

Bishop, G. D., Briede, C., Cavazos, L., Grotzinger, R., & McMahon, S. (1987). Processing illness information: The role of disease prototypes. *Basic and Applied Social Psychology, 8,* 21–43.

Bishop, G. D., & Converse, S. A. (1986). Illness representations: A prototype approach. *Health Psychology, 5,* 95–114.

Bixenstine, V. E., DeCorte, M. S., & Bixenstine, B. A. (1976). Conformity to peer sponsored misconduct at four grade levels. *Developmental Psychology, 12,* 226–236.

Bland, M. J., Bewley, B. R., & Day, I. (1975). Primary schoolboys: Image of self and smoker. *British Journal of Preventative and Social Medicine, 29,* 262–266.

Blanton, H., Gibbons, F. X., Gerrard, M., Conger, K. J., & Smith, G. E. (in press). Development of health risk prototypes during adolescence: Family and peer influences. *Journal of Family Psychology.*

Brickman, P., & Bulman, R. J. (1977). Pleasure and pain in social comparison. In J. Suls & R. L. Miller (Eds.), *Social comparison processes: Theoretical and empirical perspectives* (pp. 149–186). Washington, DC: Hemisphere.

Brown, B. B., Classen, D. R., & Eicher, S. A. (1986). Perceptions of peer pressure, peer conformity dispositions, and self-reported behavior among adolescents. *Developmental Psychology, 22,* 521–530.

Burke, P. J., & Reitzes, D. C. (1981). The link between identity and role performance. *Social Psychology Quarterly, 44,* 83–92.

Burton, D., Sussman, S., Hansen, W. B., Johnson, C. A., & Flay, B. R. (1989). Image attributions and smoking intentions among seventh grade students. *Journal of Applied Social Psychology, 19,* 656–664.

Buunk, B. P. (1994). Social comparison processes under stress: Towards an integration of classic and recent perspectives. In W. Stroebe & M. Hewstone (Eds.), *European review of social psychology* (Vol. 5, pp. 211–241). Chichester, UK: Wiley.

Buunk, B. P., & Gibbons, F. X. (1997). *Temptations: Can prototypes predict adultery?*

Manuscript in progress.
Bynner, J. M. (1970). Behavioral research into children's smoking: Some implications for anti-smoking strategy. *Royal Society of Health Journal, 90,* 159–163.
Cantor, N., Mackie, D., & Lord, C.G. (1984). Choosing partners and activities: The social perceiver decides to mix it up. *Social Cognition, 2,* 256–272.
Cantor, N., & Mischel, W. (1979). Prototypicality and personality: Effects on free recall and personality impressions. *Journal of Research in Personality, 13,* 187–205.
Chassin, L., Presson, C. C., Sherman, S. J., Corty, E., & Olshavsky, R. W. (1981). Self-images and cigarette smoking in adolescence. *Personality and Social Psychology Bulletin, 7,* 670–676.
Chassin, L., Tetzloff, C., & Hershey, M. (1985). Self-image and social-image factors in adolescent alcohol use. *Journal of Studies on Alcohol, 46,* 39–47.
Cloninger, C., Sigvardsson, S., & Bohman, M. (1988). Childhood personality predicts alcohol abuse in young adults. *Alcoholism Clinical and Experimental Research, 12,* 494–505.
Coleman, J. C. (1978). Current contradictions in adolescent theory. *Journal of Youth and Adolescence, 7,* 7–11.
Cooper, H. W., & Kohn, P. M. (1989). The social image of the young female smoker. *British Journal of Addiction, 84,* 935–941.
Cross, S., & Markus, H. (1991). Possible selves across the life span. *Human Development, 34,* 230–255.
Dreben, E. K., Fiske, S. T., & Hastie, R. (1979). The independence of evaluative and item information: Impression and recall order effects in behavior-based impression formation. *Journal of Personality and Social Psychology, 37,* 1758–1768.
Dunning, D., Perie, M., & Story, A. L. (1991). Self-serving prototypes of social categories. *Journal of Personality and Social Psychology, 61,* 957–968.
Elkind, D. (1985). Egocentrism redux. *Developmental Review, 5,* 218–226.
Ellickson, P. L., & Hays, R. D. (1991). Antecedents of drinking among young adolescents with different alcohol use histories. *Journal of Studies on Alcohol, 52,* 398–408.
Erikson, E. H. (1950). *Childhood and society.* New York: Norton.
Erikson, E. H. (1968). *Identity: Youth and crisis.* New York: Norton.
Fazio, H., Sherman, S. J., & Herr, P. M. (1982). The feature-positive effect in self perception process: Does not doing matter as much as doing. *Journal of Personality and Social Psychology, 42,* 404–411.
Fishbein, M., & Ajzen, I. (1975). *Belief, attitude, intention, and behavior: An introduction to theory and research.* Reading, MA: Addison-Wesley.
Gerrard, M., Gibbons, F. X., Benthin, A., & Hessling, R. M. (1996). The reciprocal nature of risk behaviors and cognitions: What you think shapes what you do and vice versa. *Health Psychology, 15,* 344–354.
Gerrard, M., Gibbons, F. X., & Warner, T. D. (1991). Effect of reviewing risk-relevant behaviors on perceptions of vulnerability among women marines. *Health Psychology, 10,* 173–179.
Gibbons, F. X. (1985). Social stigma perception: Social comparison among mentally retarded persons. *American Journal of Mental Deficiency, 90,* 98–106.
Gibbons, F. X. (1986). Social comparison and depression: Company's effect on misery. *Journal of Personality and Social Psychology, 51,* 140–148.
Gibbons, F. X., Blanton, H., Gerrard, M., & Eggleston, T. J. (1997). *Does social comparison make a difference? The influence of comparison level on outcome.* Manuscript submitted for publication.
Gibbons, F. X., & Boney McCoy, S. (1991). Self-esteem, similarity, and reactions to active versus passive downward comparison. *Journal of Personality and Social Psychology, 60,* 414–424.
Gibbons, F. X., & Buunk, B.P. (1996). *Development and validation of the INCOME: The*

*Iowa-Netherlands comparison orientation measure.* Manuscript in progress.

Gibbons, F. X., & Eggleston, T. J. (1996). Smoker networks and the "typical smoker": A prospective analysis of smoking cessation. *Health Psychology, 21,* 368–379.

Gibbons, F. X., & Gerrard, M. (1995). Predicting young adults' health risk behavior. *Journal of Personality and Social Psychology, 69,* 505–517.

Gibbons, F. X., Gerrard, M., Blanton, H., & Russell, D. (in press). Reasoned action and social reaction: Willingness and intention as independent predictors of health risk. *Journal of Personality and Social Psychology.*

Gibbons, F. X., Gerrard, M., & Boney McCoy, S. (1995). Prototype perception predicts (lack of) pregnancy prevention. *Personality and Social Psychology Bulletin, 21,* 85–93.

Gibbons, F. X., Gerrard, M., Lando, H. A., & McGovern, P. G. (1991). Social comparison and smoking cessation: The role of the 'typical smoker.' *Journal of Experimental Social Psychology, 27,* 239–258.

Gibbons, F. X., Gerrard, M., Ouelette, J. A., & Burzette, R. (in press). Cognitive antecedents to health risk: Discriminating between behavioral intention and behavioral willingness. *Psychology and Health.*

Goethals, G. R., & Darley, J.M. (1977). Related attributes and social comparison. In J. Suls & R. Miller (Eds.), *Social comparison theory* (pp. 259–278). Washington, DC: Hemisphere.

Goldstein, J. (1991). The stigmatization of smokers: An empirical investigation. *Journal of Drug Education, 21,* 167–182.

Goosens, L. (1984). Imaginary audience behavior as a function of age, sex, and formal operational thinking. *International Journal of Behavioral Development, 7,* 77–93.

Graham, J. W., Marks, G., & Hansen, W. B. (1991). Social influence processes affecting adolescent substance use. *Journal of Applied Psychology, 76,* 291–298.

Hansen. W. B., & Graham, J. W. (1991). Preventing alcohol, marijuana and cigarette use among adolescents: Peer pressure resistance training versus establishing conservative norms. *Preventive Medicine, 20,* 414–430.

Harrison, J. A., Mullen, P. D., & Green, L. W. (1992). A meta-analysis of studies of the health belief model with adults. *Health Education Research, 7,* 107–116.

Hooker, K. (1992). Possible selves and perceived health in older adults and college students. *Journal of Gerontology, 47,* 85–95.

Hooker, K., & Kaus, C. R. (1992). Possible selves and health behaviors in later life. *Journal of Aging and Health, 4,* 390–411.

Hooker, K., & Kaus, C. R. (1994). Health-related possible selves in young and middle adulthood. *Psychology and Aging, 1,* 126–133.

Janz, N. K., & Becker, M. H. (1984). The Health Belief Model: A decade later. *Health Education Quarterly, 11,* 1–47.

Jessor, R., & Jessor, S. L. (1977). *Problem behavior and psychosocial development: A longitudinal study of youth.* New York: Academic Press.

Kandel, D. (1980). Drug and drinking behavior among youth. *Annual Review of Sociology, 6,* 235–285.

Leventhal, H. (1970). Findings and theory in the study of fear communications. *Advances in Experimental Social Psychology, 5,* 119–186.

Leventhal, H., & Cleary, P. D. (1980). The smoking problem: A review of the research and theory in behavioral risk modification. *Psychological Bulletin, 88,* 370–405.

Markus, H., & Nurius, P. (1986). Possible selves. *American Psychologist, 41,* 954–969.

Marques, J. M., Robalo, E. M., & Rocho, S. A. (1992). Ingroup bias and the 'black sheep effect': Assessing the impact of social identification and perceived variability on group judgments. *European Journal of Social Psychology, 22,* 331–352.

Marques, J. M., Yzerbyt, V. Y., & Leyens, J. P. (1988). The "black sheep effect": Extremity of judgments towards ingroup members as a function of group identification. *European Journal of Social Psychology, 18,* 1–16.

McKennell, A. C., & Bynner, J. M. (1969). Self images and smoking behaviour among school boys. *British Journal of Educational Psychology, 39,* 27–39.

Mervis, C. B., & Rosch, E. (1981). Categorization of natural objects. *Annual Review of Psychology, 32,* 89–115.

Meyer, D., Leventhal, H., & Gutmann, M. (1985). Common sense models of illness: The example of hypertension. *Health Psychology, 39,* 115–135.

Mosbach, P., & Leventhal, H. (1988). Peer group identification and smoking: Implications for intervention. Special Issue: Models of addiction. *Journal of Abnormal Psychology, 97,* 238–245.

Moss, M. K., & Frieze, I. H. (1993). Job preferences in the anticipatory socialization phase: A comparison of two matching models. *Journal of Vocational Behavior, 42,* 282–297.

Niedenthal, P. M., Cantor, N., & Kihlstrom, J. F. (1985). Prototype matching: A strategy for social decision making. *Journal of Personality and Social Psychology, 48,* 575–584.

Niedenthal, P. M., & Mordkoff, J. T. (1991). Prototype distancing: A strategy for choosing among threatening situations. *Personality and Social Psychology Bulletin, 17,* 483–493.

Pennebaker, J. W. (1982). *The psychology of physical symptoms. New York: Springer-Verlag.*

Perloff, L. S., & Fetzer, P. A. (1986). Self-other judgments and perceived vulnerability. *Journal of Personality and Social Psychology, 50,* 502–510.

Prentice, D. A., & Miller, D. T. (1993). Pluralistic ignorance and alcohol use on campus: Some consequences of misperceiving the social norm. *Journal of Personality and Social Psychology, 64,* 243–256.

Rosch, E. H. (1978). Principles of categorization. In E. Rosch & B. B. Lloyd (Eds.), *Cognition and categorization.* Hillsdale, NJ: Lawrence Erlbaum Associates.

Sebald, H. (1989). Adolescents' peer orientation: Changes in the support system during the past three decades. *Adolescence, 24,* 937–946.

Sherman, S. J., Chassin, L., Presson, C. C., & Agostinelli, G. (1984). The role of the evaluation and similarity principles in the false consensus effect. *Journal of Personality and Social Psychology, 47,* 1244–1262.

Sherman, S. J., Presson, C. C., & Chassin, L. (1984). Mechanisms underlying the false consensus effect: The special role of threats to the self. *Personality and Social Psychology Bulletin, 10,* 127–138.

Sherman, S. J., Presson, C. C., Chassin, L., Corty, E., & Olshavsky, R. (1983). The false consensus effect in estimates of smoking prevalence: Underlying mechanisms. *Personality and Social Psychology Bulletin, 9,* 197–207.

Simmons, R. G., Rosenberg, F., & Rosenberg, M. (1973) Disturbance in the self-image at adolescence. *American Sociological Review, 38,* 553–568.

Skowronski, J. J., & Carlston, D. E. (1989). Negativity and extremity biases in impression formation: A review of explanations. *Psychological Bulletin, 105,* 131–142.

Snortum, J. R., Kremer, L. K., & Berger, D. E. (1987). Alcoholic beverage preference as a public statement: Self concept and social image of college drinkers. *Journal of Studies on Alcohol, 48,* 243–251.

Stokols, D., Ohlig, W., & Resnick, S. M. (1978). Perception of residential crowding, classroom experiences, and student health. *Human Ecology, 6,* 233–252.

Sussman, S., Dent, C. W., Stacy, A. W., Burciaga, C., Raynor, A., Turner, G. E., Charlin, V., Craig, S., Hansen, W. B., Burton, D., & Flay, B. R. (1990). Peer-group association and adolescent tobacco use. *Journal of Abnormal Psychology, 99,* 349–352.

Taylor (1991). Asymmetrical effects of positive and negative events: The mobilization-minimization hypothesis. *Psychological Bulletin, 110,* 67–85.

Taylor S. E., & Lobel, M. (1989). Social comparison activity under threat: Downward evaluation and upward contacts. *Psychological Review, 96,* 569–575.

Taylor, S. E., Wood, J.V., & Lichtman, R. R. (1983). It could be worse: Selective evaluation as a response to victimization. *Journal of Social Issues, 39,* 19–40.

Warshaw, P. R., & Davis, F. D. (1985). Disentangling behavioral intention and behavioral expectations. *Journal of Experimental Social Psychology, 21,* 213–228.
Weinstein, N. D. (1980). Unrealistic optimism about future life events. *Journal of Personality and Social Psychology, 39,* 806–820.
Weinstein, N. D. (1987). Unrealistic optimism about susceptibility to health problems: Conclusions from a community-wide sample. *Journal of Behavioral Medicine, 10,* 481–500.
Weinstein, N. D., & Klein, W. M. (1995). Resistance of personal risk perceptions to debiasing interventions. *Health Psychology, 14,* 132–140.
Wills, T. A. (1981). Downward comparison principles in social psychology. *Psychological Bulletin, 90,* 245–251.
Wills, T. A. (1987). Downward comparison as a coping mechanism. In C. R. Snyder & C. Ford (Eds.), *Coping with negative life events: Clinical and social-psychological perspectives* (pp. 243–268). New York: Plenum.
Wills, T. A. (1991). Similarity and self-esteem in downward comparison. In J. Suls & T. A. Wills (Eds.), *Social comparison: Contemporary theory and research* (pp. 51–78). Hillsdale, NJ: Lawrence Erlbaum Associates.
Wills, T. A., Baker, E., & Botvin, G. J. (1989). Dimensions of assertiveness: Differential relationships to substance use in early adolescence. *Journal of Consulting and Clinical Psychology, 57,* 473–478.
Wills, T. A., Duhamel, K., & Vaccaro, D. (1995). Activity and mood temperament as predictors of adolescent substance use: Test of self-regulation mediational model. *Journal of Personality and Social Psychology, 68,* 901–916.

# CHAPTER 4

# Social Comparison Processes and AIDS Risk and AIDS Preventive Behavior

Stephen J. Misovich
Jeffrey D. Fisher
*University of Connecticut*

William A. Fisher
*University of Western Ontario*

AIDS has rapidly become a major global public health threat. By the mid-1990s, 4.5 million people worldwide had been diagnosed with AIDS, and 19.5 million persons were infected with HIV (World Health Organization, 1995), the agent that causes AIDS (Lifson, 1990). In the United States, approximately 500,000 persons had been diagnosed with AIDS (Centers for Disease Control, 1995), and AIDS had the leading cause of death among U.S. adults between the ages of 25 to 44 (National Center for Health Statistics, 1994). HIV has had devastating effects on gay men in the United States (Centers for Disease Control, 1995; Kelly, 1994; Kelly & Murphy, 1992), minorities (Centers for Disease Control, 1995; J. Jemmott & Jemmott, 1994), and injection drug users (Centers for Disease Control, 1995; Friedman, DesJarlais, & Ward, 1994; Kelly & Murphy, 1992). Evidence is also converging to indicate that the general heterosexually active public is increasingly at risk as well (Centers for Disease Control, 1995; Edlin, Keeling, Gayle, & Holmeberg, 1994; Winslow, Franzini, & Hwang, 1992).

Because HIV is communicated behaviorally, it can be prevented by behavioral change; for example, people can avoid risky behaviors such as unprotected intercourse and can begin practicing preventive behaviors like using condoms. Nevertheless, risky behaviors remain relatively common and preventive behaviors are inconsistently practiced even among high-risk groups such as gay men (D'Augelli, 1992; Ekstrand 1992; Kelly, 1994; McCusker, Stoddard, McDonald, Zapka, & Mayer,

1992), minorities (Catania, Coates, Fullilove, Peterson, Marin, Siegel, & Hulley, 1992; Catania, Coates, Peterson, Dolcini, Kegeles, Siegel, Golden, & Fullilove, 1993; J. Jemmott & Jemmott, 1994), injection drug users and their partners (Friedman et al., 1994; Simpson, Knight, & Ray, 1993), and among the heterosexually active public (Catania et al., 1992; Catania et al., 1993; J. D. Fisher, Misovich, & Fisher, 1992) in the U.S.

## PSYCHOLOGICAL FACTORS UNDERLYING AIDS RISK AND AIDS PREVENTIVE BEHAVIORS

Several explanations have been put forth for the striking levels of AIDS risk behavior that continue to characterize diverse populations. Some explanations have invoked information deficits, suggesting that a lack of knowledge about AIDS may be inhibiting AIDS prevention (e.g., Crawford, Thomas & Zoller, 1993; Trinkaus, 1992), even though it is now widely accepted that information per se is generally not sufficient to produce AIDS preventive behavior change (e.g., J. D. Fisher & Fisher, 1992; Trad, 1994). Several motivational factors are also commonly suggested as barriers to the performance of AIDS preventive behavior. These include negative attitudes toward safer behaviors (e.g., the beliefs that condoms are uncomfortable and that using them has negative implications for perceived trust within relationships; Corby, Wolitski, Thornton-Johnson, & Tanner, 1991; W. A. Fisher, Fisher, & Rye, 1995), as well as antiprevention social norms (e.g., that important referent others view condom use negatively, and that such use may even lead to sanctions from referent others; J. D. Fisher, 1988; J. D. Fisher, Misovich, & Fisher, 1992; W. A. Fisher et al., 1995; Galligan & Terry, 1993; Kashima, Gallois, & McCamish, 1993). An additional motivational obstacle to prevention is the fact that across populations whose behavior poses HIV risk, many individuals do not feel personally vulnerable to HIV infection (e.g., Van der Pligt, Otten, Richard, & Van der Velde, 1993). Finally, deficits in AIDS prevention behavioral skills (e.g., inability to negotiate safer sex with a partner) and in perceptions of self-efficacy regarding the performance of these behaviors, have been implicated as causes of the failure to engage in AIDS prevention (e.g., Bandura, 1994; Catania et al., 1992; Walter, Vaughan, Ragin, Cohall, & Kasen, 1994).

The assertion that deficits in AIDS prevention information, motivation, and behavioral skills are associated with AIDS risk behavior and that strengths in these areas are associated with AIDS preventive behaviors has been widely espoused (Coates, 1990; J. D. Fisher & Fisher, 1989; J. D. Fisher & Fisher, 1992; Winett, Altman, & King, 1990). These views have been formalized in the Information–Motivation–Behavioral Skills (IMB) model of AIDS-risk behavior change, which holds that AIDS prevention information, motivation, and behavioral skills are fundamental determinants of AIDS preventive behavior (J. D. Fisher & Fisher, 1992; W. A. Fisher & Fisher, 1993). According to the model, *information* that is directly relevant to AIDS transmission and prevention is an initial prerequisite of AIDS preventive behavior. *Motivation* to engage in AIDS preventive behavior, including personal motivation (attitudes toward AIDS preventive acts), social motivation (perceived social support for performing these acts), and perceptions of personal vulnerability to AIDS, is a second critical prerequisite of AIDS preventive behavior. Finally, *behavioral skills* for performing specific AIDS preventive acts effectively, including objective skills at performing these behaviors and a sense of self-efficacy in doing so, are a third critical prerequisite of AIDS preventive behavior (Bandura, 1994; W. A. Fisher, 1990; Kelly & St. Lawrence, 1988).

The IMB model specifies that AIDS prevention information and AIDS prevention motivation work largely through AIDS prevention behavioral skills to affect the initiation and maintenance of AIDS preventive behavior (see Fig. 4.1). An individual's information and motivation are expected to be expressed primarily through the application of his or her behavioral skills, and therefore information and motivation work through, and are limited by, behavioral skills. Information and motivation may also have direct effects on AIDS preventive behavior when complicated or novel behavioral skills are unnecessary to effect prevention. An example of a direct effect of information on AIDS preventive behavior would be an individual switching from using ordinary lubricated condoms to condoms that are lubricated with Nonoxynol-9 after learning that the latter may be more effective at preventing HIV. An example of a direct effect of motivation on behavior might involve a highly motivated individual simply maintaining a sexually abstinent pattern—which may not require sophisticated behavioral skills—rather than being sexually active but safe, which would likely require such skills. In addition, the model regards information and motivation as generally independent constructs (J. D. Fisher, W. A. Fisher, Williams,

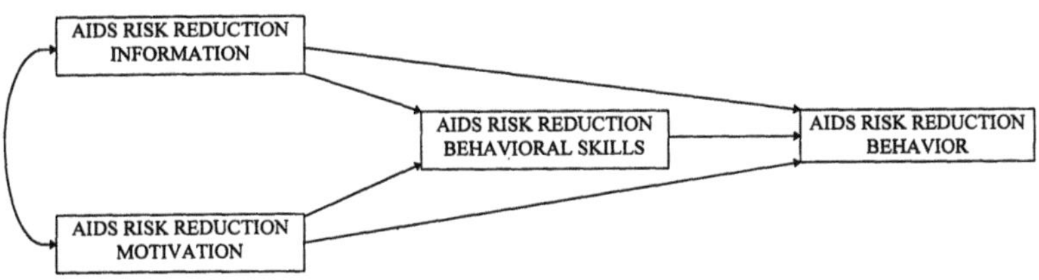


FIG. 4.1. The Information-Motivation-Behavioral Skills Model for HIV/AIDS risk reduction. Adapted from "Changing AIDS Risk Behavior," by J. D. Fisher and W. A. Fisher, 1992, *Psychological Bulletin, 111,* p. 465.

& Malloy, 1994), insofar as well-informed individuals are not necessarily well motivated to practice prevention, and well-motivated individuals are not necessarily well informed about prevention. To date, tests of the relationship between information and motivation (e.g., J. D. Fisher et al., 1994) have indicated that information and motivation are generally independent of one another, although it is possible that the two may be related under some circumstances.

The assertions of the IMB model concerning AIDS prevention information, motivation, behavioral skills, and behavior and the relationships among these constructs have been confirmed in structural equation tests with gay men, college students, and minority high school students (J. D. Fisher et al., 1994; W. A. Fisher et al., 1996). The model has also been used as the conceptual basis for an effective AIDS risk behavior change intervention (J. D. Fisher, W. A. Fisher, Misovich, Kimble, & Malloy, 1996). In this intervention, deficits in college students' levels of AIDS prevention information, motivation, and behavioral skills were identified and remediated, resulting in sustained increases in AIDS preventive behavior.

## SOCIAL COMPARISON AND AIDS PREVENTION

For present purposes, we define *AIDS prevention social comparison* as the process of evaluating one's AIDS prevention information, motivation, behavioral skills, and behavior through comparison with actual or imagined others. It is the thesis of this chapter that social comparison processes (see, e.g., Festinger, 1954) affect individuals' levels of AIDS prevention information, motivation, and behavioral skills, and thus their levels of AIDS preventive behavior, in critical ways. Under some conditions, social comparison processes act to decrease levels of AIDS prevention information, motivation, and behavioral skills, and thus inhibit AIDS preventive behavior. On the other hand, under some conditions social comparison processes act to increase the determinants of AIDS preventive behavior, and consequently, increase AIDS prevention itself. In this chapter, we employ the IMB model as a framework for discussing the possible effects of social comparison processes on individuals' AIDS risk and AIDS preventive behaviors. We draw on previously published research that is relevant to social comparison and AIDS prevention (e.g., Bandura, 1994; Dearing, Meyer, & Rogers, 1994; Kelly, 1994), and we report relevant findings of new research on this topic. As we discuss here, classic social comparison theory (e.g., Festinger, 1954) predicts that individuals in general prefer to seek out objective sources of information to assess the validity of their perceptions about AIDS prevention. In the case of AIDS prevention, however, concerns about the truthfulness of the "objective" sources of AIDS information (e.g., Barr, Waring, & Warshaw, 1992; Herek & Capitanio, 1994), or the need to validate one's beliefs or existing practices, may motivate individuals to engage in social comparison.

## SOCIAL COMPARISON PROCESSES

For the purposes of the present chapter we focus on two processes of social comparison. First, we consider *constructive social comparison* (e.g., Goethals, Messick, & Allison, 1991)—also termed *implicit social comparison* (Suls, Marco, & Tobin, 1991)—which involves social comparison that occurs in the imagination, often with a stereotyped or prototypical comparison other, and in the absence of any objective external comparison activity. In essence, with constructive social comparison, an individual who experiences some uncertainty regarding his or her opinions or abilities (or experiences some other motive for comparing) engages in a comparison with a "constructed" social comparison other that may not actually exist.

The second comparison process we consider involves more "classic" social comparison, or what has been termed *realistic comparison* by Goethals et al. (1991). This type of social comparison takes place when an individual, experiencing uncertainty regarding his or her opinions or abilities, makes use of social information elicited from comparisons with actual others to assess these beliefs or abilities.

### Constructive Social Comparison

Examples of constructive comparison abound in the literature on social comparison, health and coping. This literature frequently focuses on a form of downward comparison (e.g., Gibbons & Gerard, chapter 3, this volume; Gibbons, Gerard, Lando, & McGovern, 1991; Wills, 1991), involving the cognitive construction of "worse-off" comparison others who permit the comparer to feel better about his or her own health and risk of future negative outcomes. For instance, Suls et al. (1991) suggested that elderly people often improve their own health self-perceptions by comparing themselves with a stereotyped, generalized elderly person who is relatively unhealthy. In the literature on coping with breast cancer, women who undergo surgery have frequently been found to cope by imagining worse-off women who have had more extensive surgery (e.g., Wood, Taylor, & Lichtman, 1985; Wood & VanderZee, chapter 10, this volume). Similarly, when individuals assess their risk for negative outcomes, they may imagine others with more risk factors, compare their own risk with these stereotypical others, and arrive at confident but inaccurate judgments of personal invulnerability (e.g., Klein & Weinstein, chapter 2, this volume; Perloff & Fetzer, 1986; Weinstein, 1980). As we discuss later, this phenomenon has been observed among a wide range of participants in research on perceived vulnerability to HIV infection. However, constructive comparison is not invariably associated with increased riskiness. For instance, individuals may distance themselves from an imagined prototype of the "typical" at-risk person, using this as a comparison point for what not to do, and as a result may change their behavior to become safer (e.g., Gibbons & Gerrard, 1991).

The process of constructive comparison may also take place when people seek to create consensus to validate their AIDS prevention information (e.g., whether or not "seeing only one person" makes condom use unnecessary), their assessments of the desirability of engaging in preventive behavior (i.e., attitudes toward AIDS prevention), and their assessments of normative support for prevention. Furthermore, research on constructive comparison and false uniqueness (e.g., Goethals et al., 1991) suggests that constructive comparisons may lead individuals to overestimate their own AIDS prevention behavioral skills. This overestimation may interfere with their development of necessary objective skills.

In summary, the process of implicit or constructive comparison (e.g., Goethals et al., 1991) consists of the self-generation of comparison others to test one's beliefs and abilities, as opposed to engaging in comparisons with actual others. In the present context, constructive comparison is likely to produce consensus for one's current HIV-relevant information, attitudes, and perceptions of social norms, and to produce relatively low assessments of one's risks for various negative outcomes as well as unrealistically high assessments of one's abilities. Such outcomes would appear to bode poorly for subsequent AIDS preventive behavior. It is also possible, however, that constructive comparisons with a proprevention referent could lead to increases in prevention, or that distancing oneself from an antiprevention referent could have the same effect. Although relatively little research to date has addressed these issues in specific relation to HIV prevention, we consider the possible effects of such comparisons in this chapter, and draw on relevant research when possible.

### Realistic Social Comparison

Under some circumstances, realistic social comparison may involve comparing with a specific social comparison other (e.g., a particular friend or influential group member; Festinger, 1954; Goethals et al., 1991). It may also involve comparison with one's reference group as a whole (e.g., J. D. Fisher, 1988), or with selected members of one's reference group. In such cases, communication and comparison with multiple reference group members may affect one's beliefs and behaviors. In realistic comparison processes, individuals observe, communicate with, and are otherwise influenced by similar others. This type of social comparison often occurs naturalistically in the social environment (Wheeler & Miyake, 1992). Additionally, opportunities for such comparisons may be created or manipulated by individuals attempting to increase AIDS preventive behavior in a target audience (see J. D. Fisher et al., 1996; W. A. Fisher & Fisher, 1992; Kelly, 1994). This may occur through the presentation of the behavior of referent others in the media, or in settings such as peer-led workshops or interventions. In such settings, social comparison others for a target group are trained to communicate proprevention beliefs and to model proprevention behaviors, thus to some extent imposing social comparison on the study participants, who are forced to compare their own opinions, performance, and outcomes with those of the peer leaders.

In realistic social comparison, individuals are likely to affiliate and compare with similar others (Buunk & Ybema, chapter 12, this volume; Festinger, 1954; Miller & Suls, 1977). They are also likely to perceive the feedback they receive from similar others with respect to their levels of AIDS risk-reduction information, motivation, behavioral skills, and behavior as being especially credible, relevant, and useful, in comparison with these phenomena in extremely dissimilar others (Festinger, 1954; Suls et al., chapter 7, this volume). To the extent that similar social comparison others validate an individual's correct information, correct an individual's misinformation, express positive attitudes and norms for behavior, and act as role models for the development of behavioral skills, realistic social comparison will act to facilitate AIDS preventive behavior. Consequently, it is likely that AIDS prevention interventions that make use of similar (e.g., peer) leaders will be more effective than interventions without such leaders (e.g., Rickert, Jay, & Gottleib, 1991; Stevenson & Davis, 1994). Interventions using peer leaders have in fact been found to be effective in changing a wide range of adolescent risk behaviors including smoking, drinking, and drug use (e.g., Botvin & Eng, 1982, Botvin, Baker, Filazzola, & Botvin, 1990; Luepker, Johnson, Murray, & Pechacek, 1983; Murray, Davis-Hearn, Goldman, Pirie, & Luepker, 1988; Telch, Miller, Killen, Cooke, & Maccoby, 1990; Wiist & Snider, 1991), as well as in reducing AIDS risk behavior among gay men (e.g., Kelly, 1994).

### Choosing a Comparative Process

As Fig. 4.2 suggests, uncertainty regarding an aspect of AIDS prevention may lead either to constructive social comparison (e.g., Goethals et

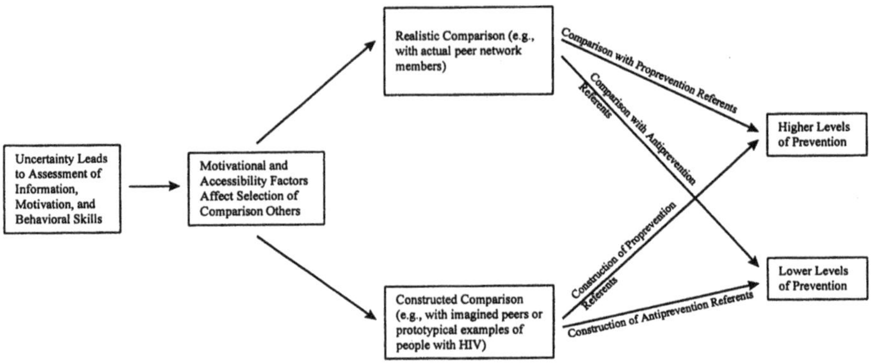


FIG. 4.2. Social comparison processes and AIDS risk and AIDS preventive behavior.

al., 1991), or to realistic social comparison with referent others (e.g., J. D. Fisher, 1988; Goethals et al., 1991). The choice of comparison process depends on several factors (Goethals et al., 1991). Individuals who are most concerned with ensuring that they validate their extant beliefs with respect to their lack of need for AIDS prevention, may engage solely in constructive social comparisons. Alternately, the desire to obtain accurate comparison information (e.g., to ascertain whether one's knowledge is correct, or one's perception of reference group norms is accurate) may be more likely to lead a person to engage in realistic comparison (Festinger, 1954; Goethals et al., 1991). Additionally, individuals who are most interested in conforming with their reference group's attitudes and norms to gain rewards and avoid sanctions regarding their preventive practices may engage primarily in realistic comparison, and communicate and compare with members of their reference group (J. D. Fisher, 1988). The differential accessibility of sources of social comparison will also affect the individual's choice. In many instances (e.g., when one is either alone and deciding whether or not to buy condoms before going on a date), the only comparison others available may be self-generated. When an individual is among his or her peers (e.g., when discussing the topic of HIV in a group of friends or in a health class) he or she may have immediate reference group-based sources for use in realistic comparisons. On the whole, however, HIV prevention and sexual behavior in general are uniquely private, more difficult to discuss with others than many other topics (e.g., Williams et al., 1992). For these reasons, less realistic social comparison and more constructive comparison may occur with HIV prevention than in other domains.

Once a modality for one's social comparison has been established, the individual engages in a comparison with an actual or constructive social comparison other or others. To the extent that these comparisons lead an individual to conclude that AIDS preventive behavior is necessary and possible, he or she may act to reduce risky behaviors. However, these realistic or constructive comparisons may instead produce in individuals confirmation of inaccurate information, reinforcement of low motivation, and even an unrealistic assessment of their ability to engage in preventive behaviors. In the remaining sections of this chapter we discuss how constructive and realistic social comparisons may affect an individual's AIDS prevention information, motivation, and behavioral skills, and how social comparison processes may be harnessed to increase preventive behavior.

## SOCIAL COMPARISON PROCESSES AND AIDS PREVENTION INFORMATION, MOTIVATION, AND BEHAVIORAL SKILLS

### Information

Having enough accurate AIDS prevention information is a prerequisite for engaging in AIDS preventive behavior. Such information includes knowledge about how HIV is transmitted (e.g., that HIV is spread through unprotected sexual contact with an infected person) and about how HIV transmission is prevented (e.g., that using condoms consistently greatly reduces the likelihood of HIV transmission). AIDS prevention information also involves the decision rules people use to judge whether or not to practice safer sex with a given individual. These decision rules include implicit personality theories of AIDS risk and AIDS risk reduction (e.g., the belief that "nice" partners with positive characteristics are unlikely to be HIV infected and do not require condom use) and AIDS prevention heuristics (e.g., the belief that sex with a partner one knows well is safe and does not necessitate condom use). Such implicit personality theories and heuristics often constitute "misinformation" that is strongly associated with risky behavior (Misovich, Fisher, & Fisher, 1996).

***Social Comparison Influences on Information.*** Social comparison influences an individual's level of AIDS prevention information when that individual, experiencing some uncertainty about a piece of AIDS information (e.g., whether condom use effectively reduces the transmission of HIV), uses social comparison processes to evaluate that information, either by constructively imagining a consensus among his or her referent others regarding the information (e.g., Goethals et al., 1991), or by realistically comparing it with actual referent others' information (e.g., Festinger, 1954; Gordon, 1966).

For the most part, individuals probably do not question the correctness of their own beliefs, and assume that others agree with their store of AIDS information. Under some circumstances, however, individuals may not be content to assume that their AIDS information is correct and is supported by referent others. This may occur when some aspect of this information is profoundly disconfirmed, or when new scientific reports are released and covered in the media, or when unexpected circumstances occur, as when a public figure like Earvin "Magic" Johnson discloses that he has become HIV positive (e.g., Kalichman & Hunter, 1992). Classic social comparison theory (e.g., Festinger, 1954) would predict that individuals who are uncertain about the validity of their AIDS prevention information would assess its validity by comparing it with information from presumably objective sources (i.e., "experts" such as physicians, or public health experts). Only in the absence of objective, expert information are people expected to turn to social comparison processes to evaluate their information. Indeed, research on health information seeking finds a general preference for information from objective, medical sources when such information is available (e.g., Barr & Warshaw, 1994; Molleman, Pruyn, & van Knippenberg, 1986; Suls, Martin, & Leventhal, chapter 7, this volume).

People may reject objective data from experts under some circumstances, however; for example, they may perceive "expert" information as *biased* in some way, as irrelevant to themselves and their situation, or as actually untrue. In the case of AIDS prevention information, the literature suggests that many individuals may reject "objective" information provided by expert sources, viewing it as inaccurate, a manifestation of social control, irrelevant, or not yet substantiated by adequate research (e.g., Barr, Waring, & Warshaw, 1992; Herek & Capitanio, 1994). When they reject expert sources for these kinds of reasons, individuals may decide to engage in realistic social comparison and seek out similar others (e.g., gay men may consult other gay men; Kelly, 1995) who they may view as being truly informative with respect to evaluating and increasing their information (e.g., Goethals & Darley, 1977; Weary, Marsh, & McCormick, 1994).

In contrast to seeking what they may perceive to be accurate information through social comparison, people may be motivated to compare with others who simply validate their own beliefs (e.g., Kruglanski & Mayseles, 1987). Under these circumstances, individuals may be motivated to seek confirmatory (but not necessarily accurate) information from social comparison others who are likely to provide it, rather than seek accurate (but not necessarily confirmatory) information from more objective sources. For example, a person who wants to continue practicing unsafe sex despite the exhortations of health experts may seek information from people who agree with him or her to support this practice. Although social comparison in this context may often lead to exposure to misinformation, under some circumstances social comparison with one's social group may lead to a beneficial reassessment of misinformation (e.g., when other group members do possess expertise and convey accurate prevention information that one lacks). However, an individual consulting social comparison others rather than expert sources in assessing his or her AIDS information is relatively likely to have many incorrect beliefs confirmed and even augmented. Such reinforcement of misinformation may result in the strengthening of potentially harmful implicit personality theories of HIV risk (e.g., Williams et al., 1992), such as the belief that HIV is a risk only for gay men (e.g., Nyamathi, Flaskerud, Bennett, Leake, & Lewis, 1994), or, if one is a gay man, the belief that HIV is an issue only for older gay men (e.g., Kelly, 1995).

***Increasing AIDS Prevention Information.*** Social comparison theory suggests several tasks for AIDS prevention advocates seeking to increase information among at-risk individuals. One is to encourage people who typically reject information from expert sources to seek and accept such information (e.g., Dearing et al., 1994). Field research has shown that having social comparison others (e.g., "Magic" Johnson, for African-American men) announce that they are HIV-positive can increase information-seeking from experts *and* from social comparison others, among individuals who are generally unlikely to seek out information from expert sources. "Magic" Johnson's announcement that he was HIV positive led African-American men who generally distrusted "expert" information to seek information from expert sources such as AIDS hotlines. Johnson's announcement also had the effect of increasing AIDS-related information seeking from social comparison others. Although this may have had a beneficial or a harmful effect, depending on the outcome of the information seeking (i.e., whether proprevention or antiprevention information was finally accepted), overall, concern about HIV increased, especially among those who had no previous contact with HIV-positive people. A social comparison interpretation of these findings is strengthened by the fact that the effects were generally strongest among African-American men similar to "Magic" Johnson in age and sexual orientation (Kalichman & Hunter, 1992; Kalichman, Russell, Hunter, & Sarwer, 1993). Research with adolescents has also suggested that using social comparison others in leadership roles within AIDS prevention interventions may encourage participants to seek more information, compared with participants in interventions run by dissimilar others (e.g., Rickert, Jay, & Gottleib, 1991; Stevenson & Davis, 1994), suggesting that similar others are regarded as especially valuable sources of information.

For individuals who generally reject expert or mass media suggestions to practice safer sex, social comparison others who are also experts on AIDS prevention may be the most effective change agents (cf. Dearing et al., 1994). To break down the mistrust that has typically prevented disenfranchised groups from accepting accurate expert information, it may be useful to recruit experts from the disenfranchised groups themselves. Through elicitation research involving focus groups, open-ended questionnaires, and interviews (J. D. Fisher & Fisher, 1992), it may be possible to identify individuals who are perceived as highly credible social comparison experts within a given population and to have such individuals participate in informative public service announcements or to appear personally before a target population. For instance, for African-American adults, an African-American physician or public health expert may be highly effective at disseminating information. Another way to use social comparison others to disseminate accurate AIDS information is to train such people and deploy them as AIDS educators or outreach workers in real-world settings (e.g., "shooting galleries," gay bars, housing projects, high schools). Across many populations, selecting high-status community members and having them occupy an advocate role for AIDS prevention may be especially effective (Kelly, 1994). Choosing individuals who have had the same problem as an addicted target population and having them disseminate AIDS prevention information may also be highly effective (e.g., former drug abusers may work with intravenous drug users; see Chitwood et al., 1990).

## Motivation

Motivation to engage in AIDS preventive behavior is a second prerequisite of AIDS prevention behavior change. According to the IMB model, this construct includes personal motivation to perform AIDS preventive behaviors (i.e., attitudes toward AIDS preventive acts), social motivation to perform AIDS preventive behaviors (i.e., perceived social support for performing these acts), and perceptions of personal vulnerability to HIV. Each of these elements may be affected by social comparison processes that may validate one's current motivation levels or may lead one to change one's attitudes, perceptions of norms, and perceived vulnerability.

***Social Comparison Influences on Attitudes and Norms.*** With respect to AIDS prevention, in order to be able to perceive their attitudes as valid and their behavior as normative, individuals may assume consensus among others regarding such attitudes and norms. Such a constructive process may be especially common in the case of AIDS risk and AIDS preventive behaviors, given that others' practice or failure to practice such behaviors is not usually visible and actual consensus information may not be available, leaving more room for construction (Goethals et al., 1991). However, under some circumstances (e.g., an actual discussion of safer sexual practices within a proprevention friendship group that leads to a realization that others have begun to practice safer sex), earlier constructive comparisons may be disconfirmed through realistic comparison. Realistic comparisons, such as an individual's observation of the incidence of AIDS preventive behavior among their social comparison others, and other feedback from comparison others, may have a strong impact on one's attitudes and perceived norms. Research on related issues (e.g., Suls, Wan, & Sanders, 1988; Suls, Martin, & Leventhal, chapter 7, this volume) suggests that when an individual perceives that social comparison others engage in AIDS preventive behavior frequently, he or she may be more confident in the validity of that behavior, and may generally develop more favorable attitudes toward it. Alternatively, when people see that others rarely engage in AIDS preventive behavior they may take this as evidence that such behavior is not useful or necessary. Similarly, if people do not observe many social comparison others advocating for or engaging in AIDS prevention, they may well decide that the behavior is not normative and that they may incur sanctions from their peer group if they engage in it (J. D. Fisher, 1988).

Research on peer influence on AIDS prevention has shown that social comparison others do exert a strong effect on individuals' AIDS prevention attitudes and norms (e.g., Fishbein, Middlestadt, & Hitchcock, 1994; J. D. Fisher & Misovich, 1990; W. A. Fisher et al., 1995; Kelly, 1994). When one's important referent others have positive attitudes toward AIDS preventive behavior and engage in AIDS prevention, one is more likely to have positive attitudes toward AIDS preventive behavior, to perceive normative support for its practice, and to actually practice preventive behavior (e.g., W. A. Fisher et al., 1995). The reverse is true when important referent others have negative attitudes toward prevention and fail to practice it. Some descriptive evidence illustrating college students' beliefs about the impact of social comparison others' AIDS prevention attitudes, norms, and behavior on their own behavior emerged in our focus group research involving groups of such students. Many students believed that HIV testing was uncommon among their social comparison others, and felt that this prevented them from being tested themselves. One student said, "if more people did it I think it would be easier to [be tested]. Everyone will just go and give blood, but it's not like 'oh, let's all go and get tested for AIDS.'" Other students did perceive positive attitudes and normative support for HIV testing from social comparison others, which seemed to facilitate testing behavior. One student said, "my friends kind of helped motivate me because when I told them I was going to get tested their reaction wasn't like 'ugh, you have to get AIDS tested,' they were like 'oh, that's a good idea.' My girlfriend, too, was happy we were going to do it, so all their attitudes were positive, which made it easy to do." Overall, it appears that social comparison others can have a significant impact on individuals' AIDS prevention attitudes and norms.

***Improving Attitudes and Social Norms.*** Research suggests that social comparison others can also be used effectively to change negative attitudes and social norms with respect to AIDS preventive behavior (Dearing et al., 1994; J. D. Fisher et al., 1996; Kelly, 1994). Such individuals may act as "natural opinion leaders" (e.g., Kelly, 1994), who may exert substantial normative influence on the behaviors of network members. Having natural opinion leaders portray AIDS prevention as "the right thing to do" may elicit proprevention changes in AIDS prevention attitudes and perceived norms (J. D. Fisher et al., 1996;; Kelly, 1994), especially because with arousal-producing issues like AIDS, similar others may be more sought after and more influential than dissimilar others (e.g., Cottrell & Epley, 1977; Misovich, Colby, & Welch, 1973; Schachter, 1959). To date, most interventions using social comparison others to increase prevention have trained them to espouse positive attitudes toward AIDS prevention, and to indicate that they are engaging in AIDS preventive behavior themselves (e.g., Kelly, 1994). This is typically done in natural settings such as gay bars or housing projects. Additional use of social comparison others who are natural opinion leaders to change attitudes and norms more broadly could involve social marketing or advertising techniques (e.g., Winett, 1995). Unfortunately, at the moment we are limited in the United States in our ability to air advertisements that are explicit in their AIDS prevention message (e.g., ads in which natural opinion leaders personally endorse the use of condoms).

***Social Comparison Influences on Perceived Vulnerability to HIV.*** The perception that one is personally at risk for HIV may be an important factor in increasing AIDS preventive behavior, in conjunction with necessary AIDS prevention information, other motivational factors, and actual and perceived behavioral skills (e.g., Bandura, 1994; J. D. Fisher & Fisher, 1992; Ijzer et al., 1995; Rogers, 1975; Van der Velde

& Van der Pligt, 1991). Social comparison may play a pivotal role in determining individuals' perceived vulnerability to HIV. When one is uncertain and attempting to determine one's vulnerability to a negative outcome (e.g., contracting HIV), both constructive and realistic social comparison processes may take place. First, individuals who practice risky behavior may engage in downward comparison or distancing processes (e.g., Brown & Gallagher, 1992; Gibbons & Gerrard, 1991; Gibbons & Gerrard, chapter 3, this volume; Wills, 1987) specifically to *decrease* their perceived HIV risk. In the case of perceived vulnerability to HIV, this often takes the form of constructive comparison with imagined others who are at greater risk for HIV than oneself. As a rule, individuals believe that their risk for HIV and other negative outcomes is somewhat lower than generalized others' risk (e.g., Perloff, 1987; Weinstein, 1989), and is much lower than dissimilar others' risk (e.g., J. D. Fisher & Misovich, 1990; Hoorens & Buunk, 1993). To reassure themselves that they are not at high risk, individuals may compare themselves to dissimilar people whom they assume to be at greater HIV risk (e.g., Perloff, 1987). Often, such individuals compare themselves with a stereotypical prototype of a person with HIV (e.g., a "down and out" drug abuser), decide that they are different from this prototype, and conclude that they are at low risk for HIV (e.g., Perloff, 1987; Van der Pligt et al., 1993). For instance, younger gay men appear often to compare themselves with older gay men whom they perceive as having more risk exposure, and to incorrectly assess their own risk as comparatively low (e.g., Kelly, 1995). Similarly, many individuals who are in close relationships appear to compare themselves with people who have "casual" sex and decide that they are safer and not at risk because they practice monogamy (Klein & Weinstein, chapter 2, this volume; Misovich, Fisher, J.D., & Fisher, W. A., in press). Thus, constructive social comparison with dissimilar others may be an intentional, motivated strategy to protect against unwanted feelings of vulnerability.

Nevertheless, individuals may instead engage in realistic social comparison of HIV risk, possibly by considering the apparent outcomes of social comparison others who have engaged in the risky behavior in question (e.g., Van der Pligt et al., 1993). Although people generally tend to consider themselves less vulnerable to negative outcomes than social comparison others who have engaged in the same behavior (e.g., Van der Pligt et al., 1993), the outcomes of such others may have a great impact on individuals' judgments of perceived vulnerability (Ijzer, Fisher, Siero, Bakker, & Misovich, 1995). Such realistic social comparison may frequently lead to feelings of invulnerability because individuals know that their realistic social comparison others engage in unprotected sex but appear not to be developing HIV or AIDS. Although this conclusion could be erroneous because of the long incubation period required to develop the symptoms associated with AIDS, the resulting perceived invulnerability may be likely to inhibit AIDS prevention. However, HIV is rapidly becoming a major health threat in the United States, with increasing numbers of people becoming HIV positive (e.g., Centers for Disease Control, 1995). When significant numbers of these individuals do learn their HIV antibody status and convey that information to peers who have engaged in similar levels of risky behavior, social comparison with these individuals should result in enhanced perceptions of vulnerability.

***Increasing Perceived Vulnerability.*** In our focus group research, college-student participants frequently suggested that meeting social comparison others who were HIV infected (e.g., someone "like the person in the next dorm room" or "like someone I would want to date") would be effective in increasing their perceived HIV risk and associated preventive behavior. The belief that contact with HIV-infected social comparison others can lead to increased perceived vulnerability and might consequently increase AIDS preventive behavior has been widely accepted in the AIDS prevention literature (see Dennehy, Edwards, & Keller, 1995, for a discussion). Direct contact with people infected with HIV or videos of HIV infected people are often included in AIDS prevention interventions (e.g., J. D. Fisher et al., 1996). Social comparison theory would argue that contact with an HIV positive individual would increase perceived vulnerability to HIV if people perceive the HIV positive person as extremely similar to themselves in terms of background and past AIDS risk behavior. Such contact may be predicted to *decrease* perceived vulnerability, however, if the infected person is not perceived by the audience to be similar in background and behaviors. Because people may also invoke a self-protective social comparison process when in AIDS prevention interventions, intervention exposure to dissimilar others who are HIV infected (e.g., exposing heterosexual adolescents to anyone who became HIV positive through injection drug use) may actually promote the belief that HIV infection occurs only in dissimilar others and thus reduce perceptions of vulnerability.

To test the hypothesis that social comparison with similar, HIV infected others would produce higher levels of perceived vulnerability to HIV than social comparison with dissimilar, HIV infected others, our research team modified an award winning HIV prevention video entitled *People Like Us* (J. D. Fisher, Fisher, & Marks, 1992) that depicts seven HIV positive adolescents. *People Like Us* was designed following the social comparison theory assumption that observation of individuals who have become infected with HIV and who have risk backgrounds that are similar to those of the audience, will increase perceived vulnerability to HIV (J. D. Fisher et al., 1996). *People Like Us* has been widely used to increase perceived vulnerability to HIV among adolescents, and usually produces strong emotional responses in audiences. Pilot research also suggests that it is effective in motivating individuals to be tested for HIV antibodies (W. A. Fisher & Fisher, 1992).

Two new videotapes were made by editing *People Like Us* to manipulate the interviewees' similarity to a target audience. The "similar to audience" videotape was essentially a slightly shortened version of the original version of *People Like Us*. The "dissimilar to audience" videotape was made by selectively portraying aspects of the interviewees' descriptions of their adolescence. In this condition, aspects of the interviewees' lives that were more nonnormative for the college student audience that participated in the experiment but that might be heuristically linked to HIV risk for the audience (e.g., having an extensive history of sexual encounters) were highlighted, without also portraying aspects of their lives that were more similar. Subjects viewed one of the videotapes in a small group, and then rated how likely it was that they already had HIV, and how likely it was that they would contract HIV in the future. As predicted, when subjects were shown similar HIV-positive interviewees, they evidenced significantly higher levels of perceived vulnerability to HIV than subjects who saw dissimilar interviewees.

This suggests that AIDS prevention interventions that depict people who are HIV infected may be most effective when these individuals are highly similar social comparison others. Indeed, as suggested by our study, and the literature on downward comparison and distancing (e.g., Brown & Gallagher, 1992; Gibbons & Gerrard, chapter 3, this volume; Wills, 1987), making use of HIV infected individuals who are dissimilar to the audience may actually serve to reduce individuals' perceived AIDS risk and to encourage risky behavior. Unfortunately, many AIDS prevention interventions with heterosexual audiences (e.g., adolescent high school students) involve a component in which HIV positive gay men and/or intravenous drug users are brought in to "tell their story." Such interventions could have unintended negative effects of decreasing perceived HIV risk, rather than increasing it. Finally, it should be noted that protection motivation theory (e.g., Rogers, 1975; Maddux & Rogers, 1983) and related research (Morris & Swann, 1996) suggest that increasing people's perceptions of vulnerability to HIV without also trying to support people's sense of self-efficacy with respect to performing AIDS preventive behavior may backfire and not lead to safer behavior. It appears that interventions attempting to increase perceived vulnerability to HIV should also place a premium on increasing perceived self-efficacy with respect to AIDS preventive behavior (J. D. Fisher et al., 1996; Morris & Swann, 1996) in order to maximally affect prevention. For this reason, theoretically based interventions should pair social comparison-based fear inductions quite closely with easy-to-accomplish behavior change recommendations (e.g., J. D. Fisher et al., 1996).

## Behavioral Skills

According to the IMB model, behavioral skills for performing AIDS preventive acts are a third critical prerequisite of AIDS preventive behavior (J. D. Fisher & Fisher, 1992; W. A. Fisher & Fisher, 1993). The behavioral skills component of the model involves people's objective level of skill at the behaviors necessary for AIDS prevention (e.g., purchasing condoms and negotiating condom use), and their perceived self-efficacy regarding the performance of these behaviors. According to the model, for individuals to act on their AIDS prevention information and motivation, they generally must possess, and perceive that they possess, the necessary behavioral skills to effectively engage in HIV prevention (e.g., Bandura, 1994; J. D. Fisher & Fisher, 1992). The assertion that behavioral skills are critical to the performance of AIDS preventive behavior has received consistent support. For instance, Walter et al. (1994) found that minority high school students' perceived levels of AIDS prevention self-efficacy predicted their actual performance of AIDS preventive behaviors, and this finding is common in the literature (e.g., Basen-Engquist, 1994; J. D. Fisher et al., 1994).

***Social Comparison Influences on Behavioral Skills.*** While classic social comparison theory suggests that obtaining an accurate assessment of one's abilities is a strong motivator for comparison, later research suggests that social comparison may also be used to protect one's perception of his or her abilities, or possibly to artificially inflate one's self-perceived abilities or self-esteem (e.g., Hakmiller, 1966; Wills, 1991). Research on constructive social comparison with respect to behavioral skills (or abilities) suggests that often the comparison process that takes place with abilities differs from the process that occurs with opinions (Buunk & Ybema, chapter 12, this volume; Goethals et al., 1991). Specifically, although individuals are often motivated to assume similarity with others on opinions and related issues, they are likely to assume *superiority* in the case of valued skills, especially if little feedback is available regarding the range or average level of ability (Goethals et al., 1991). Further, individuals are often motivated to engage in forms of social comparison, such as downward comparison with real or constructed others, that will enhance their perceived abilities and produce feelings of relative superiority. These processes of downward comparison (e.g., seeking out less capable others, or imagining them) may often lead individuals to think that they are superior to their peers on many dimensions (Goethals et al., 1991). As a result, individuals may assume that they are extremely competent in safer sexual practices such as the ability to negotiate safer sex with their partners (e.g., J. D. Fisher & Fisher, 1989), and this assumption may interfere with their development of necessary objective skills. However, when actual negative feedback regarding skills becomes available (e.g., when a person unsuccessfully attempts to insist on condom use with a partner, or when one observes a member of one's social network confidently buying condoms when one cannot do so oneself), individuals may not be able to simply assume their superiority to others. Under these circumstances, an individual may be motivated to engage in further constructive or realistic downward comparison with lower ability others to preserve his or her self-perceived superiority.

Alternately, individuals who have had their AIDS prevention abilities questioned may decide that it is necessary to improve their AIDS prevention behavioral skills. This may be especially likely to occur if they possess proprevention information and the motivation to carry out AIDS preventive behavior (e.g., J. D. Fisher & Fisher, 1992). To some extent, constructive social comparison may be used to improve an individual's performance (Bandura, 1994); for example, a person may visualize a social comparison role model effectively performing AIDS preventive behaviors and attempt to emulate the model's performance. A person seeking to improve his or her performance may also engage in realistic social comparison, seeking similar others as models for their own behavior (e.g., Bandura, 1994). Although realistic social comparison may lead to an overassessment of one's abilities when one engages in downward comparison, individuals who are motivated to improve their performance may make use of realistic upward comparison and affiliation to gain both inspiration and information about how to perform better (Helgeson & Taylor, 1993; Taylor & Lobel, 1989). In the latter case, social comparison may provide individuals with "real-life" models who display the objective skills needed to learn to engage in AIDS preventive behavior more effectively (Bandura, 1994). Realistic social comparison may also serve other purposes for an individual who seeks to increase his or her AIDS prevention behavioral skills. Individuals who are in the process of learning how to perform a task may attempt to determine, through observation of more competent others' performance, the specific behaviors involved in the enactment of the task (Butler, 1992; Molleman et al., 1986; Ruble & Frey, 1991).

*Increasing Behavioral Skills.* Social comparison can provide individuals with AIDS prevention behavioral skills both through their observation of social comparison role models, and through their affiliation with social comparison others (e.g., Bandura, 1994; J. D. Fisher, 1988). For many populations, deficits are found in behavioral skills associated with many aspects of AIDS preventive behavior, such as the ability to negotiate safer sexual practices. Minority women (e.g., Fullilove, Fullilove, Haynes, & Grass, 1990), minority adolescents (e.g., Overby & Kegeles, 1994), and young gay men (e.g., Hays, Kegeles, & Coates, 1990) have all been found to be weak in safer sex negotiation skills. For instance, Nyamathi et al. (1994) found low negotiation self-efficacy among Latino women, who believed that they would have great difficulty negotiating safer sex with close relationship partners. Furthermore, when people do engage in safer sex discussions, the discussions often tend to be too vague and often do not result in safer sexual practices (e.g., Cline, Johnson, & Freeman, 1992). Observation of films or roleplays of social comparison others negotiating safer sexual practices in situations that are relevant to the individual may serve the purpose of defining what behaviors and skills are necessary. For instance, in a recent intervention conducted with college students, a film depicting social comparison couples negotiating safer sexual practices in a range of situations, including a brief sexual encounter, a new relationship, and an ongoing relationship in which safer sexual practices had been abandoned over time, was used to increase college students' behavioral skills and perceived self-efficacy regarding AIDS prevention (J. D. Fisher et al., 1996). In conjunction with intervention role-plays and other exercises, such films of social comparison others may be useful in increasing both self-efficacy and actual behavioral skills (J. D. Fisher et al., 1996).

In general, individuals with proprevention reference groups will be exposed naturally to social comparison others who effectively model AIDS prevention behavioral skills, but this will not be the case for individuals with antiprevention reference groups (J. D. Fisher, 1988). Because individuals are highly likely to model similar, social comparison others' (e.g., reference group members') behavior (Bandura, 1986), and because perceptions of self-efficacy are affected by such modeling and by the outcomes of similar others' behavior (Bandura, 1994), having a proprevention reference group will lead to relatively high levels of objective behavioral skills and to relatively high perceptions of self-efficacy. Therefore, individuals with proprevention reference groups should possess greater AIDS risk reduction behavioral skills and greater perceptions of self-efficacy regarding their performance than those with antiprevention reference groups (J. D. Fisher, 1988). Individuals with antiprevention reference groups are likely to observe models who practice risky behavior rather than models who practice safer behaviors, and thus may become skilled in AIDS risk behavioral skills (e.g., talking a partner into risky sex against his or her will).

This suggests that one task for AIDS prevention researchers would be to promote upward comparison with proprevention social comparison others, in order to increase individuals' actual behavioral skills and perceived self-efficacy (e.g., Bandura, 1994; J. D. Fisher & Fisher, 1992). For instance, Basen-Engquist (1994) reported that an efficacy-based intervention for college students using trained peers as role models of safer sex negotiation was effective in increasing behavioral skills. Because of the critical role that actual behavioral skills and perceived self-efficacy play in determining individuals' levels of AIDS preventive behavior (e.g., Bandura, 1994; J. D. Fisher & Fisher, 1992), interventions that incorporate the modeling of AIDS prevention by more competent or experienced social comparison others are especially likely to be effective in increasing AIDS prevention (Bandura, 1994; J. D. Fisher et al., 1996; Kelly, 1995; Kirby et al., 1994). In addition to simply exposing people to more competent social comparison role models in the context of the intervention, AIDS prevention interventions may find other uses of social comparison role models helpful. For example, they might incorporate a "buddy system" in which people who purchase condoms regularly and who are comfortable doing so accompany others who have lower condom purchasing skills, helping them make their purchases.

Data we have collected at the University of Connecticut suggest that lower levels of behavioral skills may indeed be associated with a preference for upward affiliation. To investigate individuals' preferences to affiliate with others who are more or less competent with regard to AIDS prevention, we distributed a questionnaire designed to assess the extent to which individuals would prefer to purchase condoms alone or with friends who varied in levels of condom purchasing skills. Specifically, as part of a larger survey (for details on our measurement instruments, see Misovich, Fisher, W. A., & Fisher, J. D., in press), students were asked to indicate whether they would like to purchase condoms with a friend who was more or less confident in his or her own ability to perform this behavior (rated on a 5-point scale ranging from 1 [*much more confident than you*] to 5 [*much less confident than you*]. They were also asked to indicate the degree to which they would prefer to buy condoms alone (rated on a 5-point scale ranging from 1 [*very much*] to 5 [*not at all*], and, also on a 5-point scale ranging from (*very difficult*) to (*very easy*), their perceived condom purchasing behavioral skills (i.e., how difficult or easy it would be for them to purchase condoms). For both men and women, lower self-perceived behavioral skills were associated with a higher preference to affiliate during condom purchasing, and a stronger preference to affiliate upward. For women, respondents who thought condoms were more difficult to purchase also wanted more to purchase them in the company of a friend, as opposed to alone ($r = .40$, $n = 113$, $p < .001$), and preferred to purchase them with a friend who was more confident than they were ($r = .47$, $n = 113$, $p < .001$). The same pattern of results occurred for men. The more difficult a male respondent thought buying condoms was the more he wanted to buy them with a friend, instead of alone ($r = .18$, $n = 128$, $p < .046$), and the more he wanted to purchase them with a more confident, as opposed to less confident, friend ($r = .36$, $n = 124$, $p < .001$). This pattern of results suggests that for AIDS preventive behaviors for which individuals may lack behavioral skills, people may prefer to seek out more capable friends with whom to affiliate.

In summary, individuals may often decide, through constructive comparison with imaginary, less capable others, that they possess high levels of AIDS prevention behavioral skills. When these beliefs are disconfirmed through experiences of failure or by observation of more competent performances by social comparison others, people may attempt to preserve their levels of perceived behavioral skills either through continued constructive comparison or through other forms of downward comparison. Alternatively, they may engage in a process of realistic comparison with more capable others and, through observation, define the actual behaviors necessary to properly perform a preventive act and use others as models for inspiration and instruction.

## SUMMARY AND CONCLUSIONS

The process of evaluating one's own levels of AIDS prevention information, motivation, behavioral skills, and AIDS preventive behavior through comparison with real or imagined others may have a strong influence on whether one decides that AIDS preventive behaviors are necessary, desirable, and possible, or unnecessary, unpleasant, and probably too difficult to be worth the effort. Often, individuals may make use of constructive social comparison to validate their preexisting AIDS prevention information, provide them with a supportive consensus regarding AIDS prevention attitudes and norms, allow them to feel uniquely invulnerable to HIV, and uniquely skilled at HIV prevention. Alternatively, individuals may engage in realistic social comparison and affiliate with similar others in order to assess the validity of their AIDS prevention information, to determine the degree to which their AIDS prevention attitudes and perceived norms are actually representative of their social group, to assess their actual levels of AIDS risk, and to evaluate and potentially improve their behavioral skills. Although constructive comparisons are probably most likely to result in a maintenance of the status quo for an individual, realistic comparisons have the potential to facilitate or inhibit AIDS preventive behavior, depending on whether the realistic social comparison others provide proprevention or antiprevention feedback.

Finally, social comparison processes may be harnessed by prevention researchers to increase AIDS preventive behavior, by using social comparison others who are trained to advocate preventive behavior in settings that approximate naturalistic social comparison situations. The potential for changing AIDS risk behavior by providing individuals with comparison targets who are proprevention appears increasingly to be gaining support and acceptance from AIDS prevention researchers (cf. Dearing et al., 1994; J. D. Fisher et al., 1996; Kelly, 1994). Future research using social comparison processes to increase prevention across other behavioral domains (e.g., breast self-examination for breast cancer prevention among young women) may prove to be successful as well.

## ACKNOWLEDGMENTS

This research was supported by a grant from the National Institute of Health (MH 522010) to the second and third authors, and by a National Health Scientist (AIDS) award from Health Canada and a Janssen-Ortho award to the third author.

## REFERENCES

Bandura, A. (1986). *Social foundations of thought and action: A social cognitive theory.* Englewood Cliffs, NJ: Prentice-Hall.

Bandura, A. (1994). Social cognitive theory and exercise of control over HIV infection. In R. DiClemente & J. L. Peterson (Eds.), *Preventing AIDS: Theories and methods of behavioral interventions* (pp. 25–59). New York: Plenum.

Barr, J. K., Waring, J. M., & Warshaw, L. J. (1992). Knowledge and attitudes about AIDS among corporate and public service employees. *American Journal of Public Health, 82,* 225–228.

Barr, J. K., & Warshaw, L. J. (1994). Worksite AIDS education: A case study of the New York City police. *AIDS Education and Prevention, 6,* 53–64.

Basen-Engquist, K. (1994). Evaluation of a theory-based HIV prevention intervention for college students. *AIDS Education and Prevention, 6,* 412–424.

Botvin, G. J., & Eng, A. (1982). The efficacy of a multicomponent approach to the prevention of cigarette smoking. *Preventive Medicine, 11,* 199–211.

Botvin, G. J., Baker, E., Filazzola, A. D., & Botvin, E. M. (1990). A cognitive-behavioral approach to substance abuse prevention: one-year follow-up. *Addictive Behaviors, 15,* 47–63.

Brown, J. D., & Gallagher, F. M. (1992). Coming to terms with failure: Private self-enhancement and public self-effacement. *Journal of Experimental Social Psychology, 28,* 3–22.

Butler, R. (1992). What young people want to know when: Effects of mastery and ability goals on interest in different kinds of social comparisons. *Journal of Personality and Social Psychology, 62,* 934–943.

Catania, J. A., Coates, T. J., Fullilove, M. T., Peterson, J., Marin, B., Siegel, D., & Hulley, S. (1992). Condoms use in multi-ethnic neighborhoods of San Francisco: The population-based AMEN (AIDS in Multi-Ethnic Neighborhoods) study. *American Journal of Public Health, 82,* 284–287.

Catania, J. A., Coates, T. J., Peterson, J., Dolcini, M. M., Kegeles, S., Siegel, D., Golden, E., & Fullilove, M. T. (1993). Changes in condom use among Black, Hispanic, and White heterosexuals in San Francisco: The AMEN cohort study. *The Journal of Sex Research, 30,* 121–128.

Centers for Disease Control. (1995, May). *HIV/AIDS Surveillance Report.* Atlanta, GA: Center for Infectious Diseases, Centers for Disease Control and Prevention.

Chitwood, D. D., McCoy, C. B., Inciardi, J. A., McBride, D. C., Comerford, M., Trapido, E., McCoy, H. V., Page, J. B., Griffin, J., Fletcher, M. A., & Ashman, M. A. (1990). HIV seropositivity of needles from shooting galleries in south Florida. *American Journal of Public Health, 80,* 150–152.

Cline, R. W., Johnson, S. J., & Freeman, K. E. (1992). Talk among sexual partners about AIDS: Interpersonal communication or risk enhancement? *Health Communication, 4,* 39–56.

Coates, T. J. (1990). Strategies for modifying sexual behavior for primary and secondary prevention of HIV disease. *Journal of Consulting and Clinical Psychology, 58,* 57–69.

Corby, N. H., Wolitski, R. J., Thornton-Johnson, S., & Tanner, W. M. (1991). AIDS knowledge, perception of risk, and behaviors among female sex partners of injection drug users. *AIDS Education and Prevention, 3,* 353–366.

Cottrell, N. B, & Epley, S. W. (1977). Affiliation, social comparison, and socially mediated stress reduction. In J. M. Suls & R. L. Miller (Eds.), *Social comparison processes: theoretical and empirical perspectives* (pp. 43–68). New York: Wiley.

Crawford, I., Thomas, S., & Zoller, D. (1993). Communication and levels of AIDS knowledge among homeless African-American mothers and their children. *Journal of Health and Social Policy, 4,* 37–53.

D'Augelli, A. R. (1992). Sexual behavior patterns of gay university men: Implications for preventing HIV infection. *Journal of American College Health, 41,* 25–29.

Dearing, J. W., Meyer, G., & Rogers, E. M. (1994). Diffusion theory and HIV risk behavior change. In R. DiClemente & J. L. Peterson (Eds.) *Preventing AIDS: Theories and methods of behavioral interventions* (pp. 79–93). New York: Plenum.

Dennehy, E. B., Edwards, C. A., & Keller, R. L. (1995). AIDS education intervention utilizing a person with AIDS: Examination and clarification. *AIDS Education and Prevention, 7,* 124–133.

Edlin, B. R., Keeling, R. P., Gayle, H. D., & Holmberg, S. D. (1994). *Prevalence of human immunodeficiency virus infection among U.S. college students.* Unpublished manuscript, Division of HIV/AIDS, National Center for Infectious Diseases, Centers for Disease Control and Prevention, Atlanta, GA.

Ekstrand, M. L. (1992). Safer sex maintenance among gay men: Are we making any progress? *AIDS, 6,* 875–877.

Festinger, L. (1954). A theory of social comparison processes. *Human Relations, 7,* 117–140.

Fishbein, M., Middlestadt, S. E., & Hitchcock, P. J. (1994). Using information to change sexually transmitted disease-related behaviors: An analysis based on the theory of reasoned action. In R. J. DiClemente & J. L. Peterson (Eds.), *Preventing AIDS: Theories and methods of behavioral interventions* (pp. 61–78). New York: Plenum.

Fisher, J. D. (1988). Possible effects of reference group-based social influence on AIDS-risk behavior and AIDS prevention. *American Psychologist, 43,* 914–920.

Fisher, J. D., & Fisher, W. A. (1989). *A general technology for AIDS risk behavior change.* Unpublished manuscript, University of Connecticut, Storrs.

Fisher, J. D., & Fisher, W. A. (1992). Changing AIDS risk behavior. *Psychological Bulletin, 111,* 455–474.

Fisher, J. D., & Fisher, W. A. (Producers), & Marks, D. (Director). (1992). *People like us* [Videotape]. (Available from AIDS Risk Reduction Project, Department of Psychology, University of Connecticut, Storrs.

Fisher, J. D., Fisher, W. A., Misovich, S. J., Kimble, D. L., & Malloy, T. (1996). Changing AIDS risk behavior: Effects of an intervention emphasizing AIDS risk reduction information, motivation, and behavioral skills in a university student population. *Health Psychology, 15,* 114–123.

Fisher, J. D., Fisher, W. A., Williams, S. S., & Malloy, T. E. (1994). Empirical tests of an information–motivation–behavioral skills model of AIDS preventive behavior. *Health Psychology, 13,* 238–250.

Fisher, J. D., & Misovich, S. J. (1990). Social influence and AIDS-preventive behavior. In J. Edwards, R. S. Tindale, L. Heath, & E. J. Posavac (Eds.), *Social influence processes and prevention* (pp. 39–70). New York: Plenum.

Fisher, J. D., Misovich, S. J., & Fisher, W. A. (1992). The impact of perceived social norms on adolescents' AIDS-risk behavior and prevention. In R. J. DiClemente (Ed.), *Adolescents and AIDS: A generation in jeopardy* (pp. 117-136). Beverly Hills, CA: Sage.

Fisher, W. A. (1990). Understanding adolescent pregnancy and sexually transmissible disease/AIDS. In J. Edwards, R. S. Tindale, L. Heath, & E. J. Posavac (Eds.), *Social influence processes and prevention* (pp. 71-101). Beverly Hills: Plenum.

Fisher, W. A., & Fisher, J. D. (1992). Understanding and promoting AIDS preventive behavior: A conceptual model and educational tools. *The Canadian Journal of Human Sexuality, 1,* 99–106.

Fisher, W. A., & Fisher, J. D. (1993). A general social psychological model for changing AIDS risk behavior. In J. Pryor & G. Reeder (Eds.), *The social psychology of HIV infection (pp. 127–153).* Hillsdale, NJ: Lawrence Erlbaum Associates.

Fisher, W. A., Fisher, J. D., & Rye, B. J. (1995). Understanding and promoting AIDS-preventive behavior: Insights from the theory of reasoned action. *Health Psychology, 14,* 255–264.

Fisher, W. A., Williams, S. S., Fisher, J. D., & Malloy, T. M. (1996). *Understanding AIDS risk behavior among adolescents: An empirical test of the Information–Motivation–Behavioral Skills model.* Manuscript submitted for publication.

Friedman, S. R., Des Jarlais, D. C., & Ward, T. P. (1994). Social models for changing health-relevant behavior. In R. J. DiClemente & J. L. Peterson (Eds.), *Preventing AIDS: Theories and methods of behavioral interventions* (pp. 95–116). New York: Plenum.

Fullilove, M. T., Fullilove, R. E., Haynes, K., & Gross, S. (1990). Black women and AIDS prevention: A view towards understanding the gender rules. *Journal of Sex Research, 27,* 47–64.

Galligan, R. F., & Terry, D. J. (1993). Romantic ideals, fear of negative implications, and the practice of safe sex. *Journal of Applied Social Psychology, 23,* 1685–1711.

Gibbons, F. X., & Gerrard, M. (1991). Downward comparison and coping with threat. In J. Suls and T. A. Wills (Eds.), *Social comparison: Contemporary theory and research* (pp. 317–345). Hillsdale, NJ: Lawrence Erlbaum Associates.

Gibbons, F. X., Gerrard, M., Lando, H., & McGovern, P. G. (1991). Social comparison and smoking cessation: The role of the "typical smoker." *Journal of Experimental Social Psychology, 27,* 239–258.

Goethals, G. R., & Darley, J. M. (1977). Social comparison theory: An attributional approach. In J. M. Suls & R. L. Miller (Eds.), *Social comparison processes: Theoretical and empirical perspectives* (pp. 259–278). Washington, DC: Hemisphere.

Goethals, G. R., Messick, D. M., & Allison, S. T. (1991). The uniqueness bias: Studies of constructive social comparison. In J. Suls & T. A. Wills (Eds.), *Social comparison: Contemporary theory and research* (pp. 149–176). Hillsdale, NJ: Lawrence Erlbaum Associates.

Gordon, B. F. (1966). Influence and social comparison and motives for affiliation. *Journal of Experimental Social Psychology, Supplement 1,* 55–65.

Hakmiller, K. L. (1966). Threat as a determinant of downward comparison. *Journal of Experimental Social Psychology, Supplement 1,* 32–39.

Hays, R. B., Kegeles, S. M., & Coates, T. J. (1990). High HIV risk-taking among young gay men. *AIDS, 4,* 901–907.

Helgeson, V. S., & Taylor, S. E. (1993). Social comparisons and adjustment among cardiac patients. *Journal of Applied Social Psychology, 23,* 1171–1195.

Herek, G. M., & Capitanio, J. P. (1994). Conspiracies, contagion, and compassion: Trust and public reactions to AIDS. *AIDS Education and Prevention, 6,* 365–375.

Hoorens, V., & Buunk, B. P. (1993). Social comparison of health risks: Locus of control, the person-positivity bias, and unrealistic optimism. *Journal of Applied Social Psychology, 23,* 291–302.

Ijzer, M. C., Fisher, J. D., Siero, F. W., Bakker, A. B., & Misovich, S. J. (1995). *The effects of information about AIDS risk and self-efficacy on women's intentions to engage in AIDS preventive behavior.* Manuscript submitted for publication.

Jemmott, J. B., & Jemmott, L. S. (1994). Interventions for adolescents in community settings. In R. J. DiClemente & J. L. Peterson (Eds.) *Preventing AIDS: Theories and methods of behavioral interventions* (pp. 141–174). New York: Plenum.

Kalichman, S. C., & Hunter, T. L. (1992). The disclosure of celebrity HIV infection: Its effects on public attitudes. *American Journal of Public Health, 82,* 1374–1376.

Kalichman, S. C., Russell, R. L., Hunter, T. L., & Sarwer, D. B. (1993). Earvin "Magic" Johnson's HIV serostatus disclosure: Effects on men's perceptions of AIDS. *Journal of Consulting and Clinical Psychology, 61,* 887–891.

Kashima, Y., Gallois, C., & McCamish, M. (1993). The theory of reasoned action and cooperative behavior: It takes two to use a condom. *British Journal of Social Psychology, 32,* 227–239.

Kelly, J. A. (1994). HIV prevention among gay and bisexual men in small cities. In R. J. DiClemente & J. L. Peterson (Eds.), *Preventing AIDS: Theories and methods of behavioral interventions* (pp. 297–317). New York: Plenum.

Kelly, J. A. (1995). *Changing HIV risk behavior.* New York: Guilford.

Kelly, J. A., & Murphy, D. A. (1992). Psychological interventions with AIDS and HIV: Prevention and treatment. *Journal of Consulting and Clinical Psychology, 60,* 576–585.

Kelly, J. A., & St. Lawrence, J. S. (1988). AIDS prevention and treatment: Psychology's role in the health crisis. *Clinical Psychology Review, 8,* 255–284.

Kirby, D., Short, L., Collins, J., Rugg, D., Kolbe, L., Howard, M., Miller, B., Sonenstein, F., & Zabin, L. S. (1994). *School-based programs to reduce sexual risk behaviors: A review of effectiveness.* Unpublished manuscript.

Kruglanski, A. W., & Mayseles, O. (1987). Motivational effects in the social comparison of opinions. *Journal of Personality and Social Psychology, 53,* 834–842.

Lifson, A. R. (1990). The epidemiology of AIDS and HIV infection. *AIDS, 4* (Suppl. 1), S23–S28.

Luepker, R. V., Johnson, C. A., Murray, D. M., & Pechacek, T. F. (1983). Prevention of cigarette smoking: Three-year follow-up of an education program for youth. *Journal of Behavioral Medicine, 6,* 53–62.

Maddux, J. E., & Rogers, R. W. (1983). Protection motivation and self-efficacy: A revised theory of fear appeals and attitude change. *Journal of Experimental Social Psychology, 19,* 469–479.

McCusker, J., Stoddard, A. M., McDonald, M., Zapka, J. G., & Mayer, K. H. (1992). Maintenance of behavioral change in a cohort of homosexually active men. *AIDS, 6,* 861–868.

Miller, R. L., & Suls, J. M. (1977). Affiliation preferences as a function of attitude and ability similarity. In J. M. Suls & R. L. Miller (Eds.), *Social comparison processes: Theoretical and empirical perspectives* (pp. 103–123). Washington, DC: Hemisphere.

Misovich, S. J., Fisher, J. D., & Fisher, W. A. (1996). The perceived AIDS-preventive utility of knowing one's partner well: A public health dictum and individual's risky sexual behavior. *Canadian Journal of Human Sexuality, 5,* 83–90.

Misovich, S. J., Fisher, J. D., & Fisher, W. A. (in press). Close relationships and elevated HIV risk behavior: Evidence and possible underlying psychological processes. *General Psychology Review.*

Misovich, S. J., Fisher, W. A., & Fisher, J. D. (in press). A measure of AIDS prevention information, motivation, behavioral skills, and behavior. In C. M. Davis, W. H. Yarber, R. Bauserman, G. Schreer, & S. L. Davis (Eds.), *Sexuality related measures: A compendium.* Newbury Park, CA: Sage.

Misovich, S. G., Colby, J. J., & Welch, K. (1973). Similarity as a determinant of social influence in affective judgments. *Psychological Reports, 33,* 808–810.

Molleman, E., Pruyn, J., & van Knippenberg, A. (1986). Social comparison processes among cancer patients. *British Journal of Social Psychology, 25,* 1–13.

Morris, K. A., & Swann, W. B. (1996). Denial and the AIDS crisis: On wishing away the threat of AIDS. In S. Oskamp & S. C. Thompson (Eds.), *Understanding and preventing HIV risk behavior* (pp. 57–79). Thousand Oaks, CA: Sage.

Murray, D. M., Davis-Hearn, M., Goldman, A. I., Pirie, P., & Luepker, R. V. (1988). Four- and five- year follow-up results from four seventh-grade smoking prevention strategies. *Journal of Behavioral Medicine, 11,* 395–405.

National Center for Health Statistics. (1994). *Annual summary of births, marriages, divorces, and deaths: Unites States, 1993.* Hyattsville, MD: U.S. Department of Health and Human Services, Public Health Service.

Nyamathi, A. M., Flaskerud, J., Bennett, C., Leake, B., & Lewis, C. (1994). Evaluation of two AIDS education programs for impoverished Latina women. *AIDS Education and Prevention, 4,* 296–309.

Overby, K. J., & Kegeles, S. M. (1994). The impact of AIDS on an urban population of high-risk female minority adolescents: Implications for intervention. *Journal of Adolescent Health, 15,* 216–227.

Perloff, L. S. (1987). Social comparison and illusions of invulnerability to negative events. In C. R. Synder & C. E. Ford (Eds.), *Coping with negative events: Clinical and social psychological perspectives* (pp. 217–242) New York: Plenum.

Perloff, L. S., & Fetzer, B. K. (1986). Self-other judgments and perceived vulnerability to victimization. *Journal of Personality and Social Psychology, 50,* 502–510.

Rickert, V., Jay, M. S., & Gottleib, A. (1991). Effects of a peer-counseled AIDS education program on knowledge, attitudes, and satisfaction of adolescents. *Journal of Adolescent Health, 12,* 38–43.

Rogers, R. W. (1975). A protection motivation theory of fear appeals and attitude change. *The Journal of Psychology, 91,* 93–114.

Ruble, D. N., & Frey, K. S. (1991). Changing patterns of behavior as skills are acquired: A functional model of self-evaluation. In J. Suls & T. A. Wills (Eds.), *Social comparison: Contemporary theory and research* (pp. 79–113). Hillsdale, NJ: Lawrence Erlbaum Associates.

Schachter, S. (1959). *The psychology of affiliation.* Stanford, CA: Stanford University Press.

Simpson, D. D., Knight, K. & Ray, S. (1993). Psychosocial correlates of AIDS-risk drug use and sexual behaviors. *AIDS Education and Prevention, 5,* 121–130.

Stevenson, H. C., & Davis, G. (1994). Impact of culturally sensitive AIDS video education on the AIDS risk knowledge of African-American adolescents. *AIDS Education and Prevention, 6,* 40–52.

Suls, J., Marco, C. A., & Tobin, S. (1991). The role of temporal comparison, social comparison, and direct appraisal in the elderly's self-evaluation of health. *Journal of Applied Social Psychology, 21,* 1125–1144.

Suls, J., Wan, C. K., & Sanders, G. (1988). False consensus and false uniqueness in estimating the prevalence of health-protective behaviors. *Journal of Applied Social Psychology, 18,* 66–79.

Taylor, S. E., & Lobel, M. (1989). Social comparison activity under threat: Downward evaluation and upward contacts. *Psychological Review, 96,* 569–575.

Telch, M. J., Miller, L.M., Killen, J. D., Cooke, S., & Maccoby, N. (1990). Social influences approach to smoking prevention: The effects of videotape delivery with and without same-age peer leader participation. *Addictive Behaviors, 15,* 21–28.

Trad, P. V. (1994). A developmental model for risk avoidance in adolescents confronting AIDS. *AIDS Education and Prevention, 6,* 322–338.

Trinkaus, J. (1992). Some students' perceptions about AIDS: An informal look. *Perceptual and Motor Skills, 75,* 1344–1346.

Van der Pligt, J., Otten, W., Richard, R., & Van der Velde, F. (1993). Perceived risk of AIDS: Unrealistic optimism and self-protective action. In J. B. Pryor & G. D. Reeder (Eds.), *The social psychology of HIV infection* (pp. 39–58). Hillsdale, NJ: Lawrence Erlbaum Associates.

Van der Velde, F. W., & Van der Pligt, J. (1991). AIDS-related health behavior: Coping, protection motivation, and previous behavior. *Journal of Behavioral Medicine, 14,* 429–451.

Walter, H. J., Vaughan, R. D., Ragin, D. R., Cohall, A. T., & Kasen, S. (1994). Prevalence and correlates of AIDS-related behavioral intentions among urban minority high school students. *AIDS Education and Prevention, 4,* 339–350.

Weary, G., Marsh, K. L., & McCormick, L. (1994). Depression and social comparison motives. Special Issue: Affect in social judgments and cognition. *European Journal of Social Psychology, 24,* 117–129.

Weinstein, N. D. (1980). Unrealistic optimism about future life events. *Journal of Personality and Social Psychology, 39,* 806–820.

Weinstein, N. D. (1989). Perceptions of personal susceptibility to harm. In V. M. Mays, V. M. Mays, G. W. Albee, & S. F. Schneider (Eds.), *Primary prevention of AIDS: Psychological approaches* (pp. 142–167). London: Sage.

Wheeler, L., & Miyake, K. (1992). Social comparison in everyday life. *Journal of Personality and Social Psychology, 62,* 760–773.

Wiist, W. H., & Snider, G. (1991). Peer education in friendship cliques: prevention of adolescent smoking. *Health Education Research, 6,* 101–108.

Williams, S. S., Kimble, D. L., Covell, N. H., Weiss, L. H., Newton, K. J., Fisher, W. A., & Fisher, J. D. (1992). College students use implicit personality theory instead of safer sex. *Journal of Applied Social Psychology, 22,* 921–933.

Wills, T. A. (1987). Downward comparison as a coping mechanism. In C. R. Snyder & C. E. Ford (Eds.), *Coping with negative life events* (pp. 243–268). New York: Plenum.

Wills, T. A. (1991). Similarity and self-esteem in downward comparison. In J. Suls & T. A. Wills (Eds.), *Social comparison: Contemporary theory and research* (pp. 51–77). Hillsdale, NJ: Lawrence Erlbaum Associates.

Winett, R. A. (1995). A framework for health promotion and disease prevention programs. *American Psychologist, 50,* 341–350.

Winett, R. A., Altman, D. G., & King, A. C. (1990). Conceptual and strategic foundations for effective media campaigns for preventing the spread of HIV infection. *Evaluation and Program Planning, 13,* 91–104.

Winslow, R. W., Franzini, L. R., & Hwang, J. (1992). Perceived peer norms, casual sex, and AIDS risk prevention. *Journal of Applied Social Psychology, 22,* 1809–1827.

Wood, J. V., Taylor, S. E., & Lichtman, R. R. (1985). Social comparison in adjustment to breast cancer. *Journal of Personality and Social Psychology, 49,* 1169–1183.

World Health Organization (1995, January). The current global situation of the HIV/AIDS pandemic. *Global Programme on AIDS.*

# CHAPTER 5

# Future-Oriented Aspects of Social Comparisons: A Framework for Studying Health-Related Comparison Activity

Lisa G. Aspinwall
*University of Maryland at College Park*

What does the future hold? In Dickens' *A Christmas Carol* (1843/1967), Ebenezer Scrooge is visited by the ghosts of Christmas Past, Christmas Present, and Christmas Future. Although each visitor shows Scrooge vivid images of himself, his family, and his colleagues at different times in their lives, it is the ghost of Christmas Future who makes the greatest impact on Scrooge. Hooded and silent, the ghost of Christmas Future shows Scrooge a terrifying vision: Scrooge sees himself dying alone, not only unmourned, but mocked. His maid is selling his bedclothes. His colleagues attend his funeral only for the lunch. People whom he might have helped now languish in poverty and illness. Terrified, Scrooge asks, "Are these the shadows of the things that Will be, or are they shadows of the things that May be, only?" (p. 128). The unspoken answer to this question shapes Scrooge's sudden change of heart and subsequent generosity.

Whether it is perceived as threatening or full of opportunity, the future is changing and uncertain. Concerns about the future dominate people's thoughts, and people hold a richly developed set of hopes and fears about what they might be like in the future (Markus & Nurius, 1986). In particular, concerns about future health outcomes seem especially prevalent. For example, in two recent studies, 64% of young adults, 87% of middle-aged adults, and 86% of older adults who were asked to list possible future selves spontaneously listed a health-related possible self (Hooker & Kaus, 1992, 1994; see also Cross & Markus, 1991). Some of these images contained hoped-for selves (e.g., the self as physically fit or as aging well), but others were feared selves, presenting images of illness and decline. Where do such images come from? Few of us have spirit guides like Scrooge's ghost to show us what the future holds. One source of information we do have, however, is the outcomes and experiences of other people.

How do visions of the future affect our current feelings, thoughts, and behavior? Although it has been suggested that social comparisons play a major role in self-regulatory processes by influencing possible selves (cf. Markus & Nurius, 1986) and by influencing our expectancies of success in meeting a given goal (cf. Carver & Scheier, 1990), relatively little research or theory has specified ways in which particular social comparisons are sought, interpreted, and used in the service of one's future goals. This chapter presents a framework for analyzing social comparison activity with respect to its implications for future actions or outcomes. The framework analyzes two elements of social comparison activity that have received relatively little research attention: (a) properties of the dimension (attribute, belief, behavior, outcome, or emotion) on which the comparison is made,and (b) the temporal location of the comparer with respect to the development of some stressful event or the attainment of some goal state. Drawing on research on health, coping, and achievement, this chapter examines ways in which these two factors jointly influence the motives underlying social comparison activity as well as reactions to particular kinds of comparison information. Specifically, I examine the degree to which an analysis of the comparison situation and its implications for future action may explain when upward and downward comparisons may be perceived as beneficial or harmful to people who are pursuing a specific goal or coping with illness or other stressors.

First I examine the temporal aspects of social comparison activity. Of particular interest are the ways in which the motives that underly comparison activity vary as a function of whether the focal event or stressor has already occurred and whether the event will recur. My analysis suggests that comparisons made before versus after stressful events differ in terms of the kinds of information people are trying to acquire from their social environment. Next I examine properties of the comparison dimension itself that make one's likely future outcomes or beliefs about those outcomes particularly potent determinants of the meaning of a given piece of comparison information. I analyze specific health domains with respect to these properties and examine the degree to which research on comparison processes among people facing threats to mental and physical health is consistent with the predictions of the future-oriented framework.

Finally, I examine ways in which research on social comparisons and health may be expanded to address a broader range of comparison activity with respect to stressful health events and conditions than has been the case to date, and I discuss some conceptual and practical gains that such an expansion may yield. Research on physical and mental health is particularly conducive to a future-oriented analysis. The study of people facing chronic illness, surgery, and other threats to well-being has already yielded considerable insight into the nature of social comparison activity and its role in coping with stressful situations (Taylor, Wood, & Lichtman, 1983; Wills, 1981; Wood, Taylor, & Lichtman, 1985; see Gibbons & Gerrard, 1991, Kulik & Mahler, chapter 8, this volume, and Taylor, Buunk, & Aspinwall, 1990, for reviews). Health domains offer researchers a series of impactful events that may either strike acutely or evolve slowly, that involve much uncertainty about what people are facing and what they should do about it, and that have potentially threatening implications for the future. In the present context, it is important to note that these kinds of events vary a great deal in their potential for future change and in the degree of personal control people can exert over their course.

## A FRAMEWORK FOR UNDERSTANDING FUTURE-ORIENTED COMPARISON ACTIVITY

The main thesis of this chapter is that social comparison activity fundamentally depends on where people are in a course of events and what they expect to happen in the future. My analysis suggests that three factors may influence the nature of one's future engagement with an event or stressor and thus, one's reactions to relevant social comparison information: temporal development, potential for change, and perceived control (see Fig. 5.1). The first factor, the temporal location of the would-be comparer with respect to the development of the event itself, is shown on the z-axis in Fig. 5.1.[1] Studies of social comparisons have focused disproportionately on events that have already occurred (i.e., events that fall in the right half of the figure), usually assessing comparison preferences and reactions to comparison information after some experimentally delivered threat or failure or among people managing life-threatening or chronic illnesses. Relatively few studies have

[1]The comparison situation represented in Figure 1 has been simplified by characterizing stress or threat in terms of a single focal event. Although this description may apply well to some kinds of stressors and health outcomes, it is likely to be an oversimplification of most stressful experiences. Events such as chronic illness may represent continuous, rather than discrete stressors. In such cases, it might be better to view comparison activity as beginning at the onset of a stressful event and extending forward in time (cf. Stanton, 1992).

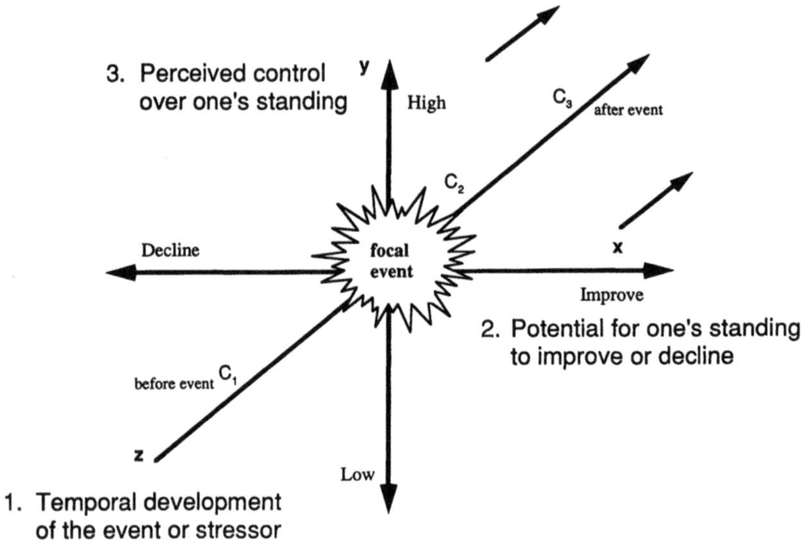


FIG. 5.1. Future-oriented aspects of social comparisons. At the origin is a focal stressor or event that has just occurred. Factor 1, on the z-axis, represents time with respect to the development of the focal event or stressor. Factor 1 ranges from well before the event (the first indication that the event might occur) to the aftermath of the event. Both the comparer and the target may vary in their placement along Factor 1. In the figure, comparer C1 is making a comparison well in advance of the focal event; C2, immediately after the event; and C3 well after the event. The location of the comparison target in the development of the stressful event is not represented in the figure.

Factors 2 and 3, shown on the x- and y-axes, respectively, represent real and perceived properties of the comparison dimension itself. Factor 2 represents the likely future course of the comparer's standing on the comparison dimension, ranging from likely decline to likely improvement. Factor 3 represents the degree of control the comparer perceives over the course of her future standing on the comparison dimension, ranging from little or no perceived control to high levels of perceived control.

examined comparison activity with respect to events that have yet to occur (events that fall in the left half of the figure), thus providing limited opportunity to examine comparisons made in the service of some future action. Moreover, many studies have examined reactions to threat or failure in situations that are single events that are known not to recur. When the event will not recur, the entire right half of the figure representing one's engagement with the event or dimension after the focal stressful event is irrelevant. Therefore, the comparison setting has limited implications for future action, and, as I discuss, comparison motives may be somewhat circumscribed.

The second factor, shown on the x-axis, is that the dimensions on which comparisons are made may vary in their potential for change over time. One's standing may be relatively fixed, may improve over time, or may decline. The third factor, shown on the y-axis, is the comparer's perceived ability to exercise control over his or her future standing, which may range from little or no control to a high level of perceived control. Together, Factors 2 and 3 are important partial determinants of what Wills (1991) termed the "future similarity" of the comparer to the target, that is, the potential for the comparer, for better or worse, to reach the target's standing on some dimension (see also Wood & VanderZee, chapter 10, this volume). As I show, these two factors may moderate the effects of comparisons once they have been made. In *A Christmas Carol*, for example, Scrooge asks whether he is seeing visions of things that will be no matter what he does or that may be if he doesn't change his ways. The point of Dickens' story is that Scrooge's future outcomes may be improved, and that Scrooge, through a change of heart and behavior, can bring about such improvement by his own efforts.

The following example illustrates how the meaning of a specific health-related social comparison may depend on the three future-oriented factors represented in the figure. Imagine a man in his 20s who learns that his father's brother, who is in his 50s, has just had coronary bypass surgery. Here, a comparison to a downward target on a potential future outcome for the self has several potential effects. First, news of the uncle's surgery might frighten and depress the younger man. Second, it might serve as a warning call about diet, exercise, and preventive health care. The three factors represented in Fig. 5.1 may play a role in determining which of these outcomes occurs. With respect to the first factor, if the nephew encounters the comparison information in young adulthood, he has time to modify his own risk and to educate himself about cardiac health. In contrast, if he acquires the same information about his family's cardiac risk at mid-life, the information would be more immediately threatening, and it would also be more difficult at that point to modify his behavior in ways that would substantially affect his risk. With respect to the second and third factors, it is likely that the young man's perceptions concerning the mutability of genetic risk for heart disease and his perceptions concerning the amount of personal control he can exercise over his risk may influence his response to his uncle's illness. Specifically, if he believes that his own genetic makeup guarantees a heart attack at mid-life (that is, that his risk is stable on Factor 2), the information about his uncle's health may be terrifying, whereas if he feels his risk is modifiable (i.e., improvement is possible on Factor 2) and he feels able to act to reduce his risk (high perceived control on Factor 3), the same information may motivate him to change his behavior. In this case, comparisons to his uncle and to others might provide information about the likely range of potential outcomes, as well as specific information useful in coping or decision making. For reasons that this chapter explores, this kind of proactive future-oriented comparison activity is likely to be quite different from the more reactive comparison activity of a man recovering from a heart attack who wishes to assess how he is doing. The next few sections examine each of the three factors of the proposed framework and their potential influence on social comparison activity in greater detail.

## TEMPORAL ASPECTS OF THE COMPARISON SITUATION

The comparison situation represented in Fig. 5.1 consists of several potentially important temporal aspects, such as the development of some event, stressor, or health condition at the time of comparison and the location of the comparison target in the development of the same event or stressor.[2] Let us focus on three aspects of the temporal development of the comparison situation with respect to their implications for social comparison activity: (a) whether the event or stressor is one in which the comparer expects some degree of future engagement; (b) the meaning of comparisons undertaken immediately after some focal event has occurred; and (c) the meaning of comparisons undertaken prior to some focal event. Two sets of contrasts are particularly important: comparisons made with or without the expectation of future engagement with the task or stressors, and comparisons made before and after focal events. An important part of this analysis is that at least two well-established influences on social comparison activity are likely to vary with the temporal development of a focal event or stressor. The first of these influences is the amount and certainty of the comparer's knowledge, both about the situation itself and about her standing with respect to its demands and challenges; the second is the comparer's degree of psychological distress. In the sections that follow I examine current research and theory concerning how these temporal factors and their correlates may jointly influence the motives underlying comparison activity, the meaning of both upward and downward comparisons, and, ultimately, responses to both upward and downward comparisons.

[2]Although it is beyond the scope of this chapter to review the social comparison literature with respect to the effects of relative placement of the comparer and the comparison target along the developmental trajectory of the event, there is some intriguing evidence from both experimental and nonexperimental studies that comparisons with someone who has been through the event are most useful to those awaiting stressful events (see Kulik & Mahler, chapter 8, this volume).

## The Effects of Future Engagement in the Comparison Domain

A review of the social comparison literature with respect to the simple question of whether the would-be comparer may reasonably expect any future engagement in the comparison domain is an important starting point for this discussion. If, as I propose, social comparisons derive much of their meaning from their implications for some future action, it is crucial to examine the degree to which a comparer may reasonably expect to encounter the event, stressor, task, situation, or comparison dimension again. Although this point may seem obvious, relatively few experimental studies of social comparisons have provided either feedback on dimensions for which subjects expect any continued involvement or additional trials of any kind on which to assess the impact of comparison activity on subsequent efforts (cf. Bandura & Jourden, 1991; Butler, 1993) or, conversely, the impact of anticipated subsequent efforts on comparison activity (cf. Jones & Regan, 1974; Testa & Major, 1990).

The degree of one's expected future involvement with a task or dimension may have a strong impact on comparison motives. If a task requires a single performance and has few implications for future action or self-evaluation, motives for acquiring information useful in self-improvement efforts may be reduced (cf. Trope, 1986). For example, studies that manipulate subjects' perceptions of a fixed skill, such as "scanning ability," are unlikely to prompt efforts to improve one's performance, especially when the performance phase of the experiment is over. Under such conditions, short-term needs to feel better about oneself and one's standing may dominate the choice of social comparison targets and reactions to comparison information. Specifically, would-be comparers may seek downward comparisons and avoid upward ones. In contrast, if one expects future engagement or if the particular threatened attribute has implications for one's future outcomes, as is the case for most health-related comparisons, one's need for both self-evaluative accuracy and self-improvement may be greater. That is, it may be more important to form a stable, accurate self-evaluation when one expects to encounter the situation or task again, and comparers may also be motivated to improve their standing. Under such conditions, one may seek lateral and upward targets instead of downward targets, because downward targets may provide relatively less information that is directly useful in the service of self-improvement.[3]

[3]It would be inaccurate to characterize downward comparisons as useless in the service of self-improvement. Many of the self-evaluative and motivational functions served by

Results from a related literature on counterfactual thinking find just this pattern of results. When an experimental task was to be repeated three additional times, subjects generated more upward counterfactuals (considerations of specific ways in which one's outcomes might have been better) and fewer downward counterfactuals (ways in which one's outcomes might have been worse) than when the task was a single trial (Markman, Gavanski, Sherman, & McMullen, 1993). When the task may be or will be repeated, both upward comparisons and upward counterfactuals may assist people in generating scripts and plans for future action (Roese, 1994). When the event is a one-time occurrence or a single trial, upward comparisons are less useful.

### Comparison Activity Immediately After Some Focal Event or Stressor

The point of departure of many social comparison studies is some focal event that has already occurred, usually just prior to a comparison opportunity or assessment. Even in situations where there is some future element to the comparison situation, the temporal placement of the comparison opportunity immediately after threat or failure may have several consequences for the motives underlying comparison activity. In particular, two well-documented influences on comparison activity may vary with the development of stressful events: psychological distress and uncertainty. Each of these influences and its respective effects on comparison motives are reviewed in turn.

***Psychological Distress and the Development of Stressful Events.*** Most stressors create the twin tasks of problem-solving and emotional regulation (cf. Lazarus & Folkman, 1984), and different kinds of comparison information may serve these coping needs differentially well at different times (Taylor et al., 1990). The amount of distress experienced by the comparer may vary considerably as a function of the develop-

---

downward comparisons—for example, understanding the range of outcomes against which one's own may be evaluated, reduction in negative mood, and increased optimism (cf. Gibbons & Gerrard, 1989, 1991; Aspinwall & Taylor, 1993; Wills, 1991)—may ultimately increase persistence or performance in a given domain. In particular, increases in positive affect, self-esteem, and optimism may facilitate more active cognitive and behavioral efforts to manage problems (see Wills, chapter 6, this volume). Additionally, downward comparisons may serve important motivational needs by creating distance between oneself and others with poor outcomes (see Gibbons & Gerrard, chapter 3, this volume), either through passive exposure to downward targets or through active derogation of others (see Gibbons & Boney-McCoy, 1991; Wills, 1981). However, despite these potential benefits, downward comparisons usually provide less direct information about successful performance itself than upward comparisons do.

ment of the event. What studies of newly diagnosed patients, failing students, and dysphoric people have in common is that immediate needs to regulate affect may be paramount. Immediately after a stressful event or experimentally manipulated failure, elevated distress may drive comparison activity downward in the service of self-enhancement (Wills, 1981). In particular, distress seems to make comparison activity diverge from an even-handed diagnostic search to more self-enhancing comparisons (cf. Pyszcsynski, Greenberg, & LaPrelle, 1985). Under such circumstances, needs for affective management and esteem-maintenance may overwhelm needs for accurate self-assessment (cf. Brown, 1990) and self-improvement (cf. Crocker & Major, 1989).

The need to regulate affect has also been shown to influence responses to particular kinds of comparisons. Consistent with Wills' (1981) analysis, there is now considerable evidence that people undergoing decreases in subjective well-being respond favorably to downward comparisons (see Gibbons & Gerrard, 1991; Taylor et al., 1990; and Wills, 1991, for reviews). In addition, studies employing either inductions of negative mood or naturally occurring dysphoria suggest that people in a negative mood respond favorably to downward comparison information (Aspinwall & Taylor, 1993; Gibbons, 1986; Gibbons & Boney-McCoy, 1991).[4] It is interesting to note that, in the absence of negative mood or an immediate threat of some kind, people do not appear to respond favorably to downward comparisons. Instead, exposure to downward comparisons may produce less positive mood, greater frustration and discouragement, and less hope for the future relative to upward comparisons (Aspinwall & Taylor, 1993; Taylor, Aspinwall, Giuliano, Dakof, & Reardon, 1993; Ybema & Buunk, 1995; see Collins, 1996, for a review).

The presence of an immediate, recent, or focal threat may moderate responses to upward comparisons as well. That is, although upward comparisons may contain information useful in self-improvement efforts (Wood, 1989), several studies suggest that upward comparisons may be especially painful when the comparer has just experienced a setback in the comparison domain (cf. Salovey & Rodin, 1984). For example, Aspinwall and Taylor (1993, Study 1) found that subjects who

[4]Although people in a negative mood do report increased subjective well-being following downward comparisons, there is some evidence that negative moods do not always prompt downward comparisons. In a daily diary study, Wheeler and Miyake (1992) found that people in a negative mood were more likely to report making upward comparisons than downward ones, a pattern that suggests mood-congruent social comparison activity rather than mood repair. Although the source of the potential discrepancy between these results and those of other studies remains to be determined, these findings highlight the immediate affective determinants of comparison activity.

reported having had an academic setback of some sort one week prior to the study reported adverse reactions to a story describing another student's highly successful adjustment to college. Among students whose setbacks were less recent, responses to upward comparisons were more favorable. If the immediacy of a threat moderates responses to upward comparisons, it would explain why studies that provide threatening failure feedback and assess comparison activity immediately after such feedback yield results suggesting that upward comparisons on self-relevant dimensions are most often harmful. Under such conditions, needs for affective management and preservation of self-esteem are high (cf. Tesser, 1988), and downward comparisons are likely to be preferred. In sum, these observations suggest that the placement of comparison opportunities or assessment of comparison preferences immediately after some focal event or stressor may provide a view of comparison activity that is slanted toward downward comparisons made in the service of self-enhancement goals.

***Uncertainty and the Development of Stressful Events.*** At the heart of social comparison theory is the hypothesis that uncertainty drives the social comparison process (Festinger, 1954); that is, when objective information is unavailable and people are uncertain about their standing, people will look to others to evaluate themselves. Uncertainty has been shown to influence both comparison and affiliation processes across a range of stressful events (see Buunk, 1994, 1995, for reviews; Molleman, Pruyn, & van Knippenberg, 1986). There are, however, two ways in which studying comparison activity immediately after some focal event or stressor may create a relatively narrow portrait of the role of uncertainty in comparison activity. First, if the event has already occurred (e.g., an experimentally manipulated failure on a task or test), there is little uncertainty about the outcome itself, especially if one has been given a score of some kind. Second, when there is little or no future engagement in the event, uncertainty is further reduced. That is, if the event has already happened and is known to be isolated, little uncertainty about the meaning of the event for one's future actions and outcomes may exist. Under such conditions, comparison information may simply be less useful. For example, Jones and Regan (1974) found that subjects desired normative information about their test performance before, but not after, making a decision that required a good understanding of their own abilities. That is, once a decision has been made or the focal event has occurred, the usefulness of the comparison information in making decisions about the event itself is necessarily lessened.

Some level of future engagement with the stressor may increase the potential of comparison activity to reduce uncertainty, even for events that have already occurred. For events with continuing implications for well-being, such as most health-related events, social comparisons have the potential to reduce uncertainty about one's situation and ways of managing it. Buunk's (1994) work on distressed marriages, professional burnout, and disability provides good examples of such events (see Buunk & Ybema, chapter 12, this volume). Comparison information may be especially useful for events that fall in the left half of Fig. 5.1. That is, for events that have yet to occur or that are early in their development, the final outcome may be uncertain and the implications of the event for future actions and outcomes unknown. Under such conditions, heightened uncertainty about the stressor and its future course may prompt more, and more varied, comparison activity than for stressors whose current nature and future course are known. A good example of such events and the comparison activity they generate is represented by research on how people interpret physical symptoms and decide whether they warrant medical attention (see Suls, Martin, & Leventhal, chapter 4, this volume). Physical symptoms are often ambiguous: They may be benign, or they may represent the early warning signs of a developing illness. People experiencing symptoms may consult or observe a wide range of other people in order to determine whether they are facing a potentially serious health problem or a temporary inconvenience, and social comparison information may play an especially great role in judgments of whether one's situation warrants medical attention (cf. Croyle, 1992). The following sections expand on these observations by examining comparison activity early in the temporal development of stressors in greater detail.

### Comparison Activity Early in the Course of Stressful Events or Prior to Their Occurrence

A stressor or potential stressor may have many stages of development, encompassing not only the focal event itself, but also a series of events beginning with the first glimmer that something stressful may occur and continuing through the aftermath of the event (cf. Aspinwall & Taylor, in press; McGrath & Beehr, 1990). The sections that follow examine what might be gained from expanding the study of comparison activity in general, and of health-related comparisons in particular, to the relatively unexplored left half of the comparison space in Fig. 5.1 that represents comparisons undertaken prior to some focal stressor. I suggest that comparisons undertaken prior to the occurrence of stressful events are different in many ways from those made after an event has occurred. In particular, I draw on the achievement literature and from my own work on proactive coping to relate the comparer's temporal location with respect to the development of a stressor to (a) interest in different kinds of comparison information, (b) the meaning of upward and downward comparisons, and (c) the potential for the comparison information to be used to alter behavior with respect to potentially stressful events in ways that influence the course of the event itself.

***Interest in Different Kinds of Comparison Information.*** One line of research that has explicitly considered the comparer's progress with respect to engagement in a particular domain is the achievement literature. Ruble and Frey (1991) presented a model of social comparison activity that tracks changes in the motives underlying social comparison activity from the perspective of the comparer's development of competence in particular domains. According to Ruble and Frey, "What one needs to extract from social comparison depends on what one already knows and can do in that domain (p. 80)." In terms of the present analysis, the potential for social comparison information to provide information about new and upcoming situations may be greatest prior to some focal event, because the range of possible outcomes is wider and because parameters of the comparison dimension, such as its likely future course and amenability to personal control, are likely to be unknown. That is, social comparison may play a useful role in yielding information not only about one's ability to manage the stressor, but also about the nature of the stressor and its likely future course (see also Kulik & Mahler, chapter 8, this volume).

Ruble and Frey's model incorporates such functions by dividing comparison activity into three distinct phases: gaining information about a task prior to engaging in it, making an assessment of one's competence, and maintaining one's competence across the lifespan. In the first phase, people use comparison information to learn about the task itself and to make a choice about whether they should pursue it. At this stage of task acquisition, Ruble and Frey argued that people are especially interested in a range of comparisons and the diagnostic information they may provide. Accurate self-assessment, even if unflattering, is desired at this stage, so that an adaptive strategy choice about future engagement may be made. Only when performance begins to decline do people engage in selective comparisons that might allow them to maintain their sense of task competence.

Ruble and Frey's (1991) analysis paints a more varied portrait of social comparison activity than does research that focuses on comparisons that occur after some decline, setback, or threat. Specifically, their model suggests that there are qualitative differences in the kind of information desired as a function of the development of the event (see also Butler,

1992, 1993). In addition, the present analysis suggests that the potential for comparers to profit from this information may also be greater early in the course of their engagement with a task or stressor. When a focal stressor has not yet occurred, the comparison process may not be dominated by needs for distress reduction and self-enhancement. Under such conditions, comparisons undertaken earlier in the course of events may be directed toward those that provide information about one's competence (cf. Trope, 1986) and one's future prospects for success in that domain (Ruble & Frey, 1991).

Understanding how people use comparison activity to gather information about upcoming events may provide considerable insight into people's decisions to undertake or to fail to undertake preventive health behaviors. A good example of this kind of comparison-driven search for information may be represented by situations in which people may compare themselves to similar others, or to older individuals one expects to resemble later in life, to identify behaviors that may be effective in preventing illness and those that are likely to increase risk. Consider an active young woman who is trying to gauge her risk for breast cancer and osteoporosis. She may mentally survey the behavior and outcomes of older women in her family (What is the family's risk history? How much exercise did Auntie Em get? What role did her daily consumption of Scotch and butter cookies play in her development of breast cancer?). The results of such a search are likely to inform the comparer's view of whether her risk is high and under her control. Such judgments are likely to bear important relations to preventive behavior (Rosenstock, 1974; Weinstein, 1988; see Salovey, Rothman, & Rodin, in press, for a recent review).

***The Meaning of Upward and Downward Comparisons.*** In addition to affecting the motives underlying comparison activity and the comparer's degree of knowledge about the comparison dimension and his or her standing on it, the comparer's location with respect to the development of a particular stressful event may also affect the meaning of a given piece of comparison information. Specifically, the meaning of upward and downward comparisons may be different to a person who is not yet irrevocably engaged in an event, but is simply considering it. Imagine a person with cancer who, against his physician's advice, chooses an unproven surgery or treatment. The procedure is a failure, and the person's health is further compromised, making him ineligible for other forms of treatment. The meaning of this example would be very different to a patient who has not yet made a decision concerning his treatment than to one who has and who is dissatisfied with his treatment outcome. For the person contemplating such a decision, the comparison holds information about what can go wrong, the lower boundary of outcomes, and what not to do. For the person whose decision has already been made and whose outcome is not as good as he desired, the story may be comforting in some ways, because his own outcome is already better than the target's. This analysis may also be applied to upward comparisons. Responses to the outcomes of a person who undergoes succesful surgery or treatment might also vary as a function of whether the outcome of one's own treatment is known. If it is, someone else's success story may provide an aversive benchmark for one's own outcomes. However, if one has yet to undergo surgery, the successful outcome could increase one's expectations regarding the success of one's own treatment.

As these examples illustrate, the implications of social comparison information for future action and outcomes may depend on the comparer's location with respect to the focal event. When the focal events of choosing and undergoing a surgical procedure have not yet occurred, both upward and downward comparisons—in these examples, the successful and unsuccessful treatment outcomes—"could be me." At this early junction, both upward and downward comparisons may serve an important proactive function by providing information about one's prospects. Specifically, an upward comparison may serve as a standard for what might be achieved (cf. Ruble & Frey, 1991), whereas a downward comparison may represent the lower boundary of possible outcomes and may provide information about what not to do. Additionally, these proactive comparisons may be useful not only in decision making, but also in emotional regulation. One may use the outcomes of others to anticipate and mentally simulate one's own emotional response to different outcomes (e.g., "How would I feel if this happened to me? What would I do?"). In this way, the information provided by other people's actions, outcomes, and emotional responses may facilitate the development of action plans and of mental simulations of how one would cope with different possible outcomes and their affective consequences. Such simulations may foster coping efforts in a variety of ways (cf. Taylor & Schneider, 1989).

As suggested earlier, it is important to note that comparisons made in advance of a focal event may not be driven downward by self-enhancement needs or by the lack of actual or anticipated future engagement in the event. Therefore, people may be able to use information from a range of available comparisons. Once one has undergone the procedure, however, and it is in the past, responses to comparison information may become reactive. When the focal event is over, the implications of social comparison information for future actions with respect to the event are potentially reduced, although social comparisons may still provide information useful in self-evaluation and the regulation of affect. At this point, dissatisfaction with one's own outcomes may drive comparison activity downward, and, in cases in which subsequent improvement is unlikely, upward comparisons may be especially aversive.

***Potential for Comparisons to Alter Behavior With Respect to Stressful Events.*** Our discussion of the distinctions between proactive and reactive comparisons has focused on the differences between responses to comparisons undertaken prior to some focal event and responses to comparisons after such an event. However, it is not only the temporal location of the comparison information vis-à-vis the stressful event but also the potential to alter one's behavior in response to this information that distinguishes proactive from reactive comparisons. As an illustration of this distinction, consider the classic Mr. Clean/Mr. Dirty study. Morse and Gergen (1970) exposed subjects to either an upward or downward comparison target immediately prior to a job interview. Subjects exposed to the sloppy, unprepared Mr. Dirty felt better about themselves, while those exposed to the impeccable Mr. Clean reported decreased estimates of their own abilities. In terms of the time dimension diagrammed in Fig. 5.1, this study would fall slightly to the left of the center of the figure, because the comparison information was delivered just prior to the focal event (the job interview). However, because the subject was already in the waiting room, the information gleaned from the comparison could not motivate him to prepare better for the interview. Rather, the comparison could only alter the subject's perception of how well prepared he was.

In contrast, imagine a scenario in which the subject encounters Mr. Clean at the job placement service 1 week prior to the interview and learns they are both applying for the same job. At this point, the subject could do several things in response to Mr. Clean's obvious superiority. First, he could increase his preparation for the interview, wear a suit, and compete more successfully for the job. Alternatively, he could cancel his own interview, saving time and effort, because he knows that Mr. Clean has a lock on the job. This potential to change the course of events or to reduce their subsequent impact in response to new information is what distinguishes proactive comparison activity from reactive comparison activity.

In more general terms, proactive coping involves gathering information about potential stressors early in their development and using this information to alter the course of stressful events or to reduce their impact (Aspinwall & Taylor, in press; Folkman & Lazarus, 1985). As in the earlier examples of the young man facing his uncle's heart attack and the young woman gauging her risk of breast disease, proactive comparisons may be made in cases in which it is uncertain (a) whether one's own situation will develop into a stressful one, and (b) exactly how the stressor will evolve if it does occur. Such situations may prompt a wider range of comparison activity than situations in which future engagement with the stressor is both certain and imminent. Instead of being primarily directed toward managing negative affect, proactive comparison activity may be directed toward managing the potential stressor itself. Specifically, proactive activity may be directed toward understanding the likely range of possible outcomes, whether control is possible, and other parameters of the situation.

As in the example of the young man and his uncle, proactive comparisons may be especially useful when one can compare to someone at a later stage of adjustment than the self. There is some evidence that these kinds of comparisons may be especially impactful. In Kulik and Mahler's (1987) study of patients undergoing heart surgery, patients assigned preoperatively to a roommate who had already undergone surgery and was recovering (even if it was from a different kind of surgery) reaped a number of benefits: They were less anxious, engaged in twice as much post-surgical ambulation, and were discharged from the hospital sooner than patients who had been assigned a roommate who was also awaiting surgery. It is possible that exposure to the postoperative roommate provided both evidence that one can survive surgery and information about how to deal with discomfort following surgery. Both kinds of information may have improved patients' problem-focused and emotion-focused coping with the stress of major surgery (see also Kulik & Mahler, chapter 8, this volume). Interestingly, roommate assignment following surgery had no effect on patients' outcomes. Like other kinds of reactive comparisons, postoperative comparison information may come too late in the course of events to influence their outcome. That is, although reactive comparison information may be quite useful in changing the way people think about their outcomes, proactive comparisons may be unique in their potential to provide information useful in modifying actual outcomes.

The fact that a comparison is proactive, however, is no guarantee that it will be constructive. It will be important to study proactive comparisons that may interfere with preventive health behavior and other future-oriented behaviors. For example, many people know a healthy 70-year-old life-long smoker. If a smoker chooses such a person as a basis for comparison for her own future health outcomes, she is unlikely to initiate or maintain preventive behaviors like quitting. Additionally, a proactive search for risk factors may be biased (cf. Klein & Weinstein, chapter 2, this volume; Weinstein, 1984). The young man digesting the news of his uncle's heart attack could search for risk factors that apply to the uncle but that do not apply to him, thus falsely inflating his sense of his relative health. A biased search such as this would have little constructive implication for future action and would likely interfere with preventive behavior.

These examples raise the possibility that proactive comparisons, like their reactive counterparts, may be biased or selective in ways that hinder adaptation to threatening circumstances. Returning to the analysis of factors that vary with the temporal development of stressful events, I suggest that there are two reasons to believe that proactive comparisons may be more "honest" than reactive ones. Proactive comparisons are more likely to be made when distress is relatively low (the focal event hasn't happened yet) and opportunity for improvement is relatively high (the outcome of the situation isn't written in stone). It will be important for future research to examine the conditions under which comparisons made in advance of focal stressors and health-related events are informed by a wide range of relevant comparisons or whether, like more reactive comparisons, they turn out to be frequently biased in self-serving or defensive ways.

## FUTURE-ORIENTED ASPECTS OF COMPARISON DIMENSIONS

In the preceding sections we have treated social comparison dimensions as if they were interchangeable, focusing mostly on the temporal aspects of one's engagement in events or activities. This section considers the other two factors in the framework—the potential for the comparer's standing on the comparison dimension to improve, to remain stable, or to decline, and the degree to which the comparer perceives that the course of her future standing is amenable to personal control—as important determinants of the implications of any given comparison for some future action or outcome (cf. Buunk & Ybema, chapter 12, this volume; Major, Testa, & Bylsma, 1991; Wills, 1991; Wood & VanderZee, chapter 10, this volume). In addition to their utility in understanding social comparison activity, it is important to note that these two factors have been identified as important secondary appraisals of stressful events more generally; that is, research on stress and coping has shown that people use their judgments of the likely future course of their situations and their degree of personal control over them to determine, in part, whether they are stressed or challenged by demanding events (Folkman, 1984; Smith & Lazarus, 1990).

Before reviewing of the effects of these factors on comparison activity, it is necessary to consider in some detail how these factors may be related to one another. First, although these two factors may seem similar, potential for change in one's standing and perceptions of personal control over one's standing are not necessarily correlated. For example, it may be possible to improve one's level of physical fitness, but one may feel powerless to do so. Second, although the two factors are portrayed as orthogonal in the figure, they may be initially positively correlated and may influence each other over time. For example, if one feels powerless to improve one's fitness level, one might come to believe that one's standing is relatively fixed at some low level. In this case, responses to comparisons may resemble those for fixed dimensions, even though potential for change in one's standing may exist. In turn, as I illustrate, perceptions that a given situation is immutable (for whatever reason) may lead people to rely on downward comparisons and avoid upward comparisons that would inform their judgments about the amenability of the situation to control or expose them to higher standards that would raise their expectations for their own outcomes (cf. Gibbons, Gerrard, Blanton, & Eggleston, 1996). A good example of this process comes from Major's (1989) work on pay equity. Her findings suggest that women avoid making potentially painful upward comparisons to men's salaries and compare themselves primarily to other women, thus remaining satisfied with their inferior compensation. In this way, comparison activity may itself shape perceptions of the likely future course of one's standing. For these reasons, we suggest that even though these two factors may covary highly in some settings, they are distinct and important determinants of the implications of social comparisons for future actions and outcomes.

### A Future-Oriented Model of the Comparison Space for Health Domains

Figure 5.2 presents an expanded view of the influence of potential for improvement or decline in one's standing on the comparison dimension and perceived control over one's standing as joint influences on social comparison processes. To illustrate the potential joint effects of these two factors, I identified several aspects of mental and physical health that may vary in terms of these two factors. In the sections that follow I use these specific examples to examine the implications of the future-oriented framework for understanding health-related social comparison activity. Let us first examine comparisons made on dimensions perceived to be fixed or stable. Next, we can consider some hypotheses about the ways in which the potential for change in one's standing on the comparison dimension and perceptions of personal control over

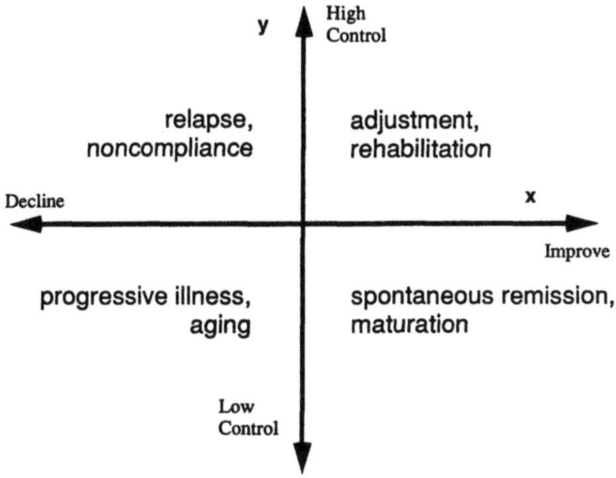


FIG. 5.2. A future-oriented model of the comparison space for health domains. Illnesses and other threats to mental and physical health are used to illustrate the joint effect of the potential for change in the comparer's standing on the comparison dimension (x-axis) and the comparer's degree of perceived control over her standing (y-axis).

one's standing may moderate comparison preferences and reactions to both upward and downward comparisons. Specifically, we suggest that an examination of these two aspects of the comparison dimension may explain some apparent inconsistencies in the social comparison literature. For example, although dozens of studies find that upward comparisons are frustrating and that downward comparisons improve subjective well-being, recent evidence suggests that the affective consequences of comparisons may not be intrinsic to their direction (Buunk, Collins, Taylor, VanYperen, & Dakof, 1990; Buunk & Ybema, chapter 12, this volume). Under certain circumstances, upward comparisons may be inspiring, rather than daunting (Collins, 1996; Taylor & Lobel, 1989; Taylor et al., 1993; Ybema & Buunk, 1995). Similarly, downward comparisons may not always be comforting. Instead, they may frighten the comparer when they provide examples of failure or deterioration (Brickman & Bulman, 1977; Gibbons & Gerrard, 1991; Wills, 1991). The entire section examines the utility of a future-oriented analysis of comparison dimensions to account for these differences.

***Comparisons on Fixed or Stable Dimensions.*** The majority of experimental studies of social comparisons fall at or near the center of the model presented in Figure 5.2. These studies provide failure feedback on a dimension that is unlikely to change and over which subjects may have little perceived personal control. As noted earlier, studies of downward comparison activity among threatened persons often experimentally manipulate levels of threat by providing low scores on personality inventories, such as scanning ability (Brickman & Bulman, 1977), social sensitivity (Pyszczynski et al., 1985), and social awareness (Gibbons & Boney-McCoy, 1991). If subjects perceive their standing on such traits to be fixed, they may perceive little chance for improvement or decline in their status (cf. Major et al., 1991). When one's standing is fixed and one has little personal control over one's outcomes, the role of social comparisons with respect to one's future actions or outcomes may be somewhat circumscribed: Downward comparisons may provide the welcome information that one is, at least, better off than someone else, whereas upward comparisons provide the unwelcome information that someone who is currently superior to the self always will be.

Fixed-attribute situations may circumscribe the effects of comparison activity in other ways as well. Specifically, in fixed-attribute situations, the risks of downward comparisons are reduced, and the benefits of upward comparisons are nearly eliminated. If one's standing on the comparison dimension is fixed, one need not fear declining to the level of the downward target. If one cannot improve, there is little point in seeking superior models. Under these conditions, there is little cost to making comparisons that bolster mood or self-esteem. For these reasons, experiments that manipulate threat by providing false feedback on relatively stable attributes may create just the set of circumstances likely to prompt predominantly favorable responses to downward comparisons and unfavorable responses to upward comparisons. For these reasons, comparison activity in fixed-attribute situations may resemble comparison activity in situations with little expected future engagement.

A final impediment to using comparison information on fixed dimensions in the service of some future action or outcome is the meaning of the task itself. As Trope (1986) pointed out, if one's performance on a task is fixed at some level, the task itself loses both its diagnostic value and its self-enhancement value, because one's performance on the task provides little ability-relevant information. However, if change in either direction is possible, one's task performance and associated comparison activity may have implications for the self and for future actions and outcomes.

***Comparisons on Changing Dimensions.*** As one moves away from the center of Fig. 5.2, the likely future course of one's standing on the comparison dimension may affect the meaning of both upward and downward comparisons. That is, the implications of such comparisons may be quite different for someone who fears decline than for someone who hopes for improvement. In the upper right quadrant of the figure are comparison dimensions that are both subject to improvement and amenable to personal control, such as temporary setbacks, adjustment to new situations, and rehabilitation from injury or accident. In this case, neither upward nor downward comparisons hold much psychological risk for the would-be comparer, because his or her situation is likely to improve and the pace and quality of that improvement may depend on his or her own efforts.

In the lower right quadrant are situations, such as maturation (e.g., adolescent difficulties) or healing (e.g., a clean fracture) that are subject to improvement, but not amenable to personal control. To the person who expects improvement, a downward comparison may provide some comfort and has fewer risks, because the person expects to improve over time. If the situation is understood to be likely to improve one day, people making downward comparisons may confidently assert, "At least *that* didn't happen to me." In this case, comparison activity in any direction may be generally useful when it provides information about the likely time course of one's condition and a frame of reference for understanding one's own outcomes.

Other quadrants of the figure have received far less research attention, and it is here that research on health outcomes may continue to be especially informative. In the lower left quadrant are dimensions on which one's health status is likely to decline and in which objective levels of control over one's outcomes are relatively low, such as progressive illness. Under such circumstances, downward comparisons have the potential to be frightening because one can decline to the level of the downward target (Wills, 1991; see Wood & VanderZee, chapter 10, this volume), and upward comparisons are unlikely to be inspiring because one is unlikely ever to attain the target's superior standing. It is possible that people managing health threats that fall in this quadrant may switch their comparison activity to dimensions other than disease progression,[5] such as coping, adjustment, or other attributes on which they may be relatively advantaged (cf. Taylor et al. 1983; Wills, 1991) and

[5]It is important to note that favorable affective reactions to downward comparisons have been reported among people with illnesses that fall in this quadrant of the figure. In a survey study by Hemphill and Lehman (1991), patients with multiple sclerosis reported both favorable and unfavorable affective reactions to downward comparisons on the physical disability–prognosis dimension. Patients' beliefs about personal control over the course of their illness were not assessed, so it is impossible to test whether high levels of such beliefs accounted for favorable responses to downward comparisons. Interestingly, a measure of specific beliefs about the future course of the illness did not moderate affective responses to downward comparisons in this sample. One potential explanation for this null result is that there may have been a restricted range of such beliefs among people managing a progressive illness.

that afford greater possibility of improvement or personal control (cf. Hemphill & Lehman, 1991; Ybema & Buunk, 1995).

Finally, in the upper left quadrant of the figure are situations in which decline is possible but amenability to control is potentially high. For behaviors such as abstinence from drugs or alcohol and treatment compliance, one's status can improve or decline depending on one's actions (e.g., health maintenance behaviors, treatment adherence, self-monitoring); therefore, the implications of other people's outcomes for one's own behavior may be especially important. To the recovering alcoholic, a downward comparison to someone who has "fallen off the wagon" may provide valuable information about the kinds of situations that might promote relapse. If the person perceives some level of personal control over avoiding such situations herself, the comparison may not be perceived as aversive. On the other hand, because decline is possible, exposure to a lapsing alcoholic could be terrifying, depending on one's perceived degree of personal control over one's drinking. Similarly, responses to upward comparisons—for example, to recovering alcoholics with several years of sobriety—may be inspiring instead of discouraging only if the person believes she can achieve such an outcome. Of particular importance for dimensions that fall in this quadrant is the observation that when decline is possible, neither upward nor downward comparisons may be made without some potential cost. Conversely, neither upward nor downward comparisons may be safely ignored by people facing threats in this quadrant, because both kinds of comparisons have the potential to provide information useful in improving one's lot, either by achieving desired outcomes or avoiding undesirable ones. It is possible that research in this under-studied quadrant of the comparison space may prove to be especially fruitful, because comparisons made by people in such circumstances may be critical in understanding the success or failure of efforts to maintain long-term change in behavior or to adhere to treatments required to manage chronic illness.

### Empirical Evidence for the Role of Perceived Control and Potential for Improvement or Decline in Social Comparison Activity

In the following sections, we review research on both upward and downward comparisons with respect to perceived control and potential for improvement or decline and suggest that the future-oriented framework affords good predictive value in understanding reactions to comparison information among people under stress.

***Future-Oriented Aspects of Downward Comparison Dimensions.*** Only a few published studies have explicitly examined either the relation of potential for change in one's outcomes or perceptions of control over one's outcomes to responses to downward comparison information, and these have generated seemingly contradictory results. In an interesting demonstration of the ability of information about future outcomes to moderate responses to comparison information, Testa and Major (1990) operationalized control over one's outcomes in terms of the level of performance perceived possible on a future task. Subjects who received failure feedback about their performance on an essay task were told that performance on a second (different) task was either highly related or unrelated to performance on the first task. As predicted, subjects who thought their initially low level of performance was unlikely to change on the second task sought more downward comparison information about their relative performance on the first task than subjects who believed they could improve on the second task. This pattern of results led Testa and Major to speculate that downward comparisons might alleviate some of the negative consequences of low control perceptions.

Studies in patient populations have yielded seemingly different results. In a structured interview study, Buunk and his colleagues (1990) found that cancer patients who reported high levels of perceived control over the course of their illness reported more favorable responses to downward comparisons than did patients with low perceived control. Additionally, patients with low perceived control were more likely to report that downward comparisons had negative implications for the self. Jensen and Karoly (1992) obtained similar results in a cross-sectional study of chronic pain patients. Contrary to their predictions, higher levels of perceived control over pain predicted greater self-reports of the frequency of use comparative self-evaluation strategies, such as downward comparisons and the construction of hypothetical worse worlds. The use of such strategies was associated with lower levels of depression, controlling for measures of pain.

On the surface, these two sets of findings appear to be contradictory. In Testa and Major's experiment, subjects in the low-control condition sought downward comparison information, whereas in the two patient samples, respondents with low perceived control reported adverse reactions to such comparisons and lower levels of such comparisons. Although these studies differ in many respects, a critical difference among them is the likely future course of subjects' standing on the comparison dimension. In the Testa and Major study, subjects in the "low control" condition had their performance on the second task virtually fixed at the level of the first task. Subjects could improve on the second task or perform at the same low level, but it was unlikely that their performance would decline. Under such conditions, downward comparison information may provide comfort at little risk to the self. In contrast, respondents in the two patient samples faced the possibility that their health status might decline. For patients with low perceived control over the course of their illness, downward comparisons might be frightening rather than reassuring.

The hypothesis that the likely future course of one's standing on a comparison dimension moderates responses to downward comparison information was tested in a recent experiment (Aspinwall & Kissam, 1995). Two weeks prior to the final exam in an upper level psychology course, we provided college students with false feedback indicating that they had received a score of 4 out of 10 on a practice test for the final exam. We then told subjects that the actual final exam was easier than the practice exam (subsequent improvement likely), of the same difficulty (same low performance likely), or harder than the practice exam (subsequent decline likely). Subjects then overheard a confederate who received a lower score—2 out of 10. The results showed that responses to the downward target depended on the potential for the actual final exam to be more difficult than the practice exam. In the condition in which subjects were told that the final exam would be just as difficult as the practice test, subjects exposed to the low-scoring confederate reported more positive mood and more favorable self-evaluation, compared to a no-comparison baseline. As predicted, the results were quite different when subjects were told that the final exam would be more difficult than the practice test. Subjects in this condition who were exposed to the downward confederate reported more negative affect than subjects in the no-comparison baseline condition. In addition, subjects in the declining condition reported higher perceptions of similarity to the downward target than subjects in the other conditions.

These results suggest that the likely future course of one's standing on the comparison dimension moderates whether one will respond favorably or unfavorably to the news that someone else is worse off. When one's situation has the potential to decline, the implications of downward comparisons for the self may shift from "At least that's not me" to "That could be me." If this is the case, the downward comparison target may seem more similar to the self (cf. Molleman et al., 1986; Ybema & Buunk, 1995), and the poor performance of a similar other may raise the spectre of one's own failure. That is, one may identify with, rather than contrast one's situation to, a downward target under these conditions (see Wood & VanderZee, chapter 10, Buunk & Ybema, chapter 12, this volume, for extended discussions of this issue).

A final note about our study concerns the responses of subjects who were told the final exam would be easier than the practice exam. Although we had expected subjects in the improving condition to respond at least somewhat favorably to the downward comparison information, these subjects reported no gains in mood or self-evaluation over baseline. These results are consistent with those of other experimental investigations. In Testa and Major's (1990) study, subjects who thought they could improve their performance on the second task showed no preference for downward comparisons. It seems, therefore, that threatened people who are told they can expect to improve neither seek exposure to worse-off others, nor profit from it when it is provided. It is possible that making potential improvement salient might orient threatened persons away from downward targets and toward upward targets in the service of self-improvement (cf. Taylor & Lobel, 1989; Testa & Major, 1990).

***Future-Oriented Aspects of Upward Comparison Dimensions.*** A similar analysis may be applied to responses to upward comparisons. Considerable research has assumed that the ideal and preferred comparison target for a stable, accurate self-evaluation is a similar other doing slightly better than the self (see Wood, 1989, for a review). A common finding, however, is that upward comparisons produce negative affects, such as jealousy (Salovey & Rodin, 1984), hostility (Testa & Major, 1990), and frustration (Martin, 1986), as well as lowered self-evaluations (Marsh & Parker, 1984; Morse & Gergen, 1970). Because of their potential utility in self-improvement efforts, it is important to understand when upward comparisons may provide information and encouragement and when they may prove discouraging.

In interpreting the results of classic upward comparison studies, it is important to consider beliefs subjects may have had about their likely future standing on the comparison dimension. In general, studies showing adverse responses to upward comparisons have provided comparison information about subjects' abilities. If performance on such dimensions is perceived to be stable or fixed, upward comparisons provide the unwelcome information that an upward target is not only better than the self at the present time, but will always be superior. For example, in Salovey and Rodin's (1984) study of social comparison jealousy, subjects were outperformed on a personality measure said to assess aptitude or ability in their chosen field. Comments from debriefing support the interpretation that subjects felt inferior to the target on the ability in question and that such feelings affected their beliefs about their future outcomes. One subject given false feedback on his medical science aptitude commented, "I was feeling a bit worried and very sensitive about my own abilities. Then, when I read the other guy's story, I hated him and envied him at the same time because he seemed so good at his work, while I was beginning to doubt my ability to ever become a doctor" (p. 790). Similarly, Tesser's studies of self-evaluation maintenance have also employed dimensions that may have been perceived to represent fixed abilities (e.g., "cognitive perceptual integration," Tesser & Paulhus, 1983; and social sensitivity and creativity, Tesser, Millar, & Moore, 1988). The tendency for subjects who are outperformed on a self-relevant attribute to downgrade the importance of that attribute may be exacerbated by subjects' perceptions that they cannot improve to the level of the superior target. Other attributes, such as attractiveness, may also be viewed as fixed properties and so generate adverse responses to upward comparisons (cf. Kenrick, Montello, Gutierres, & Trost, 1993).

In contrast to the findings for fixed dimensions or abilities, studies in which subjects are given information suggesting that they might improve their performance find that such information seems to offset the adverse effects of upward comparisons and to create interest in information useful in self-improvement. Specifically, Testa and Major (1990) found that subjects given failure feedback on an initial task who expected to improve on a second task reported lower levels of depression and hostility in response to upward comparison information than subjects who did not expect to improve on a second task. Ybema and Buunk (1993) manipulated subjects' beliefs about whether performance on a written test of leadership ability could be improved through training or was fixed. Subjects who had received below average scores preferred to see the tests of subjects who had outperformed them, and this preference for upward information was especially strong for subjects who had been told that improvement was possible.

Interest in self-improvement information seems also to depend on subjects' goals. In a series of studies, Butler (1992, 1993) manipulated subjects' goals for undertaking a task and measured subsequent interest in different kinds of information. In one study, sixth-grade students performed a creativity task under either mastery or ability instructions (Butler, 1992). In the mastery condition, students were told that the task . . . "can help you express your imagination, and develop new ways of looking at everyday things" (p. 936). In the ability condition, students were told that some people were more creative than others and that the task would test their creativity. After completing the task, students were given the opportunity to review different kinds of information. Subjects in the ability condition spent less time viewing task-relevant information and more time viewing normative information about other children's performance than subjects in the mastery condition. Interestingly, more than one third of the children in the ability condition avoided task-relevant information altogether. In a conceptually similar study with college students, Butler (1993) found that the provision of ability goals for an analytic thinking task created strong interest in normative performance information, to the exclusion of task information. In contrast, subjects given mastery goals requested information about other students' superior solutions and subsequently outperformed the ability-focus subjects. One implication of these studies for the present analysis is that studies that focus on testing fixed abilities may serve to heighten interest in normative information and may do so at the expense of information useful in completing the task. Mastery goals, in contrast, may communicate the idea that improvement is possible and thus create or preserve interest in self-improvment.

From the preceding review, it seems that upward comparisons are less likely to be perceived as aversive when improvement is possible. Strikingly consistent results have been obtained in studies that consider perceptions of control over one's standing on a comparison dimension. In an experiment in which people receiving disability benefits were exposed to a fictitious interview with another disabled person, Ybema and Buunk (1995) found greater positive affect following exposure to upward information than to downward comparison information and greater levels of identification with the successful target among respondents with high levels of perceived control over their disability, its consequences, and their ability to cope with it. In contrast, respondents with low perceived control identified more with the struggling downward target. Other studies (see Buunk, 1995, for a review) have compared interest in affiliation and comparison information for dimensions that seem more or less amenable to personal control and found stronger preferences for upward information on dimensions that seem more controllable (e.g., coping) than for dimensions that seem less controllable (e.g., problem severity).

In sum, several recent studies suggest that upward comparisons may be most beneficial to people undergoing stress when some future similarity to the upward target is possible; that is, when improvement is possible or when perceived control is high. Under such conditions, one may derive benefits from identifying with an upward target (Buunk & Ybema, chapter 12, this volume). One potential limitation to these findings is that favorable responses to upward comparisons may be restricted to settings in which the upward comparison contains some information useful in self-improvement. Although positive responses to upward comparisons can occur independently of the informativeness of the comparisons (Taylor et al., 1993), upward comparisons that contain information about successful performance—for example, not only the upward target's superior score, but also the target's answers and the reasoning behind them—seem to be rated especially favorably (Butler, 1993; Kulik & Mahler, chapter 8, this volume; Nosanchuk & Erickson, 1985; Ybema & Buunk, 1993).

### Directions for Future Research on Conceptions and Perceptions of Comparison Dimensions

It is, perhaps, appropriate to conclude this discussion of future-oriented aspects of comparison dimensions by identifying directions for future research on human developmental and individual differences. This section focuses, in particular, on how people conceptualize the likely future course of important life domains and on how such research might provide insight into social comparison activity across the life span.

***Developmental Expectations About Future Standing on Dimensions.*** The observation that perceptions of the potential for change in one's standing on a comparison dimension may moderate people's responses to social comparison information suggests that developmental research on whether people view dimensions such as personality and health as fixed entities or as incremental talents that can be developed in some way (cf. Dweck & Leggett, 1988) may have important implications for comparison activity. To the person with an entity conception of important life domains like intelligence or health, upward comparisons are likely to be frustrating; however, the same upward comparisons may be motivating to the person who believes he can develop such attributes through effort, education, or practice (Anderson, 1994). Butler's (1992, 1993) studies suggest that interventions designed to increase perceptions of skills as attributes to be developed rather than fixed abilities to be assessed might offset aversive reactions to upward comparisons in school, work, and health settings. For example, it would seem important for modeling interventions in health settings not only to expose patients to successful models but to make sure that critical therapeutic goals—for example, successful coping, adjustment to chronic illness, dietary change, exercise adoption, recovery from addiction, relapse prevention, and rehabilitation—are seen as specific skills that must be developed, rather than as tasks requiring fixed abilities, such as will power or athleticism. Consistent with this point, interventions that promote mastery goals instead of ability goals may serve to reduce the adverse consequences of upward comparisons and so allow people to profit from the information such comparisons provide (cf. Butler, 1993).

***Applications to Aging.*** The foregoing analysis may also have some implications for the study of social comparison and aging. Increasing evidence suggests that social comparisons may play an important role in maintaining well-being as people confront age-related declines in health (cf. Brandstadter & Greve, 1994; Heidrich & Ryff, 1993; Suls, Marco, & Tobin, 1991). Specifically, although elderly people report more feared possible selves in the health domain than younger respondents (Cross & Markus, 1991) and perceive greater decline in their physical health and ability, they do not report lower levels of self-esteem, higher levels of depression, or a lesser quality of life (see Brandstadter & Greve, 1994, for a review). In fact, recent studies have identified comparison processes as strong moderators of the relation between perceived physical health and psychological well-being. Among elderly people who make favorable comparisons to other elderly people, those with poorer physical health report levels of psychological well-being equal to those with better physical health (Brandstadter & Greve, 1994; Heidrich & Ryff, 1993). In addition, comparisons to some generalized image of the frail elderly seem to be especially useful in maintaining favorable health perceptions among the elderly (Brandstadter & Greve, 1994; Suls et al., 1991).

Studies that examine beliefs about the mutability of personality and intelligence over the lifespan may offer additional insight into the role that social comparisons may play in how people think about themselves as they age. For example, Heckhausen and Krueger (1993) surveyed a large sample of German adults about their beliefs concerning changes in central personality traits, such as agreeableness, extraversion, and emotional stability, over the lifespan. Respondents generally expected to peak at age 30 and to show declines in desirable traits and increases in undesirable traits as they aged. However, these expected declines co-occurred with high perceptions of personal control over their standing on these dimensions. Put simply, respondents expected to decline, but to do so less rapidly than other people. These results prompt the speculation that high perceptions of personal control over important aspects of functioning (or comparisons based on the rate of decline when decline is inevitable) may offset the negative consequences of perceptions or expectations of decline that may accompany aging.

***Understanding Individual Differences in Responses to Comparison Information.*** The observation that perceptions of one's likely future improvement or decline and perceptions of personal control over the course of one's improvement may moderate responses to social comparison information suggests that understanding individual differences in such perceptions may provide some insight into comparison activity. For example, both dispositional optimism and beliefs about personal control may influence such appraisals of comparison dimensions, especially in situations that are changing and uncertain (see Taylor & Aspinwall, 1996, for a review). Specifically, by definition, dispositional optimists expect good future outcomes. This tendency may bias optimists' assessments of their likely future standing on specific dimensions toward the "improve" end of the continuum. Tendencies to see oneself as likely to improve much of the time may make social comparison information of either direction beneficial: for example, a woman may profit from upward comparisons because she believes she will attain good future outcomes; moreover, she may be protected from the adverse effects of downward comparisons because she believes her standing is unlikely to decline. Support for these predictions about responses to downward comparisons comes from Hemphill and Lehman's (1991) survey of people with multiple sclerosis. Respondents who were high in dispositional optimism reported more favorable affective reactions to downward comparisons on the physical health dimension and fewer unfavorable reactions than people low in optimism.

A similar argument may be made about people with strong beliefs in personal control. Such people may be buffered from adverse responses to comparison information because they believe that by personal effort they can achieve the good standing of an upward comparison target or avoid the poor standing of a downward target. These speculations raise the possibility that people with pessimistic beliefs or low perceived control may be especially vulnerable to the adverse effects of both upward and downward comparisons (cf. Buunk et al., 1990). In particular, depressed or dysphoric people may be especially vulnerable (see Lyubomirsky & Ross, 1996, for related evidence), because of their characteristically dim view of the future and the certainty with which they may hold such views (cf. Andersen, Spielman, & Bargh, 1992) and/or reduced perceptions of personal control over important life domains. In such cases, people may perceive both upward and downward comparisons as aversive because they may not believe they can improve to the level of the upward target, but may believe that they can, and inevitably will, decline to the level of the downward target.

For these reasons, continued research examining the degree to which stressed populations appear to develop increased optimism and perceptions of control (Taylor, 1983; Taylor et al., 1992) and to maintain perceptions of control by shifting control efforts away from disease progression to more controllable aspects of chronic illness (Affleck, Tennen, Pfeiffer, & Fifield, 1987; Thompson, Sobolew-Shubin, Galbraith, Schwankovsky, & Cruzen, 1993) may provide important insight into how people facing threats to health and well-being maintain beliefs that may allow them to profit from different kinds of social comparisons and to be protected from some of the negative implications of such comparisons. It remains to be seen, of course, whether high levels of control beliefs and optimism render people immune to potentially useful negative information that may be contained in both upward and downward comparisons (see Aspinwall & Brunhart, 1996; Aspinwall & Taylor, in press; Taylor, Collins, Skokan, & Aspinwall, 1989, for discussions of such issues). That is, it may sometimes be adaptive to conclude from exposure to an upward target that one cannot achieve the target's superior level of performance if, in fact, this conclusion is true. Such decisions may be essential to adaptive early disengagement from goals that are inappropriate, that cannot be achieved, or that are not worth the effort required to reach them. As noted earlier, it is often necessary for people with chronic illnesses to disengage from efforts to control their prognosis and to switch their control efforts to aspects of the illness that are more amenable to personal control to maintain psychological well-being. Interestingly, the same individual differences that may protect people from the adverse effects of social comparisons—optimism and control beliefs—seem also to be associated with the ability to accomplish the transfer of problem-solving effort from uncontrollable to relatively controllable aspects of stressful situations (Aspinwall & Richter, 1996; Scheier, Weintraub, & Carver, 1986; Vitaliano, Russo, & Maiuro, 1987). Longitudinal studies that track the relations among such individual differences and shifts in the domain and direction of comparison activity should provide insight into adjustment to chronic illness and other stressors.

## SUMMARY AND CONCLUSIONS

This chapter presents a framework for analyzing social comparison activity with respect to its implications for future actions and outcomes. Most comparison situations, especially those involving mental and physical health, represent ongoing events in various stages of development. People are somewhere in a course of action with respect to a stressful event, with corresponding variations in the psychological distress and uncertainty surrounding that event, and they have expectations about the likely future course of that event and their ability to influence what that course may be. This review suggests that these factors may jointly influence the motives underlying both people's comparison activity and their reactions to particular kinds of comparison information. These discussions also suggest that an analysis of the comparison situation and its implications for future action may help to explain when upward and downward comparisons may be perceived as beneficial or harmful to people coping with illness and other stressors.

This concluding section examines the conceptual yield of a future-oriented analysis of social comparison activity and suggests ways in which research in health settings may be ideal for understanding more future-oriented and proactive forms of social comparison activity.

## A Future-Oriented Perspective on the Costs and Benefits of Upward and Downward Comparisons

In general, in contrast to the idea that upward and downward comparisons are either inherently beneficial or inherently harmful, the present analysis suggests that the psychological impact of social comparisons may depend in part on their implications for some future action or outcome. That is, to predict the effects of exposure to upward or downward comparison information in a given situation, we need to know where the comparer is in the course of events and what the comparer expects to be doing in the future.

What are the implications of a future-oriented analysis for understanding comparison activity among people under stress? First, my analysis raises the possibility that the preponderance of self-enhancing comparisons among threatened persons found in the social comparison literature may be a partial function of a focus on immediate or focal threats to fixed abilities or traits. In particular, many studies have examined a fairly restricted part of the comparison space—comparisons made immediately after some threat to well-being on dimensions in which subjects' standing is fixed and in which they may not expect to engage in any future activity. In this case, comparison activity is likely to be somewhat static, because the situation itself is a dead end and the person's relative standing is unlikely to change. Under such circumstances, affective needs—specifically, an individual's need to feel better about his low standing—are likely to drive comparison activity downward and to reduce interest in upward comparisons. In addition, if a person expects little future involvement with the comparison dimension, she has little to lose by focusing exclusively on comparison information that would allow her to feel better. Under such conditions, there would be little constructive information to gain from upward comparisons, and much comfort in knowing that others did worse. As a result, studies of comparison processes among threatened persons yield overwhelming evidence that downward comparisons are preferred and that upward comparisons are experienced as aversive.

The present review suggests that comparison activity is likely to be quite different as one moves away from the focal stressful event. When one's standing on the dimension has the potential to change, and as one acquires more information about the stressor, more varied responses to upward and downward comparisons may emerge. Specifically, when the event has yet to occur or its impact has yet to be fully realized, comparison activity may not be driven toward downward targets by needs to regulate affect and maintain self-esteem. Instead both upward and downward comparisons may provide important—and welcome—information about the nature of the event, its likely future course, and ways of managing it or even preventing it. In one recent study of people awaiting sweeping changes in their disability benefits (Buunk, 1995), upward affiliation and information-seeking preferences were strongest among the most distressed respondents, a finding that would be difficult to interpret without considering what people hoped to gain from such contact and information (cf. Buunk & Ybema, chapter 12; Kulik & Mahler, chapter 8, this volume; Taylor & Lobel, 1989).

Along these lines, a future-oriented analysis of comparison activity may provide insight into how people learn about stressful situations. To this point, my review has assumed that would-be comparers already know quite a bit about the parameters of a given stressful situation, such as its likely future course and its amenity to personal control. In many laboratory studies, these questions are a moot point, because the dimension on which false feedback is provided doesn't exist and subjects may not necessarily be concerned about their future performance in that domain. In naturalistic settings, however, social comparison activity may play a useful role in yielding information about the nature and likely course of potential stressors (cf. Kulik & Mahler, chapter 8, this volume; Ruble & Frey, 1991). Specifically, gathering information about other people's experiences and outcomes may provide information not only about the magnitude of potential threats to well-being, but also about their likely duration, their impact on other life domains, and ways of coping with them.

Taken together, these observations suggest that much experimental research on comparison processes among threatened people may have both underestimated some of the potential benefits of upward comparisons and artificially limited some of the potential risks of downward comparisons. First, experimental studies that focus on threats to fixed abilities may dampen interest in upward comparisons (cf. Major et al., 1991; Testa & Major, 1990) and reduce the motivation to weather their affective costs. In contrast, in situations in which one's performance may improve (for whatever reason), people may welcome upward comparisons, particularly when a comparison target's superior performance provides information useful in self-improvement. In situations where people have many trials in which to learn a task, in which individual mastery goals are emphasized over normative ability goals, and in which people perceive some degree of control over their outcomes, people appear to seek and to profit from upward information (cf. Butler, 1993; Roese, 1994; Taylor et al., 1993; Ybema & Buunk, 1995), even when they have failed or are otherwise distressed (Buunk, 1995; Markman et al., 1993; Ybema & Buunk, 1993).

Finally, experimental studies to date may have also underestimated some of the risks of downward comparisons. Although downward comparisons clearly provide affective, self-evaluative, and perhaps also motivational benefits to people experiencing threats to well-being (cf. Aspinwall & Taylor, 1993; Wills, 1981, 1991), they may also have some costs, depending on the situation. If a person's standing is fixed or he or she does not expect to encounter the situation again, there is little cost to focusing on the outcomes of those who did worse than he or she did. However, in situations in which a person has ongoing involvement with the comparison dimension, downward comparisons may impede self-improvement efforts in a given domain over time (Crocker & Major, 1989; Gibbons et al., 1996; Taylor, Wayment, & Carillo, 1995). Although the mechanisms underlying such effects have yet to be identified, it is likely that such effects may be partially due to the inability of downward comparisons, relative to upward ones, to provide information directly useful in self-improvement efforts. Downward comparisons may also decrease expectations of success under some conditions (Gibbons et al., 1996). Finally, in situations with potential future engagement and the potential for decline, downward comparisons may provide a frightening vision of the future (Brickman & Bulman, 1977) and may produce more negative affect than no comparison information at all (Aspinwall & Kissam, 1995).

### Using Health Settings to Expand the Research Base of Social Comparison Theory

Throughout the chapter, I have tried to highlight ways in which most health-related comparisons capture the critical elements of future-oriented comparison activity. In particular, most health-related comparisons simultaneously involve some degree of future engagement with the comparison dimension and some degree of uncertainty about the future. Moreover, many health decisions are made in the service of some future goal, usually either to achieve or to avoid some future outcome. Unlike many other kinds of dimensions, health-related dimensions offer a range of situations that vary in terms of their likely improvement or decline and in the degree of actual or perceived control they afford. For these reasons, the continued study of social comparison activity in health settings has the potential to capture a broad range of future-oriented comparison activity.

The current review suggests that such potential has yet to be fully realized for several reasons. First, researchers have oversampled comparison dimensions that either are fixed or are both subject to improvement and amenable to personal control, such as adjustment to college (cf. Aspinwall & Taylor, 1993) and task acquisition (cf. Butler, 1992, 1993; Ruble & Frey, 1991). One potentially important limitation of such studies, and by implication, of our analysis of proactive comparison activity, is that comparison activity on such dimensions may not be easily generalized to coping with stressors that do not match this profile. In the achievement context, for example, the expected trajectory of task acquisition is one of predictable linear improvement, followed perhaps by plateaus or declines in performance with age (Ruble & Frey, 1991). That is, as we learn things, we usually get better at them, or at least expect to. Comparisons undertaken in health settings may only sometimes have such a profile. Instead, the future course of events may be uncertain, with decline possible or even likely. Continued study of comparison activity undertaken among people facing terminal or progressive illnesses, such as cancer and multiple sclerosis, will provide additional insight into such processes (cf. Hemphill & Lehman, 1991; Wood & VanderZee, chapter 10, this volume).

For these reasons, the continued examination of social comparison processes among people facing health threats and other stressors has considerable potential to expand the research base of social comparison theory. Conditions such as progressive illness, depression, and addiction simultaneously present the challenge of improvement and the possibility of decline in health and functioning. Moreover, some aspects of chronic conditions are amenable to control, whereas others are not. For these reasons, illness and other stressors are likely to evoke comparison processes that are varied and that serve many motives over time. Studies that track the relation of comparison activity to changes in perceptions of control over different aspects of chronic illness and other stressors may continue to provide insight into how people manage the affective and practical implications of both upward and downward comparisons, even as their situations worsen (cf. Buunk et al., 1990).

Health research has the potential to broaden our understanding of social comparison activity in other ways. For example, another potentially important difference between achievement settings and health settings that may affect responses to comparison information is whether the situation has the potential for selective disengagement. In many learning and performance situations, if we fail to improve, we have the option of quitting and choosing other activities (cf. Aspinwall & Richter, 1996; Crocker & Major, 1989). As many authors have noted, comparisons undertaken in health settings rarely afford the possibility of disengagement. One cannot decide whether to be a breast cancer patient, to forego a heart attack, or refuse to age when comparison activity yields unfavorable results in the same way that one can abandon one's Wimbledon hopes in the face of overwhelming evidence of mediocre tennis ability. If one cannot disengage from a comparison domain, one may have to be quite creative in selecting or creating aspects of comparison information on which one is relatively advantaged (cf. Brandstadter & Greve, 1994; Taylor et al., 1983; Wood & VanderZee, chapter 10, this volume).

Finally, a future-oriented approach to social comparisons and health may broaden our understanding of social comparison activity by calling attention to how people conceptualize dimensions, such as stress and health, and the relation of such beliefs to psychological outcomes and health behaviors. For example, understanding whether people conceptualize entities such as physical and mental health as fixed or incremental may provide insight into whether people undertake behaviors designed to improve or maintain their current good health and how they respond to conditions that threaten or compromise their health. It is also possible that our views of such dimensions may be influenced by available social comparison information. The grandmother who takes up mountain biking may change our beliefs about the mutability of physical fitness later in life, whereas the yo-yo dieter who never achieves his goal may make us believe that our weight has an inherent setpoint from which it will not deviate, regardless of our behavior.

A rich literature on adjustment to chronic illness and other threats to mental and physical health has demonstrated that social comparisons play an important role in how we feel about ourselves following adversity. Taking a more proactive and future-oriented view of social comparison activity may highlight ways in which people facing stressful circumstances use comparison information not only for the purposes of self-evaluation but also for the purposes of self-regulation. That is, social comparisons may provide information that is useful both in adjustment to current outcomes and in the prediction and control of future outcomes. In this way, future-oriented social comparisons may function like Dickens' Ghost of Christmas Future: they may sound alarms of future danger as well as provide models of future achievements. Expanding the research base of social comparison theory to take advantage of the future-oriented nature of health domains and developmental phenomena, such as aging, may provide additional insight into the varied mechanisms through which information about other people is used both to understand the events of our lives and to alter them.

## ACKNOWLEDGMENTS

I acknowledge the support of the Department of Psychology of the University of Maryland at College Park in the preparation of this chapter, and I thank Kyra Kissam for her assistance in this work. I also thank Tom Wills and the editors of this volume for many helpful comments on an earlier version of this chapter.

## REFERENCES

Affleck, G., Tennen, E., Pfeiffer, C., & Fifield, J. (1987). Appraisals of control and predictability in adapting to a chronic disease. *Journal of Personality and Social Psychology, 53,* 273–279.

Andersen, S. M., Spielman, L. A., & Bargh, J. A. (1992). Future-event schemas and certainty about the future: Automaticity in depressives' future-event predictions. *Journal of Personality and Social Psychology, 63,* 711–723.

Anderson, C. (1994, August). *Increasing positive interpretations of social comparison: The effect of conception of ability.* Poster session presented at the annual meeting of the American Psychological Association, Los Angeles.

Aspinwall, L. G., & Brunhart, S. M. (1996). Distinguishing optimism from denial: Optimistic beliefs predict attention to health threats. *Personality and Social Psychology Bulletin, 22,* 993–1003.

Aspinwall, L. G., & Kissam, K. D. (1995). *From bad to worse: Potential for decline moderates the effects of downward comparisons.* Manuscript in preparation.

Aspinwall, L. G., & Richter, L. (1996). *Positive beliefs and nonproductive persistence: Optimism and self-mastery predict rapid disengagement from insoluble tasks.* Manuscript submitted for publication.

Aspinwall, L. G., & Taylor, S. E. (1993). The effects of social comparison direction, threat, and self-esteem on affect, self-evaluation, and expected success. *Journal of Personality and Social Psychology, 64,* 708–722.

Aspinwall, L. G., & Taylor, S. E. (in press). A stitch in time: Self-regulation and proactive coping. *Psychological Bulletin.*

Bandura, A., & Jourden, F. J. (1991). Self-regulatory mechanisms governing the impact of social comparison on complex decision-making. *Journal of Personality and Social Psychology, 60,* 941–951.

Brandstadter, J., & Greve, W. (1994). The aging self: Stabilizing and protective processes. *Developmental Review, 14,* 52–80.

Brickman, P., & Bulman, R. J. (1977). Pleasure and pain in social comparison. In J. M. Suls & R. L. Miller (Eds.), *Social comparison processes: Theoretical and empirical perspectives* (pp. 149–186). Washington, DC: Hemisphere.

Brown, J. D. (1990). Evaluating one's abilities: Shortcuts and stumbling blocks on the road to self-knowledge. *Journal of Experimental Social Psychology, 26,* 149–167.

Butler, R. (1992). What young people want to know when: Effects of mastery and ability goals on interest in different kinds of social comparisons. *Journal of Personality and Social Psychology, 62,* 934–943.

Butler, R. (1993). Effects of task- and ego-achievement goals on information seeking during task engagement. *Journal of Personality and Social Psychology, 65,* 18–31.

Buunk, B. P. (1994). Social comparison processes under stress: Towards an integration of classic and recent perspectives. In W. Stroebe & M. Hewstone (Eds.) *European review of social psychology* (Vol. 5, pp. 212-241). Chichester: Wiley.

Buunk, B. P. (1995). Comparison direction and comparison dimension among disabled individuals: Toward a refined conceptualization of social comparison under stress. *Personality and Social Psychology Bulletin, 21,* 316–330.

Buunk, B. P., Collins, R. L., Taylor, S. E., VanYperen, N. W., & Dakof, G. A. (1990). The affective consequences of social comparison: Either direction has its ups and downs. *Journal of Personality and Social Psychology, 59,* 1238–1249.

Carver, C. S., & Scheier, M. F. (1990). Principles of self-regulation: Action and emotion. In E. T. Higgins & R. M. Sorrentino (Eds.), *Handbook of motivation and cognition* (Vol. 2, pp. 3–52). New York: Guilford.

Collins, R. L. (1996). For better or worse: The impact of upward social comparison on self-evaluations. *Psychological Bulletin, 119,* 51–69.

Crocker, J., & Major, B. (1989). Social stigma and self-esteem: The self-protective properties of stigma. *Psychological Review, 96,* 608–630.

Cross, S., & Markus, H. (1991). Possible selves across the life span. *Human Development, 34,* 230–255.

Croyle, R. T. (1992). Appraisal of health threats: Cognition, motivation, and social comparison. *Cognitive Theory and Research, 16,* 165–182.

Dickens, C. (1843/1967). *A Christmas carol: A facsimile of the manuscript in the Pierpont Morgan Library.* New York: Heineman.

Dweck, C. S., & Leggett, E. L. (1988). A social-cognitive approach to motivation and personality. *Psychological Review, 95,* 256–273.

Festinger, L. (1954). A theory of social comparison processes. *Human Relations, 7,* 117–140.

Folkman, S. (1984). Personal control and stress and coping processes: A theoretical analysis. *Journal of Personality and Social Psychology, 46,* 839–852.

Folkman, S., & Lazarus, R. S. (1985). If it changes, it must be a process: Study of emotion and coping during three stages of a college examination. *Journal of Personality and Social Psychology, 48,* 150–170.

Gibbons, F. X. (1986). Social comparison and depression: Company's effect on misery. *Journal of Personality and Social Psychology, 51,* 140–148.

Gibbons, F. X., Gerrard, M., Blanton, H., & Eggleston, T. (1996). *Does social comparison make a difference? The influence of comparison level on outcome.* Manuscript submitted for publication.

Gibbons, F. X., & Boney-McCoy, S. (1991). Self esteem, similarity, and reactions to active versus passive downward comparison. *Journal of Personality and Social Psychology, 60,* 414–424.

Gibbons, F. X., & Gerrard, M. (1989). Effects of upward and downward social comparison on mood states. *Journal of Social and Clinical Psychology, 8,* 14–31.

Gibbons, F. X., & Gerrard, M. (1991). Downward comparison and coping with threat. In J. Suls & T. A. Wills (Eds.), *Social comparison: Contemporary theory and research* (pp. 317–345). NJ: Lawrence Erlbaum Associates.

Heckhausen, J., & Krueger, J. (1993). Developmental expectations for the self and most other people: Age grading in three functions of social comparison. *Developmental Psychology, 29,* 539–548.

Heidrich, S. M., & Ryff, C. D. (1993). The role of social comparison processes in the psychological adaptation of elderly adults. *Journal of Gerontology: Psychological Sciences, 48,* 127–136.

Hemphill, K. J., & Lehman, D. R. (1991). Social comparisons and their affective consequences: The importance of comparison dimension and individual difference variables. *Journal of Social and Clinical Psychology, 10,* 372–394.

Hooker, K., & Kaus, C. R. (1992). Possible selves and health behaviors in later life. *Journal*

*of Aging and Health, 4,* 390–411.
Hooker, K, & Kaus, C. R. (1994). Health-related possible selves in young and middle adulthood. *Psychology and Aging, 9,* 126–133.
Jensen, M. P., & Karoly, P. (1992). Comparative self-evaluation and depressive affect among chronic pain patients: An examination of selective evaluation theory. *Cognitive Therapy and Research, 16,* 297–308.
Jones, S. C., & Regan, D. T. (1974). Ability evaluation through social comparison. *Journal of Experimental Social Psychology, 10,* 133–146.
Kenrick, D. T., Montello, D. R., Gutierres, S. E., & Trost, M. R. (1993). Effects of physical attractiveness on affect and perceptual judgments: When social comparison overrides social reinforcement. *Personality and Social Psychology Bulletin, 19,* 195–199.
Kulik, J. A., & Mahler, H. I. (1987). Effects of preoperative roomate assignment on preoperative anxiety and recovery from coronary bypass surgery. *Health Psychology, 6,* 525–543.
Lazarus, R. S., & Folkman, S. (1984). *Stress, appraisal and coping.* New York: Springer.
Lyubomirsky, S., & Ross, L. (1996). *Hedonic consequences of social comparison: A contrast of happy and unhappy people.* Manuscript submitted for publication.
Major, B. (1989). Gender differences in comparisons and entitlement: Implications for comparable worth. *Journal of Social Issues, 45*(4), 99–115.
Major, B., Testa, M., & Bylsma, W. H. (1991). Responses to upward and downward social comparisons: The impact of esteem-relevance and perceived control. In J. Suls & T. A. Wills (Eds.), *Social comparison: Contemporary theory and research* (pp. 237–259). NJ: Lawrence Erlbaum Associates.
Markman, K. D., Gavanski, I., Sherman, S. J., & McMullen, M. N. (1993). The mental simulation of better and worse possible worlds. *Journal of Experimental Social Psychology, 29,* 87–109.
Markus, H., & Nurius, P. (1986). Possible selves. *American Psychologist, 41,* 954–969.
Marsh, H. W., & Parker, J. W. (1984). Determinants of student self-concept: Is it better to be a relatively large fish in a small pond even if you don't learn to swim as well? *Journal of Personality and Social Psychology, 47,* 213–231.
Martin, J. (1986). The tolerance of injustice. In J. M. Olsen, C. P. Herman, & M. P. Zanna (Eds.), *Relative deprivation and social comparison: The Ontario Symposium* (Vol. 4, pp. 217–242). NJ: Lawrence Erlbaum Associates.
McGrath, J. E., & Beehr, T. A. (1990). Time and the stress process: Some temporal issues in the conceptualization and measurement of stress. *Stress Medicine, 6,* 93–104.
Molleman, E., Pruyn, J., & van Knippenberg, A. (1986). Social comparison processes among cancer patients. *British Journal of Social Psychology, 25,* 1–13.
Morse, S., & Gergen, K. J. (1970). Social comparison, self-consistency, and the concept of the self. *Journal of Personality and Social Psychology, 36,* 148–156.
Nosanchuk, T. A., & Erickson, B. H. (1985). How high is up? Calibrating social comparison in the real world. *Journal of Personality and Social Psychology, 48,* 624–634.
Pyszczynski, T., Greenberg, J., & LaPrelle, J. (1985). Social comparison after success and failure: Biased search for information consistent with a self-serving conclusion. *Journal of Experimental Social Psychology, 47,* 780–792.
Roese, N. J. (1994). The functional basis of counterfactual thinking. *Journal of Personality and Social Psychology, 66,* 805–818.
Rosenstock, I. M. (1974). The health belief model and preventive behavior. *Health Education Monographs, 2,* 354–386.
Ruble, D. N., & Frey, K. S. (1991). Changing patterns of comparative behavior as skills are acquired: A functional model of self-evaluation. In J. Suls & T. A. Wills (Eds.), *Social comparison: Contemporary theory and research* (pp. 79–113). NJ: Lawrence Erlbaum Associates.

Salovey, P., & Rodin, J. (1984). Some antecedents and consequences of social-comparison jealousy. *Journal of Personality and Social Psychology, 47,* 780–792.
Salovey, P., Rothman, A. J., & Rodin, J. (in press). Social psychology and health behavior. In D. Gilbert, S. Fiske, & G. Lindzey (Eds.), *Handbook of social psychology* (4th ed.). New York: McGraw-Hill.
Scheier, M. F., Weintraub, J. K., & Carver, C. S. (1986). Coping with stress: Divergent strategies of optimists and pessimists. *Journal of Personality and Social Psychology, 51,* 1257–1264.
Smith, C. A., & Lazarus, R. L. (1990). Emotion and adaptation. In L. A. Perrin (Ed.), *Handbook of personality: Theory and research* (pp. 609–637). New York: Guilford.
Stanton, A. L. (1992). Downward comparison in infertile couples. *Basic and Applied Social Psychology, 13,* 389–403.
Suls, J., Marco, C., A., & Tobin, S. (1991). The role of temporal comparison, social comparison, and direct appraisal in the elderly's self-evaluations of health. *Journal of Applied Social Psychology, 21,* 1125–1144.
Taylor, S. E. (1983). Adjustment to threatening events: A theory of cognitive adaptation. *American Psychologist, 38,* 1161–1173.
Taylor, S. E., & Aspinwall, L. G. (1996). Mediating and moderating processes in psychosocial stress: Appraisal, coping, resistance and vulnerability. In H. B. Kaplan (Ed.) *Psychosocial stress: Perspectives on structure, theory, life-course, and methods* (pp. 71–110). Orlando, FL: Academic Press.
Taylor, S. E., Aspinwall, L. G., Giuliano, T. A., Dakof, G. A., & Reardon, K. (1993). Storytelling and coping with stressful events. *Journal of Applied Social Psychology, 23,* 703–733.
Taylor, S. E., Buunk, B. P., & Aspinwall, L. G. (1990). Social comparison, stress and coping. *Personality and Social Psychology Bulletin, 16,* 74–89.
Taylor, S. E., Collins, R. L., Skokan, L. A., & Aspinwall, L. G. (1989). Maintaining positive illusions in the face of negative information: Getting the facts without letting them get to you. *Journal of Social and Clinical Psychology, 8,* 114–129.
Taylor, S. E., Kemeny, M. E., Aspinwall, L. G., Schneider, S. G., Rodriguez, R., Herbert, M., & Dudley, J. (1992). Optimism, coping, psychological distress, and high-risk sexual behavior among men at risk for Acquired Immunodeficiency Syndrome (AIDS). *Journal of Personality and Social Psychology, 63,* 460–473.
Taylor, S. E., & Lobel, M. (1989). Social comparison activity under threat: Downward evaluation and upward contacts. *Psychological Review, 96,* 569–575.
Taylor, S. E., & Schneider, S. K. (1989). Coping and the simulation of events. *Social Cognition, 7,* 176–196.
Taylor, S. E., Wayment, H. A., & Carrillo, M. A. (1995). Social comparison and self-regulation. In R. M. Sorrentino & E. T. Higgins (Eds.), *Handbook of motivation and cognition* (pp. 3–27). New York: Guilford.
Taylor, S. E., Wood, J. V., & Lichtman, R. R. (1983). It could be worse: Selective evaluation as a response to victimization. *Journal of Social Issues, 39*(2), 19–40.
Tesser, A. (1988). Toward a self-evaluation maintenance model of social behavior. In L. Berkowitz (Ed.), *Advances in experimental social psychology* (Vol. 21, pp. 181–227). Orlando, FL: Academic Press.
Tesser, A., Millar, M., & Moore, J. (1988). Some affective consequences of social comparison and reflection processes: The pain and pleasure of being close. *Journal of Personality and Social Psychology, 54,* 49–61.
Tesser, A., & Paulhus, D. (1983). The definition of self: Private and public self-evaluation management strategies. *Journal of Personality and Social Psychology, 44,* 672–682.
Testa, M., & Major, B. (1990). The impact of social comparisons after failure: The moderating effects of perceived control. *Basic and Applied Social Psychology, 11,* 205–218.

Thompson, S. C., Sobolew-Shubin, A., Galbraith, M. E., Schwankovsky, L., & Cruzen, D. (1993). Maintaining perceptions of control: Finding perceived control in low-control circumstances. *Journal of Personality and Social Psychology, 64,* 293–304.

Trope, Y. (1986). Self-assessment, self-enhancement, and achievement behavior. In R. M. Sorrentino & E. T. Higgins (Eds.), *Handbook of motivation and cognition* (pp. 350–378). New York: Guilford.

Vitaliano, P. O., Russo, J., & Maiuro, R. D. (1987). Locus of control, type of stressor, and appraisal within a cognitive-phenomenological model of stress. *Journal of Research in Personality, 21,* 224–237.

Weinstein, N. D. (1984). Why it won't happen to me: Perceptions of risk factors and illness susceptibility. *Health Psychology, 3,* 431–457.

Weinstein, N. D. (1988). The precaution adoption process. *Health Psychology, 7,* 355–386.

Wheeler, L., & Miyake, K. (1992). Social comparison in everyday life. *Journal of Personality and Social Psychology, 62,* 760–773.

Wills, T. A. (1981). Downward comparison principles in social psychology. *Psychological Bulletin, 90,* 245–271.

Wills, T. A. (1991). Similarity and self-esteem in downward comparison. In J. Suls & T. A. Wills (Eds.), *Social comparison: Contemporary theory and research* (pp. 51–78). NJ: Lawrence Erlbaum Associates.

Wood, J. V. (1989). Theory and research concerning social comparisons of personal attributes. *Psychological Bulletin, 106,* 231–248.

Wood, J. V., Taylor, S. E., & Lichtman, R. R. (1985). Social comparison in adjustment to breast cancer. *Journal of Personality and Social Psychology, 49,* 1169–1183.

Ybema, J. F., & Buunk, B. P. (1993). Aiming at the top? Upward social comparison of abilities after failure. *European Journal of Social Psychology, 23,* 627–645.

Ybema, J. F., & Buunk, B. P. (1995). Affective responses to social comparison: A study among disabled individuals. *British Journal of Social Psychology, 34,* 279–292.

# CHAPTER 6

# Modes and Families of Coping: An Analysis of Downward Comparison in the Structure of Other Cognitive and Behavioral Mechanisms

Thomas Ashby Wills
*Ferkauf Graduate School of Psychology and Albert Einstein College of Medicine*

The purpose of this chapter is to consider the place of social comparisonas a coping mechanism within the structure of other coping mechanisms. It is known that social comparison may be used to cope with uncertainty, threats to self-esteem, and negative life events (e.g., Affleck & Tennen, 1991; Affleck, Tennen, Pfeiffer, & Fifield, 1988; DeVellis, Holt, Renner, Blalock, Blanchard, Cook, Klotz, Mikow, & Harring, 1990; DeVellis, Blalock, Holt, Renner, Blanchard, & Klotz, 1991; Gibbons, 1986; Gibbons, Benbow, & Gerrard, 1994; Helgeson & Taylor, 1993; Pelham, 1991, 1993; Pyszczynski, Greenberg, & LaPrelle, 1985; Spencer, Josephs, & Steele, 1993; Suls & Wan, 1987; Wood, Taylor, & Lichtman, 1985). Theories of comparison-oriented coping have posited that through selective use of information from the social environment, an individual can obtain a relatively favorable comparison with one or more target others and that favorable comparison situation then produces an increase in subjective well-being for the comparer (Wills, 1981, 1987). On this view, social comparison fits criteria for definition as a coping mechanism; moreover, earlier studies have provided evidence of its use in a range of life contexts, including but not limited to physical health problems (Gibbons & Gerrard, 1991).

A number of other coping mechanisms can be distinguished empirically (Carver, Scheier, & Weintraub, 1989; Lazarus & Folkman, 1984; Stone, Helder, & Schneider, 1988). I have proposed that several specific coping mechanisms (modes) may be grouped together under higher-order domains (families) of coping mechanisms that share essential similarities. These include domains characterized as *behavioral coping,*

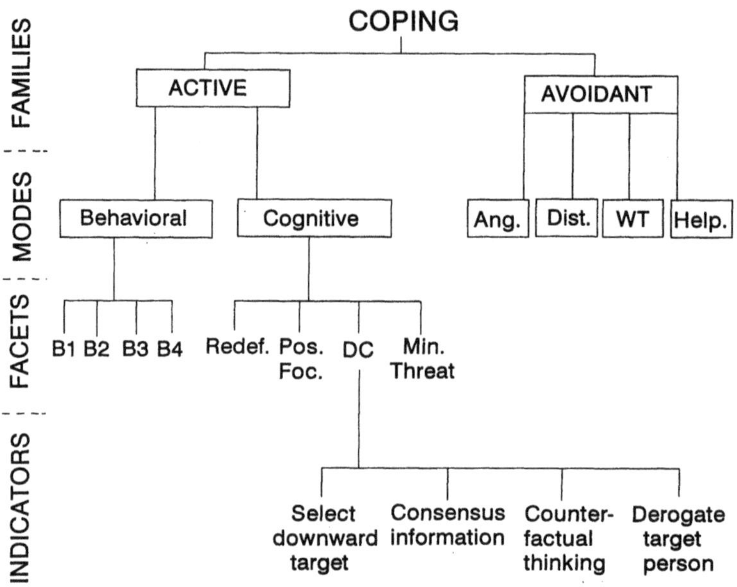


FIG. 6.1. Theoretical model for structure of modes and families of coping. Indicated are families of Active Coping and Avoidant Coping. Modes of Behavioral and Cognitive Coping are listed under Active family. Four modes of Avoidant Coping are listed under Avoidant family; these are ang. = anger coping; dist. = distraction coping; WT = wishful thinking; help. = helplessness. Four unnamed facets are listed under behavioral coping (B1, B2, B3, B4). Four facets are listed under cognitive coping (Redef. = situation redefinition, Pos. Foc. = focus on positives, DC = downward comparison, Min. threat = threat minization). Four indicators are listed under facet of downward comparison (selection of downward target person, selective processing of social consensus information, use of counter-factual thinking, derogation of target).

mechanisms in which an active approach is taken to solving the problem; domains characterized as *cognitive coping,* mechanisms in which cognitive strategies are used to perceive the problem situation in a more favorable light; and domains characterized as *avoidant coping,* involving mechanisms for coping with problems in ways that avoid dealing with the problematic issue. This kind of hierarchical model is outlined in Fig. 6.1. The prevailing viewis that behavioral and cognitive coping both represent adaptive types of coping and will be negatively correlated with the avoidant domain, which is posited as a maladaptive way of coping with problems.[1]

[1]I recognize that in traditional coping theory, no given type of coping is assumed to be universally effective or ineffective, and the situational context of the problem and the coping implementation should always be considered. For example, distraction may be

Research on social comparison has usually focused on comparison-oriented coping, studied alone as a coping mechanism. Although this research has provided information on how people may use social comparison as a coping strategy, it has not considered how coping through social comparison is related to coping through mechanisms that may be pursued concurrently. This oversight could lead to restricted theoretical perspectives that miss connections between social comparison and other types of coping. A single-mechanism focus could also lead to inappropriate analytic strategies that fail to control for correlations among different types of coping.

## LOCATING DOWNWARD COMPARISON IN THE STRUCTURE OF COPING MECHANISMS

This chapter considers the question of where downward comparison is located within the structure of other coping mechanisms.[2] It could be argued that because downward comparison involves selective use of information, it is cognitive in nature and thus a member of a large group of cognitive coping mechanisms. However, an alternative position would construe downward comparison as a means of avoiding rather than actively confronting a problem; this would put it in the group of avoidant coping mechanisms. A third position proposes that social comparison may be used in concert with behavioral mechanisms to mobilize an effort for actively dealing with the problem; on this view it would be classified as a type of coping that shares essential attributes with both cognitive and behavioral mechanisms (Wills, 1991a).

It is important to determine where social comparison falls within the structure of coping mechanisms in order to identify its similarities to or differences from other coping mechanisms, to predict the situations in which comparison-oriented coping would be most effective in enhancing adjustment, and to suggest statistical procedures for analyses that recognize the multivariate nature of coping efforts. Unfortunately, the theoretical approaches to this question yielded by the coping literature are by no means straightforward. A variety of two- and

---

most effective for coping with short-term physical stressors (McCaul & Malott, 1984; Suls & Fletcher, 1985). However our prior studies with adolescents, with substance use as an outcome, generally find that behavioral coping is adaptive and avoidant coping maladaptive.

[2]The focus of the this chapter is on downward comparison as a coping mechanism. The question of how downward comparison and upward comparison may be used in different situations or for different coping goals is considered in detail elsewhere (see, e.g., Taylor & Lobel, 1989; Tigges, Wills, & Link, 1996; Wills, 1991a; Wood, 1989).

three-dimension classification systems have been proposed, including approach versus avoidance (Roth & Cohen, 1986), problem-focused versus emotion-focused coping (Compas, Malcarne, & Fondacaro, 1988), active coping versus avoidant coping (Moos & Schaefer, 1993; Rohde, Lewinsohn, Tilson, & Seeley, 1990), and engagement versus disengagement (Carver, Scheier, & Weintraub, 1989). However, these approaches all involve rather different concepts of the structure of coping, they define coping mechanisms classified under their various rubrics differently, they have not drawn explicit linkages to social comparison research, and their originators generally have not conducted empirical analyses to support the proposed structures.

In this chapter I take a combined theoretical–empirical approach to the question. First, I present current theory about the hierarchic structure of coping processes. Next I discuss the theory of how downward comparison may be employed as a coping mechanism and consider theoretical arguments about how comparison-oriented coping may be classified within the structure of other domains of coping. Then I report some analyses of data from studies of adolescents' coping mechanisms that bear on the question. In a final section I draw some conclusions and suggest directions for further research on coping through social comparison. I conclude that downward comparison may be classified with cognitive and behavioral mechanisms in the "active" category but that ambiguities in the data suggest that downward comparison may have avoidant aspects; thus, this type of coping may have both positive and negative aspects. For future research I suggest that cognitive coping is quite complex and deserves detailed attention in both assessment and analysis.

## PROPOSED HIGHER-ORDER STRUCTURE OF COPING

Theorizing about a possible higher-order structure of coping mechanisms was motivated by the large number of distinct coping mechanisms found in community samples. For example, studies of adult samples indicated that somewhere between 8 and 12 distinct coping mechanisms could be identified (e.g., Pearlin & Schooler, 1978; McCrae, 1984; Stone & Neale, 1984). Similar results have been obtained in studies of adolescents; for example, Wills (1985) factor analyzed a 54-item coping inventory administered to an adolescent sample and found 11 coping dimensions. Although there were positive correlations among some measures, the studies showed that various coping dimensions could be extracted independently. The number of observed dimensions led to several proposals for a higher-order structure in which several modes of coping that were positively correlated with each other could be classified under a few higher order families, with minimal correlations between families.

Proposals for two-domain systems are based on the notion that most all coping mechanisms either involve investment of effort in actively confronting and dealing with a problem or represent a failure to invest any effort in trying to cope, and instead represent various ways of disengaging from dealing with the problem. This had led to systems contrasting active vs. avoidant coping (Carver et al., 1989; Moos & Shaefer, 1993). A coping approach that involves getting information, considering alternatives, and formulating and implementing a plan of action to solve the problem (behavioral coping) would be classified as active or engagement coping because of the effort invested. Approaches in which the person dealt with a problem by getting angry at other people (anger coping), trying to avoid thinking about it (avoidant coping), just wishing the problem would go away (wishful thinking), or taking the attitude that he/she couldn't deal with it (helpless coping), would all be classified as avoidant because no effort is invested.

The use of cognitive strategies is proposed by some theorists to fall under the rubric of active coping because it is assumed that these mechanisms require extensive cognitive effort and would serve to prepare a person to confront the problem in other ways (Carver et al., 1989). For example, trying to see the situation in a more positive light (situation redefinition in Lazarus' terms) involves cognitive efforts to see alternative views and could serve to reduce distress. Other cognitive strategies such as minimization of threat, or focusing on positive aspects, also involve cognitive effort and could serve to prepare the person for other types of effortful coping.

Among the domains, or families,of coping mechanisms that have been suggested, seeking social support is the most relevant to the present discussion, as we will see later. On one view, social support represents another domain because it involves a social rather than an individual approach to coping. Thus some systems classify it as a third family, others as simply another type of active coping; all agree, however, that coping through social support is an effortful and probably benefical approach.

## DOWNWARD COMPARISON AS A COPING MECHANISM

Most researchers assume that the coping mechanism of downward comparison is evoked by a decrease in subjective well-being and that it is most likely to come into play when the individual cannot easily change or control the original problem (Wills, 1981). Downward comparison in these conditions could take any of several forms: (a) A person could attend to comparison targets who happen to be presented in daily life or through the media such as television or newspapers (e.g., Heath, 1984). (b) A person could actively select a worse-off other as a target for comparison (e.g., Gibbons, 1986). (c) A person could make supportive cognitive constructions of social consensus information; for example, she could decide that there were a great many people with negative behaviors (e.g., Suls & Wan, 1987) or that her own behaviors were less negative than those of typical others (Klein & Kunda, 1993). (d) A person could imagine worse situations than the one he currently experiences (Markman, Gavanski, Sherman, & McMullen, 1995; Roese & Olson, 1995). Finally, (e) a person could actively derogate a target person, thus increasing the perceived social distance between himself and the other (e.g., Gibbons, Gerrard, Lando, & McGovern, 1991; Gibbons & Boney McCoy, 1991).[3] Following such occurrences the person now has salient in memory the perception that there exist some (or many) individuals who are also having problems (or worse problems), that there exist potentially worse situations, or that there exist persons who possess attributes inferior to those of the self. Comparison ensues, the person emerges with the perception that his or her status is relatively more favorable, and this produces an increase in subjective well-being.

The outcome dimensions through which downward comparison helps persons to cope, in theory, are several. Downward comparison could act to reduce current negative affect (i.e., anxiety, depression, or general emotional distress) and hence enable persons simply to feel better for a while. Alternatively, the cognitive operations involved in processing comparison information could divert a person from ruminating about the problem and hence disrupt a process of depressive self-focus that otherwise could prevent her from engaging other coping mechanisms to deal with the problem. Either of these could serve to assist the coping process because the person is in a more positive affective state and could be better prepared to begin to mobilize other coping resources and mechanisms. Another possibility is that downward comparison produces at least a temporary increase in self-esteem. This could occur through a direct experience of self-enhancement,

[3]This is not meant to exclude the possibility of a more automatic process of assuming relative superiority to others (cf. Alicke, 1985; Alicke, Klotz, Breitenbecher, Yurak, & Vredenburg, 1995; Tice, 1993; Van Lange & Rusbult, 1995). However, I think the latter phenomenon differs from the motivated and effortful coping process that occurs in times of distress.

resulting from the experience of perceiving that one is in a more favorable status than another. Alternatively, the belief that one is unlike the worse-off other in essential characteristics (i.e., those to which one attributes a causal role in the person's problem) could have a favorale impact on self-esteem. Either of these could operate to assist the coping process because self-esteem is a basic resource that serves to motivate more effortful types of coping. Finally, downward comparison might give people more positive outcome expectancies, because people are more optimistic when they are less depressed and when they believe they are not like people with problems. Because optimism serves to mobilize more effortful types of coping (Scheier & Carver, 1987; Scheier et al., 1989), downward comparison could have an indirect effect on coping through this pathway.

How, then, should downward comparison be classified within the structure of coping? On the one hand it may be seen as an active-cognitive strategy: Several types of downward comparison represent an effortful cognitive process in that people must seek out particular types of information and then to process this information in a particular way (i.e., in a way favorable to the self). Because this is an effortful process with investment of effort in information search, attentional focusing, and selective processing, it could represent an active coping mechanism. This basic argument is buttressed by the suggestion that use of downward comparison reduces subjective distress, at least in the short term. An extension of the argument suggests that if use of downward comparison increases self-esteem or self-efficacy, then it would meet all the requirements of an active coping mechanism. The latter argument is conjectural, however, because there is little evidence on whether downward comparison increases efficacy or optimism. Note that the foregoing analysis does suggest a distinction between active types of comparison (e.g., seeking out information about a comparison target) and passive types of comparison (e.g., happenstance exposure to a worse-off other on television) and predicts that only the former type will have adaptive consequences. This prediction has not been tested as far as I know (but see Buunk & Ybema, chapter 12, this volume, who make a similar argument).

Downward comparison may be seen, on the other hand, as an avoidant mechanism. First, downward comparison may be construed as a process in which people don't do anything about a problem but, instead, just try to make themselves feel better. To the extent that extensive use of downward comparison might divert people from other efforts to confront and solve problems it could represent a type of avoidant coping. A second consideration is that downward comparison may undermine coping if people feel worse because they think they will become like the worse-off other; this may lead them to give up trying to cope, which ipso facto may be defined as avoidance. This aspect of comparison is predicted to occur only under certain conditions (see Major, Testa, & Bylsma, 1991; Wills, 1991a), but evidence is needed on how prevalent such conditions are. A cross-cutting issue is the type of problem: use of downward comparison may be adaptive only when a problem is essentially unchangeable, and an inappropriate application of comparison-oriented coping to problems that are changeable may undermine active coping efforts. Hence the outcome of coping, with implications for classification, could depend substantially on the type of problem and the judgment of the coper in applying downward comparison only to appropriate problems. It should be noted that there is almost no empirical evidence bearing on the validity or invalidity of the foregoing propositions; evidence of this type is greatly needed to understand more about how downward comparison actually operates in naturalistic settings (cf. Tennen & Affleck, chapter 9, this volume).

To summarize, arguments about the classification of downward comparison can be presented on both sides, one to the effect that downward comparison is an active, cognitive type of coping mechanism, another to the effect that downward comparison as actually employed may represent an avoidant mechanism. To get at this question empirically, several types of analyses can be pursued. One is to examine the correlation between comparison-oriented coping and other types of cognitive and behavioral mechanisms. Another is to test for hierarchic structure with multiple dimensions of coping. A third is to conduct multivariate predictive analyses, which control for the correlations among different coping mechanisms using various indices of adjustment as criterion variables. The following section presents some illustrative analyses of these types, using data from studies of adolescents.

## EMPIRICAL ANALYSES OF COMPARISON-ORIENTED COPING

Several studies have been conducted by our research group on stress-coping processes in adolescence (e.g., Wills, 1982, 1986, in press; Wills & Cleary, 1995; Wills & Filer, 1996; Wills, Vaccaro, & Benson, 1995). This school-based research was conducted with samples of adolescents from public school districts in the New York metropolitan area. The participants ranged in age from 12 to 15 years, and the samples have ranged in size from about 700 to about 1,800 people. The samples are multiethnic, including participants of African-American, Hispanic, and Euro-American ethnicity. The participants were also diverse in socioeconomic backgrounds, and recent data show the samples to be representative of the New York State population.

Breifly, the research procedures called for obtaining data from self-report questionnaires that trained project staff administered to students in classrooms. The staff members followed a standardized protocol in giving instructions to students and answering questions about individual items. The self-report questionnaire takes about 40 minutes to administer and includes a number of structured scales with Likert-type responses. Typically, completed questionnaires are obtained from around 90% of the eligible population.

### Conceptualization and Assessment of Coping

This research was designed based on a multidimensional conceptualization of coping processes like that outlined in Fig. 6.1. Because the research focused on predicting adolescent substance use, assessment choices and priority decisions derived from that focus. Measures were obtained to sample both behavioral and cognitive types of coping mechanisms, and a range of measures was included so as to index coping mechanisms predicted to be adaptive (e.g., behavioral and cognitive strategies) as well as mechanisms predicted to be maladaptive (e.g., avoidance and anger). A psychometric approach was employed, using multiple items (facets) aggregated together to index particular coping mechanisms (modes), which could then be grouped into related domains (families). Empirical procedures including descriptive factor analysis, internal consistency analysis, and confirmatory factor analysis were used to determine the structure of the measures. The research was initiated using available response-based coping inventories (Bugen & Hawkins, 1981; Folkman & Lazarus, 1980; Wills, 1982) and the measures were subsequently modified through ongoing research (e.g., Folkman, Lazarus, Dunkel-Schetter, DeLongis, & Gruen, 1986; Wills, 1986).

Coping was assessed in this research in two ways. In the *response-based method*, subjects are given an introductory stem ("Here are some things that people may do when they have a problem") followed by an inventory with 40 to 50 possible responses such as "Get information about the problem" or "Try to notice the good things in life." For each of the possible responses the participant is asked to indicate (typically on a 5-point scale ranging from 1 [*never*] to 5 [*usually*] how often he or she does this when facing a problem. In the *intention-based method*, the subject was presented with a given coping intention (e.g., "doing something to solve the problem," "doing something to see the problem in a different way") and asked to indicate the extent to which he or she does things with that intention when confronted with a particular type of problem. The latter approach was introduced because of concerns originally raised by Stone and Neale (1984) that response-based methods might have lower validity as an assessment approach. Our research has generally found that the two methods of coping assessment produce quite similar results in predicting substance use, so these findings are not strongly method-dependent (see, e.g., Wills & Hirky, 1996).

With regard to social comparison, the studies began with several items that were intended to index comparison-oriented coping. Analyses showed that rather than forming a separate dimension, these items factored with a diverse set of other items that represented cognitive coping strategies. For this reason the items were scored within the cognitive mode of coping (see, e.g., Wills, 1985), and for priority reasons the number of these items was reduced over time. Thus the adolescent data sets do not provide the strongest possible test of social comparison hypotheses. Nonetheless, they illustrate several points about social comparison that need to be considered in future research.

**Factor Analysis of Cognitive Coping Modes**

A first step is to characterize the structure of cognitive coping and determine where comparisons are placed within this mode. To address this question, factor analysis was performed for data from a response-based coping inventory from a sample of students ($N = 747$) who were surveyed at the beginning of grade 8. This inventory included 10 items designed to index cognitive approaches to coping and included 2 items intended to index comparison-oriented coping ("I think about others with similar problems" and "I think about how things could be worse"). To examine how these items were interrelated, the 10-item set was analyzed using the iterated principal-factor method with varimax rotation.

As Table 6.1 shows, the factoring procedure indicated that three facets could be distinguished within the mode of cognitive coping. There were appreciable correlations (about $r = .40$) among the factors, so these three scales would be termed "facets of cognitive coping" rather than orthogonal dimensions. One facet, with rather discrepant loadings, represents coping through not letting the problem affect oneself (e.g., "I just ignore the problem," "I try to put the problem out of my mind"). The second facet represents coping through strategies that represent endurance ("I tell myself the problem will be over in a short time") and downward comparison ("I remind myself that things could be worse" [counterfactual], "I think of others with similar problems" [social]). The third facet contained items representing an attempt to minimize the threatening qualities of the problem ("I tell myself it's not worth getting

TABLE 6.1
Eighth-Grade Coping Inventory, Cognitive Coping Items, Factor Analysis, and Scale Intercorrelations

*Factor Loadings for Cognitive Items*

| | *FAC1* | *FAC2* | *FAC3* | *M*[a] | *SD* | *Item* |
|---|---|---|---|---|---|---|
| Facet I: Ignoring | | | | | | |
| COP28 | .82 | .13 | .06 | 2.25 | 1.21 | I just ignore the problem. |
| COP16 | .43 | .12 | .34 | 2.87 | 1.34 | I try to put it out of my mind. |
| COP40 | .39 | .21 | .25 | 2.16 | 1.12 | I go on as if nothing had happened. |
| Facet 2: Endurance–social comparison | | | | | | |
| COP22 | .19 | .53 | .29 | 2.82 | 1.23 | I tell myself it will be over in a short time. |
| COP19 | −.02 | .50 | .20 | 3.10 | 1.25 | I remind myself that things could be worse. |
| COP20 | .26 | .49 | .16 | 3.16 | 1.25 | I wait and hope things will get better. |
| COP29 | .11 | .35 | .06 | 2.65 | 1.25 | I think about others with problems. |
| Facet 3: Minimization–positive focus | | | | | | |
| COP11 | .09 | .16 | .62 | 3.17 | 1.28 | I tell myself not to worry about it. |
| COP17 | .20 | .25 | .51 | 2.82 | 1.19 | I tell myself it's not worth getting upset. |
| COP13 | .18 | .32 | .37 | 3.07 | 1.23 | I try to notice the good things in life. |

*Note.* Tabled values are rotated factor loadings, FAC = facet. Items with loadings > .35 are underlined for emphasis.

*Intercorrelations for Facets of Cognitive Coping*

| | *Ignor* | *Endur* | *Minim* |
|---|---|---|---|
| Ignoring | – | | |
| Endurance/comparison | .37 | – | |
| Minimization | .41 | .45 | – |

[a]Mean, on 1–5 response scale (*Never do this* to *Usually do this* for all items).

upset about") together with an item on positive focus ("I try to notice the good things in life"), which had a dual loading on the second facet.

In summary, two things should be noted about this analysis. First, fairly different items on cognitive coping were substantially intercorrelated, and hence represent across-subject consistency in the use of cognitive types of coping; in other words, there is a coherent mode of cognitive coping. Second, the social comparison items were clearly identified with one facet of this mode, and thus can be located within the cognitive mode of coping. There are some ambiguities within these data, particularly the discrepant magnitudes of loadings and the dual loadings for some items, but these effects may simply derive from factoring a set of items that are substantially intercorrelated.

## Cognitive Coping in Relation to Other Modes of Coping

A second step is to determine how cognitive coping is related to other modes of coping. To address this question, another factor analysis was performed using a set of 27 items from the same sample and inventory, including the 10 cognitive items together with items designed to index behavioral coping and anger/avoidant coping.[4] The results, presented in Table 6.2, indicated a solution with cognitive coping clearly distinguished from factors of behavioral coping and anger coping. Within factors there were few discrepant loadings, indicating coherence of these dimensions. The exception is the two comparison items; one (counterfactual comparison) had a relatively low loading on the cognitive coping factor, while the other (social comparison) had low, dual loadings on both behavioral coping and cognitive coping factors. Factor analysis for another assessment with the same sample (at the end of Grade 8) indicated a replicable solution, with a 7-item cognitive coping factor distinguished from a 9-item behavioral coping factor. In this solution the item "I remind myself that things could be worse" had a loading of .54 on the cognitive factor and a loading of .28 on the behavioral factor. Thus these analyses also identify the comparison items with the cognitive mode of coping, but there was some evidence for dual loadings.

Correlations between the factors raise several other issues. First, cognitive and behavioral coping are positively correlated, providing some basis for suggesting membership in the same higher order family. However, their patterns of correlates are different: behavioral coping is inversely correlated with avoidant-type strategies, while the cognitive coping measure shows positive correlations with these strategies. This suggests that cognitive strategies of coping may have some commonality with active coping, but may share some aspects with avoidant types of coping.

In summary, these results suggest some paradoxical properties of cognitive coping in general and social comparison in particular, though it would be desirable to have more items to index the constructs. One suggestion is that comparison-oriented coping, although identified with the cognitive mode, may have some commonality with active coping. This may derive from the effortful aspects of comparison-oriented coping through conceiving worse situations and selectively focusing on cues that indicate a positive status for the self. A second suggestion is that while cognitive coping is positively correlated with behavioral coping it has some positive correlations with avoidance, suggesting that it may have aspects of both.

[4]This is not one of the best inventories for assessing avoidant coping, and subsequent measures were revised to include more items in this mode. However, it was desirable to perform the present analysis on exactly the same data as the previous one. The items listed here on the Avoidant Coping factor loaded with avoidant-type items in other data sets.

TABLE 6.2
Rotated Factor Loadings for Behavioral, Cognitive, and Anger–Avoidance Items

| *FACT1* | *FACT2* | *FACT3* | *FACT4* | *Item* |
|---|---|---|---|---|
| Factor 1: Behavioral Coping | | | | |
| .69 | −.02 | −.04 | −.00 | Think about best alternative |
| .66 | −.09 | −.09 | −.02 | Think about risk of different ways |
| .65 | −.03 | −.08 | .21 | Think about consequences of alternatives |
| .65 | .05 | −.05 | −.07 | Determine which information truthful |
| .63 | −.06 | −.16 | .06 | Think about choices before action |
| .61 | .07 | −.05 | .07 | Compromise to get something positive |
| .58 | .07 | .04 | −.10 | Get information about problem |
| .56 | .16 | −.08 | .09 | Think about what alternatives mean |
| .48 | .11 | .07 | −.07 | Think about past similar experience |
| .44 | .11 | −.03 | −.17 | Make a plan of action and follow it |
| .41 | .13 | −.12 | .16 | Change attitude that contributes to problem |
| .38 | .28 | −.05 | .15 | Promise self, things will be different next time |
| Factor 2: Cognitive Coping | | | | |
| .09 | .59 | −.08 | −.14 | Tell self, problem not worth getting upset about |
| .16 | .56 | .11 | .13 | Tell self, problem will be over in short time |
| .24 | .55 | .07 | −.19 | Try to notice good things in life |
| .05 | .53 | .06 | .24 | Wait/hope things get better |
| −.10 | .53 | .13 | .07 | Try to put problem out of mind |
| .14 | .49 | .04 | −.12 | Tell self not to worry |
| −.18 | .46 | .26 | .03 | Ignore the problem |
| −.08 | .47 | .19 | −.02 | Go on as if nothing happened |
| .16 | .36 | −.03 | .05 | Remind self that things could be worse |
| .27 | .23 | .16 | .18 | Think about others who have problems also |
| Factor 3: Anger Coping | | | | |
| −.04 | .03 | .78 | .07 | Get mad at people |
| −.09 | .07 | .58 | −.05 | Do something bad, cause trouble |
| −.10 | .15 | .53 | .11 | Blame others for the problem |
| Factor 4: Avoidant Coping | | | | |
| .05 | −.04 | .26 | .52 | Worry a lot |
| −.03 | .11 | .30 | .18 | Avoid being with people |

*Note.* Tabled values are rotated factor loadings, FACT = factor. Items with loadings > .35 are underlined for emphasis.

*Correlations for Scales*

| | *Beh* | *Cog* | *Ang* | *Avoid* |
|---|---|---|---|---|
| Behavioral | – | | | |
| Cognitive | .26 | – | | |
| Anger | −.14 | .17 | – | |
| Avoidance | −.01 | .10 | .31 | – |

## Analysis of Higher Order Structure for Families of Coping

To examine the hierarchical structure of coping, structural modeling analysis was performed with data for the response-based inventory

TABLE 6.3
Correlations Among Coping Dimensions for Study With Coping Data for Adolescents ($N = 1{,}826$)

| *Mode* | *Beh* | *Cog* | *Parent* | *Peer* | *Avoid* | *Anger* | *Helpl* |
|---|---|---|---|---|---|---|---|
| Behavioral | – | | | | | | |
| Cognitive | .48 | – | | | | | |
| Parent support | .35 | .34 | – | | | | |
| Peer support | .29 | .32 | .27 | – | | | |
| Avoidance | .09 | .23 | −.11 | .08 | – | | |
| Anger | −.21 | −.11 | −.21 | −.01 | .29 | – | |
| Helpless | −.17 | −.06 | −.18 | −.02 | .35 | .53 | – |

from a seventh-grade data set with 1,826 cases (see Wills, DuHamel, & Vaccaro, 1995, for description).[5] The zero-order correlations for these modes of coping are presented in Table 6.3.It can be seen that behavioral coping and cognitive coping are positively correlated,and both are positively related to measures of coping through social support. Conversely, anger, avoidance, and helpless coping are intercorrelated and tend to be inversely related to active types of coping. Some complexity for cognitive coping can be seen in that it is positively correlated with behavioral coping but also is positively correlated, at a lower level, with avoidance coping.

The hierarchical structure was tested with a second-order structural modeling analysis (cf. McGee & Newcomb, 1992). Higher order families are specified so as to generate values of coping modes, which in turn are indexed by several indicators that are measured variables. I specified a two-domain model in which the family of active coping mechanisms was indexed by behavioral, cognitive, and support coping, whereas the family of avoidant mechanisms was indexed by anger, avoidance, and helpless coping. This model had good fit to the data, with a comparative fit index of 0.98, and the pattern of loadings was consistent with the theoretical structure in Fig. 6.1. Loadings of behavioral, cognitive, and

[5]The cognitive scale for the response-based inventory contained the items, "I think, 'It will be over in a short time' "; "I think, 'It's not worth getting upset about' "; "I try to see the problem in a different way"; "I look for something good in what is happening"; "I say 'Things will turn out all right' ", and "I try to notice the good things in life." Instructions for the other measure defined the intention for cognitive coping as when you "Do something to see the problem in a different way, for example, you try to notice the good things in life, tell yourself the problem will be over in a short time, tell yourself it's not worth getting upset about, and look for something good in what is happening." Thus these measures place somewhat more emphasis on reinterpretation and positive focus. The avoidance measures in both scales included items about keeping away from people, wishing the problem would just go away, daydreaming, and trying not to think about the problem.

parent support coping on the active domain were 0.80, 0.83, and 0.60, respectively; whereas loadings of anger, avoidance, and helpless coping on the avoidant domain were 0.78, 0.64, and 0.92, respectively. Peer support coping had a lower loading (0.47) but was identified with the active domain. This analytic approach was applied to another data set in which coping was assessed with a different method, and results were similar (Wills, Cleary, & Shinar, 1996). Thus the results were consistent with a hierarchical structure with two families, active and avoidance, each of which comprises several modes of coping.

## Correlations with Psychosocial Criterion Measures

The prior findings have implications for analytic procedures in research on comparison-oriented coping. Given that downward comparison is correlated with other types of cognitive strategies, this interrelationship should be recognized in research on social comparison. Morever, the fact that behavioral coping and cognitive coping are positively correlated indicates that analyzing social comparison measures alone as predictors of depression–anxiety or other outcomes could be misleading, because the analysis ignores the correlation of cognitive coping with other types of coping as these occur in natural environment. This issue can be resolved statistically through partial correlation or multiple regression procedures, which analyze comparison measures together with other types of coping measures.

An illustration of these statistical issues is provided in Table 6.4 using the same data set as in Tables 6.1 and 6.2. This table presents analyses of behavioral and cognitive coping measures in relation to four psychosocial variables commonly used in health research. These are scales for internal health locus of control (from Wallston et al., 1978), global self-efficacy (from Pearlin & Schooler, 1978), global positive self-regard (Rosenberg,1965), and perceived stress (Cohen, Kamarck, & Mermelstein, 1983). The table first presents the zero-order correlations of behavioral and cognitive coping with the psychosocial variables, then presents multiple regressions where several coping measures are entered simultaneously.

The zero-order correlations suggest two conclusions. First, behavioral coping is related to better outcomes, that is, higher levels of internal control, self-efficacy and self-esteem and lower levels of subjective stress. A different pattern is noted for the mode of cognitive coping, which appears to be significantly related to more internal locus of control, unrelated to efficacy or esteem, and positively related to stress. Specific analyses for the three facets suggest that this overall effect is largely driven by the indices of ignoring and endurance–comparison; a

TABLE 6.4
Correlations and Multiple Regression Analyses, for Behavioral and Cognitive Coping Modes [with Facets], with Four Psychosocial Measures as Criterion Variables

| | *IHLC* | *Efficacy* | *Esteem* | *Stress* |
|---|---|---|---|---|
| Zero-Order Correlations | | | | |
| Behavioral coping | .21**** | .19**** | .24**** | .00 |
| Cognitive coping | .13** | −.03 | −.02 | .09** |
| [Ignore] | .03 | −.13** | −.13** | .07 |
| [Endure/compare] | .14*** | −.04 | −.05 | .14*** |
| [Minimize/focus] | .10** | .05 | .13** | −.06 |

| *Modes* | *Beta* | *With Facets* | *Beta* |
|---|---|---|---|
| Multiple Regression: Health Locus of Control as Criterion | | | |
| Behavioral | .18**** | Behavioral | .18**** |
| Cognitive | .07 | [Ignore] | .03 |
| | | [Endure/compare] | .05 |
| | | [Mininize/focus] | .03 |
| Multiple Regression: Self-Efficacy as Criterion | | | |
| Behavioral | .22**** | Behavioral | .17**** |
| Cognitive | −.08* | [Ignore] | −.16*** |
| | | [Endure/compare] | −.07 |
| | | [Minimize/focus] | .13** |
| Multiple Regression: Self-Esteem as Criterion | | | |
| Behavioral | .26**** | Behavioral | .20**** |
| Cognitive | −.09** | [Ignore] | −.16*** |
| | | [Endure/compare] | −.14** |
| | | [Minimize/focus] | .21**** |
| Multiple Regression: Perceived Stress as Criterion | | | |
| Behavioral | −.01 | Behavioral | .01 |
| Cognitive | .10** | [Ignore] | .07 |
| | | [Endure/compare] | .21**** |
| | | [Minimize/focus] | −.18**** |

*Note.* IHLC = internal health locus of control. For multiple regression analyses, tabled values are for standardized coefficients and are for models with all predictors entered simultaneously. Column 1 has two variables entered simultaneously; column 2 has four variables entered simultaneously. For multiple regressions, $R^2$s are .044, .046, .063, and .010 for four models, respectively.

$^*p < .05$. $^{**}p < .01$. $^{***}p < .001$. $^{****}p < .0001$.

different and in fact opposite pattern is suggested for the facet representing threat minimization and focus on positives.

The multiple regression results illustrate how conclusions based on zero-order correlations can be treacherous. When the correlation between behavioral and cognitive coping is partialled, these analyses indicate cognitive coping unrelated to health locus of control, negatively related to self-efficacy and self-esteem, and positively related to stress. Because the multivariate analyses consider the covariance between behavioral and cognitive coping, these results have greater statistical validity. Analyses for the three facets of cognitive coping (Table 6.4, column 3) again suggest that the overall mode effect is largely driven by the facets of ignoring and endurance–comparison; opposite findings occur for the facet of threat minimization–focus on positives, which shows significant positive relationships to efficacy and esteem and a significant inverse relationship to perceived stress.[6]

A final methodological issue is addressing the possible relation between coping and recent stressors. Several researchers (e.g., Vitaliano et al., 1985) have suggested that coping efforts are activated by stressful events and accordingly have proposed that analyses of coping–outcome relationships should control for the level of recent stressors. This data set included a measure of recent negative events, and so the regression analyses were repeated entering the negative events measure together with the coping variables, to control for any coping–activation effects. (The negative-events measure had independent significant effects in all regression analyses, inversely related to esteem and control and positively related to perceived stress.) In multiple regression analyses conducted at the facet level (Table 6.4, column 2), results were unchanged by the stress control in 4 out of 4 tests for behavioral coping and in 12 out of 12 tests for facets of cognitive coping. A replication test with the second data set (see footnote 6) indicated results unchanged in 4 out of 4 tests for behavioral coping and 11 of 12 tests for facets of cognitive coping. Thus the observed results for coping are not attributable to a correlation with current stress level.

In summary, these analyses illustrate the desirability of analyzing cognitive coping with other coping measures. When cognitive and behavioral coping were entered simultaneously, behavioral coping remained related to better outcomes but cognitive coping tended to be related to worse outcomes (e.g., lower self-efficacy and self-esteem). Although the present analyses are cross-sectional and the direction of effects cannot be conclusively demonstrated, the statistical issues are clear and show that interpretation of zero-order correlations observed for a single coping measure may not be appropriate. The results also illustrate the complexity of cognitive coping; while two facets were related to worse outcomes, the facet that represented minimizing threat and focusing on positives was consistently related to better outcomes in multivariate analyses. Thus there is evidence for the desirability of distinguishing between different types of cognitive strategies for coping.

[6]These analyses were repeated with another data set, based on data from the same group of participants assessed at the end of eight grade ($N = 675$). The results reported here for behavioral and cognitive coping (and facets of cognitive coping) were exactly replicated.

## DISCUSSION

This chapter has presented a combined theoretical–empirical discussion of the location of downward comparison within the families of coping mechanisms. I reviewed theoretical arguments about the status of comparison-oriented coping and presented empirical analyses of how particular types of social comparison are related to other cognitive and behavioral mechanisms. The analyses suggest that downward comparison can be located within the cognitive mode of coping. This is consistent with the original proposal that comparison-oriented coping involves cognitive operations aimed at reducing subjective distress, and thus shares an essential commonality with other cognitive mechanisms. This finding has both methodological and theoretical implications.

The methodological goal of this chapter was to point out that comparison-oriented coping is correlated with other mechanisms, and therefore these correlations should be partialled in predictive analyses. An illustrative set of analyses showed that the overall mode of cognitive coping had different effects in multivariate analyses than were suggested by a quick glance at the zero-order correlations. In fact these analyses tended to suggest cognitive coping as being inversely correlated with desirable outcomes and positively correlated with undesirable outcomes. Because these findings are based on cross-sectional analyses it is not possible to draw strong conclusions about causality, and extension of such analyses in further longitudinal research would certainly be desirable.

The main theoretical point of this work is that the cognitive mode of coping is complex and deserves careful attention from both psychometric and analytic standpoints. Confirmatory analyses indicated that the measures indexing behavioral coping and cognitive coping could be conceptualized as members of a higher-order family of active coping. However, when the indicators for the mode of cognitive coping were broken into specific facets including downward comparison, there was some evidence for differential effects. Indicators such as ignoring, endurance, focusing on positives, and using downward comparison may be positively correlated but can have different effects in some situations. What this suggests is that assessment of a broad range of cognitive coping strategies is essential, and that analytic approaches should carefully examine the structure of cognitive coping and its correlations with other mechanisms. However, it could well be that the apparently duality of cognitive coping is inherent in the nature of this mode of coping, just as the electron can be either a wave or a particle at different times (Lederman & Schramm, 1989).

The strengths and advantages of this research can be stated as follows. The findings are based on samples of adolescents that are representative of the general population, hence indicate the prevalence and correlates of coping as it occurs in real settings including a diverse array of ethnic and socioeconomic backgrounds. Thus the findings have greater evidential value than data from small and/or unrepresentative samples. The results are robust, replicated over two assessment methods and four studies. Empirical procedures were used to characterize the relation of comparison measures to other facets and modes of coping, and multivariate analyses controlled for the correlation among different indices of coping. Multiple outcome measures were employed so that the relation of comparison indices to a range of outcomes could be determined. Finally, the findings for behavioral coping were strong and robust, consistently indicating this type of coping related to better outcomes. Such findings have been demonstrated concurrently and prospectively (see Wills, 1986; Wills, Cleary, & Shinar, 1996). The evidence thus is reasonably clear that behavioral coping is an adaptive coping mechanism.

The constraints on conclusions drawn from these data also are apparent. The participants are younger adolescents, and it is conceivable that the ways in which adolescents cope with problems through cognitive mechanisms, and/or the types of problems they face, are less differentiated than those of adults. The findings are based on cross-sectional analyses and do not allow strong inferences about causality. (I actually did perform prospective analyses for the coping predictors, as in Table 6.4, and these were nonsignificant, which was not unexpected given the short follow-up interval and the stability of criterion variables such as self-esteem.) Finally, the indices of social comparison were two items that tapped different aspects of comparison (counterfactual thinking and social comparison). These considerations place some constraints on the conclusions that can be drawn about social comparison in general, as there are several possible types of coping through downward comparison and there is no theoretical assurance that these have equivalent effects (cf. Buunk & Ybema, chapter 12, this volume, Gibbons & Gerrard, chapter 3; Helgeson & Mickelson, 1995; Tigges, Wills, & Link, 1996; Wood, 1989).

### Directions for Further Research

A first issue for further research on social comparison and health is addressing the complex nature of downward comparison. In the present chapter I have outlined no less than five ways in which downward comparison may be used as a coping mechanism, and this does not exhaust the possibilities. Despite the extent of the theoretical framework for this question, previous research has tended to address one or two types of downward comparison, to the exclusion of other types. There are reasonable grounds for predicting that the various types of downward comparison will have different consequences. For example, theory suggests that types of downward comparison involving more effortful cognitive operations (e.g., purposive selection of a comparison person, counterfactual thinking about worse situations) would produce different effects than those involving less effort (e.g., passive exposure to a target of opportunity, or derogation of a socially acceptable target). At present, however, there is almost no evidence available on this question.

A second issue is the need for multivariate studies with several predictors and multiple outcome measures. The need for such studies is indicated by several aspects of the previous presentation. For one, it is clearly of crucial importance to control statistically for the correlation of comparison-oriented coping with other facets and modes of coping. For another, it is difficult to see what effects downward comparison really has unless a broad range of outcomes is examined. For example, a univariate study might have suggested that downward comparison was related to more internal health locus of control, but the multivariate study suggests it is related to lower self-efficacy.

A specific hypothesis is that cognitive strategies that involve focusing on positive aspects of one's situation will be more adaptive and will be related to greater feelings of optimism and efficacy. This conception is certainly consistent with the present data. Whether one or more types of downward comparison will result in increased optimism is another hypothesis for further investigation. Given some suggestions in the present data that it could lead to reductions in efficacy and esteem, this is indicated as a significant issue for further research.

Another specific hypothesis is that there may be dispositional tendencies to engage in particular types of comparison-oriented coping or other types of cognitive coping. There are some definite suggestions in prior literature of individual differences in the tendency to engage in social comparison (e.g., Gibbons & Gerrard, 1995; Hemphill & Lehman, 1991) and the present factor-analytic results are also consistent with this position. Thus it may be worthwhile for research to focus on identifying a subgroup of persons who consistently do not use social comparison (or other cognitive mechanisms) and contrasting them with the group of persons who do.

A cross-cutting issue is the goal of the coper when he or she does a particular thing to cope with a particular situation. One insight of Arthur Stone's analysis of coping was that, observed across persons or instances, a given response could be motivated by quite different intentions and could have different effects (see Stone & Neale, 1984). For example, the behavior of going shopping could have very different intentions depending on whether one was going to a store to solve a particular instrumental problem (e.g., buying a frame to put up a picture), going to the store to buy something that would make you feel better about yourself, going shopping to provide a temporary distraction from ruminating about a problem, or going to the mall to avoid problems and just hang out for a while without engaging in any productive activity. Despite a number of methodological refinements, this question has rarely been addressed in coping research or social comparison research. Research is needed that can focus on particular episodes and ask "why did you do that" questions to get at the intentionality for particular responses.

Another cross-cutting issue is the temporal course of the coping effort. A specific prediction is that coping through downward comparison will be adaptive when it is used early in the course of coping with a problem, so that setbacks to self-esteem can be countered and employment of active coping can be mobilized (e.g., "I'm not such a bad person, I'm going to go back and keep working on this problem"). The adaptive effect of downward comparison may depend on whether it is used in concert with other coping mechanisms, rather than as a replacement for them. Getting at this question would involve research that examined the time course of coping with a particular problem and could differentiate failed coping efforts—where the person remained stuck in helplessness and passivity—from successful ones. Therefore, research to provide detailed examination of the development of coping episodes would be valuable for helping to clarify how the co-occurrence of social comparison with other coping mechanisms influences the outcome of the coping effort.

A third cross-cutting issue is whether coping through social comparison is appropriately employed. The majority of coping research (my own included) has simply asked participants how frequently they used a given coping mechanism. While there are good reasons for doing this, a needed direction for further research is to study the matching of problem and coping response. Coping through social comparison may have very different consequences for coping with problems that are essentially unchangeable (e.g., chronic pain from arthritis) than for problems that are more controllable though instrumental coping (e.g., getting a bad grade on an exam). This issue is of particular significance for research in health settings, because much of the adverse impact of physical illness may derive from realistic loss of control, and efforts to restore self-esteem and perceived control assume considerable importance for the adjustment of the afflicted person (cf. Wills, 1994). Research on this question would be methodologically demanding because it involves obtaining detailed information on specific problems and specific coping responses, and moreover requires some determination (probably aside from the subject's opinion) of whether the response was appropriately matched to the problem. Getting at this kind of question probably will not be feasible with retrospective studies, and research using prospective assessments and repeated-measures designs will be necessary.

Finally there is the issue of how the other types of social comparison, lateral comparison and upward comparison, are involved in coping efforts along with downward comparison. The focus on downward comparison in the present chapter is not intended to exclude the possibility that lateral or upward comparisons also occur in the course of coping efforts (for extended discussion see Wills, 1991b). This is an area of theoretical interest because proposals have been advanced about how downward cognitive evaluations may co-occur with upward social affiliations (Taylor & Lobel, 1989) and how various social comparison processes may be selectively employed in the pursuit of different coping goals (Helgeson & Mickelson, 1995; Wood, 1989). However, there is relatively little good evidence available as to whether the different types of comparison are complementary, mutually exclusive, or situationally dependent in their occurrence and/or effects. Examination of this question in research involving persons with acute or chronic physical illness should prove most informative for both applied significance and theoretical advancement.

## Summary

The bottom line for this chapter is a mixed message. It is suggested that coping through downward comparison can be a double-edged sword: It may have some good aspects and some bad aspects. The message from the present data is a qualified one because the simple measures preclude definitive inferences. Yet there is sufficient evidence in the present data to suggest that comparison-oriented coping is a strategy with mixed effects. The possible benefit of downward comparison is that a person maintains self-esteem in times of trouble and generates a more positive outlook on the current situation while other types of coping are brought into operation; the possible drawback is that reliance on cognitive mechanisms reduces the use of active coping, encourages passivity, and deters change (Perloff, 1987; Tigges, Wills, & Link, 1996; Wills, 1992). Thus downward comparison, like fire, may be "a kind servant but a cruel master." Asking what aspects of downward comparison predominate in real-world settings, whether there are discriminable subgroups of individuals with consistent patterns of cognitive coping, and how different aspects of comparison may enhance adjustment to illness, are significant questions for further research.

## ACKNOWLEDGMENTS

Preparation of this chapter was supported by Research Scientist Development Award #K02-DA00252 from the National Insitute on Drug Abuse. Earlir collection of previous data was supported by grants #80A-23 from the Centers for Disease Control, #R01-DA05950 from the National Institute on Drug Abuse, and #S184A-00035 from the U.S. Department of Education.

In this research program, the following graduate students and professional staff members have assisted in the work: Gregory Benson, Sean D. Cleary, Kate DuHamel, Marnie Filer, Edith Friedman, A. Elizabeth Hirky, John Mariani, Grace McNamara, Freida Nesmith, Stephen Ramirez, Angela Riccobono, Daniel Schreibman, Mark Spellman, Karen Spera, Donna Spitzoff, Donato Vaccaro, Roger Vaughan, Jody Wallach, Aaron Warshawsky, and Caroline Zeoli.

## REFERENCES

Affleck, G., & Tennen, H. (1991). Social comparison and coping with major medical problems. In J. Suls & T. A. Wills (Eds.), *Social comparison: Contemporary theory and research* (pp. 369–393). Hillsdale, NJ: Lawerence Erlbaum Associates.

Affleck, G., Tennen, H., Pfeiffer, C., & Fifield, J. (1988). Social comparisons in rheumatoid arthritis: Accuracy and adaptational significance. *Journal of Social and Clinical Psychology, 6*, 219–234.

Alicke, M. D. (1985). Global self-evaluation as determined by the desirability and controllability of trait adjectives. *Journal of Personality and Social Psychology, 49*, 1621–1630.

Alicke, M. D., Klotz, M. L., Breitenbecher, D. L., Yurak, T. J., & Vredenburg, D. S. (1995). Personal contact, individuation, and the better- than-average effect. *Journal of Personality and Social Psychology, 68*, 804–825.

Bugen, L. A., & Hawkins, R. C. (1981, August). *The Coping Assessment Battery: Theoretical and empirical foundations.* Paper presented at the meeting of the American Psychological Association, Los Angeles.

Carver, C. S., Scheier, M. F., & Weintraub, J. K. (1989). Assessing coping strategies. *Journal of Personality and Social Psychology, 56*, 267–283.

Cohen, S., Kamarck, T., & Mermelstein, R. (1983). A global measure of perceived stress. *Journal of Health and Social Behavior, 24*, 385–395.

Compas, B. E., Malcarne, V. L., & Fondacaro, K. M. (1988). Coping with stressful events in older children and young adolescents. *Journal of Consulting and Clinical Psychology, 56*, 405–411.

DeVellis, R. F., Blalock, S. J., Holt, K., Renner, B. R., Blanchard, L. W., & Klotz, M. L. (1991). Arthritis patients' reactions to unavoidable social comparisons. *Personality and Social Psychology Bulletin, 17,* 392–399.

DeVellis, R., Holt, K., Renner, B., Blalock, S., Blanchard, L., Cook, H., Klotz, M., Mikow, V., & Harring, K. (1990). The relationship of social comparison to rheumatoid arthritis symptoms and affect. *Basic and Applied Social Psychology, 11,* 1–18.

Folkman, S., & Lazarus, R. S. (1980, August). *The Ways of Coping scale: A method for coping assessment.* Paper presented at the meeting of the American Psychological Association, San Francisco.

Folkman, S., Lazarus, R. S., Dunkel-Schetter, C., DeLongis, A., & Gruen, R. (1986). The dynamics of a stressful encounter: Cognitive appraisal, coping, and encounter outcomes. *Journal of Personality and Social Psychology, 50,* 992–1003.

Gibbons, F. X. (1986). Social comparison and depression: Company's effect on misery. *Journal of Personality and Social Psychology, 51,* 140–148.

Gibbons, F. X., Benbow, C. P., & Gerrard, M. (1994). From top dog to bottom half: Social comparison strategies in response to poor performance. *Journal of Personality and Social Psychology, 67,* 638–652.

Gibbons, F. X., & Boney McCoy, S. (1991). Self-esteem, similarity, and reactions to active versus passive downward comparison. *Journal of Personality and Social Psychology, 60,* 414–424.

Gibbons, F. X., & Gerrard, M. (1989). Effects of upward and downward social comparison on mood states. *Journal of Social and Clinical Psychology, 8,* 14–31.

Gibbons, F. X., & Gerrard, M. (1991). Downward comparison and coping with threat. In J. Suls & T. A. Wills (Eds.), *Social comparison: Contemporary theory and research* (pp. 317-345). Hillsdale, NJ: Lawrence Erlbaum Associates.

Gibbons, F. X., & Gerrard, M. (1995). Predicting young adults' health risk behavior. *Journal of Personality and Social Psychology, 69,* 505–517.

Gibbons, F. X., Gerrard, M., Lando, H., & McGovern, P. G. (1991). Smoking cessation and social comparison: The role of the "typical smoker." *Journal of Experimental Social Psychology, 27,* 239–258.

Heath, L. (1984). Impact of newspaper crime reports on fear of crime: A multimethod investigation. *Journal of Personality and Social Psychology, 47,* 263–276.

Helgeson, V. S., & Mickelson, K. D. (1995). Motives for social comparison. *Personality and Social Psychology Bulletin, 21,* 1200–1209.

Helgeson, V. S., & Taylor, S. E. (1993). Evaluative and affiliative comparisons and coping among cardiac patients. *Journal of Applied Social Psychology, 23,* 1171–1195.

Hemphill, K. J., & Lehman, D. R. (1991). Social comparisons and their affective consequences: The importance of comparison dimension and individual difference variables. *Journal of Social and Clinical Psychology, 10,* 372–394.

Klein, W. M., & Kunda, Z. (1993). Maintaining self-serving social comparisons: Biased reconstructions of one's past behaviors. *Personality and Social Psychology Bulletin, 19,* 732-739.

Lazarus, R. S., & Folkman, S. (1984). *Stress, appraisal and coping.* New York: Springer.

Lederman, L. M., & Schram, D. N. (1989). *From quarks to the cosmos.* New York: Scientific American Library.

Major, B., Testa, M., Bylsma, W. H. (1991). Responses to upward and downward social comparisons: The impact of esteem-relevance and perceived control. In J. Suls & T. A. Wills (Eds.), *Social comparison: Contemporary theory and research* (pp. 237–260). Hillsdale, NJ: Lawrence Erlbaum Associates.

Markman, K. D., Gavanski, I., Sherman, S. J., & McMullen, M. N. (1995). The impact of perceived control on the imagination of better and worse possible worlds. *Personality and Social Psychology Bulletin, 21,* 588–595.

McCaul, K. D., & Malott, J. M. (1984). Distraction and coping with pain. *Psychological Bulletin, 95,* 516–533.

McCrae, R. R. (1984). Situational determinants of coping responses: Loss, threat, and challenge. *Journal of Personality and Social Psychology, 46,* 919–928.

McGee, L., & Newcomb, M. D. (1992). General deviance syndrome: Expanded hierarchical evaluations at four ages from early adolescence to adulthood. *Journal of Personality and Social Psychology, 60,* 766–776.

Moos, R. H., & Schaefer, J. A. (1993). Coping resources and processes: Current concepts and measures. In L. Goldberger & S. Bresnitz (Eds.), *Handbook of stress* (2nd ed., pp. 234–257). New York: Free Press.

Pearlin, L. I., & Schooler, C. (1978). The structure of coping. *Journal of Health and Social Behavior, 19,* 2–21.

Pelham, B. W. (1991). On the benefits of misery: Self-serving biases in the depressive self-concept. *Journal of Personality and Social Psychology, 61,* 670–681.

Pelham, B. W. (1993). On the highly positive thoughts of the highly depressed. In R. Baumeister (Ed.), *Self-esteem: The puzzle of low self-regard* (pp. 183–199). New York: Plenum.

Perloff, L. (1987). Social comparison and illusions of invulnerability. In C. R. Snyder & C. Ford (Eds.), *Coping with negative life events.* New York: Plenum.

Pyszczynski, T., & Greenberg, J. (1987). Self-regulatory perseveration and the depressive self-focusing style. *Psychological Bulletin, 102,* 122–138.

Pyszczynski, T., Greenberg, J., & LaPrelle, J. (1985). Social comparison after success and failure: Biased search for information consistent with a self-serving conclusion. *Journal of Experimental Social Psychology, 21,* 195–211.

Roese, N. J., & Olson, J. M. (1995). Outcome controllability and counterfactual thinking. *Personality and Social Psychology Bulletin, 21,* 620–628.

Rohde, P., Lewinsohn, P. M., Tilson, M., & Seeley, J. R. (1990). Dimensionality of coping and its relation to depression. *Journal of Personality and Social Psychology, 58,* 499–511.

Rosenberg, M. (1965). *Society and the adolescent self-image.* Princeton, NJ: Princeton University Press.

Roth, S., & Cohen, L. H. (1986). Approach, avoidance, and coping with stress. *American Psychologist, 41,* 813–819.

Scheier, M. F., & Carver, C. S. (1987). Dispositional optimism and physical well-being: The influence of generalized outcome expectancies on health. *Journal of Personality, 55,* 169–210.

Scheier, M. F., Matthews, K. A., Owens, J. F., Magovern, G. J., Sr., Lefebvre, R. C., Abbott, R. A., & Carver, C. S. (1989). Dispositional optimism and recovery from coronary artery bypass surgery. *Journal of Personality and Social Psychology, 57,* 1024–1040.

Spencer, S. J., Josephs, R. A., & Steele, C. (1993). Low self-esteem: The struggle for self-integrity. In R. Baumeister (Ed.), *Self-esteem: The puzzle of low self-regard* (pp. 21–36). New York: Plenum.

Stone, A. A., Helder, L., & Schneider, M. S. (1988). Coping with stressful events: Coping dimensions and issues. In L. Cohen (Ed.), *Stressful life events: Theoretical and methodological issues* (pp. 182–210). Newbury Park, CA: Sage.

Stone, A. A., & Neale, J. M. (1984). A new measure of daily coping. *Journal of Personality and Social Psychology, 46,* 892–906.

Suls, J., & Fletcher, B. (1985). Relative efficacy of avoidant and nonavoidant coping strategies. *Health Psychology, 4,* 249–288.

Suls, J., & Wan, C. K. (1987). In search of the false-uniqueness phenomenon: Fear and estimates of social consensus. *Journal of Personality and Social Psychology, 52,* 211–217.

Taylor, S. E., & Lobel, M. (1989). Social comparison activity under threat: Downward evaluations and upward contacts. *Psychological Review, 96,* 569–575.

Tice, D. (1993). The social motivations of people with low self-esteem. In R. Baumeister (Ed.), *Self-esteem: The puzzle of low self-regard* (pp. 37–53). New York: Plenum.

Tigges, B. B., Wills, T. A., & Link, B. G. (1996). *Social comparison, the threat of AIDS, and adolescent condom use.* Manuscript submitted for publication.

Van Lange, P. A. M., & Rusbult, C. E. (1995). My relationship is better than—and not as bad as—yours is: The perception of superiority in close relationships. *Personality and Social Psychology Bulletin, 21,* 32–44.

Vitaliano, P. P., Russo, J., Carr, J., Maiuro, R. D., & Becker, J. (1985). The Ways of Coping checklist: Revision and psychometic properties. *Multivariate Behavioral Research, 20,* 3–26.

Wallston, K. A., Wallston, B. S., & DeVellis, R. (1978). Development of the Multidimensional Health Locus of Control scales. *Health Education Monographs, 6,* 160–170.

Wills, T. A. (1981). Downward comparison principles in social psychology. *Psychological Bulletin, 90,* 245–271.

Wills, T. A. (1982, August). Stress, coping, and substance use among adolescents. In L. Bugen (Chair), *Applications of the Coping Assessment Battery.* Symposium presented at the meeting of the American Psychological Association, Los Angeles.

Wills, T. A. (1985). Stress, coping, and tobacco and alcohol use in early adolescence. In S. Shiffman & T. A. Wills (Eds.), *Coping and substance use* (pp. 67–94). Orlando, FL: Academic Press.

Wills, T. A. (1986). Stress and coping in early adolescence: Relationships to substance use in urban school samples. *Health Psychology, 5,* 503–529.

Wills, T. A. (1987). Downward comparison as a coping mechanism. In C. R. Snyder & C. E. Ford (Eds.), *Coping with negative life events: Clinical and social-psychological perspectives* (pp. 243–268). New York: Plenum.

Wills, T. A. (1991a). Similarity and self-esteem in downward comparison. In J. Suls & T. A. Wills (Eds.), *Social comparison: Contemporary theory and research* (pp. 51–78). Hillsdale, NJ: Lawrence Erlbaum Associates.

Wills, T. A. (1991b). Social comparison processes in coping and health. In C. R. Snyder & D. R. Forsyth (Eds.), *Handbook of social and clinical psychology* (pp. 376–394). Elmsford, NY: Pergamon.

Wills, T. A. (1992). Social comparison and self-change. In J. D. Fisher, J. Chinsky, Y. Klar, & A. Nadler (Eds.), *Self-change: Social-psychological and clinical perspectives* (pp. 231–252). New York: Springer-Verlag.

Wills, T. A. (1994). Self-esteem and perceived control in adolescent substance use: Comparative tests in concurrent and prospective analyses. *Psychology of Addictive Behaviors, 8,* 223–234.

Wills, T. A. (in press). Coping relates to important external criteria. In T. Pickering (Ed.), *Concepts and controversies in behavioral medicine.* Mahwah, NJ: Lawrence Erlbaum Associates.

Wills, T. A. , & Cleary, S. D. (1995). Stress-coping model for alcohol-tobacco interactions in adolescence. In J. B. Fettig & J. P. Allen (Eds.), *Alcohol and tobacco: From basic science to clinical practice* (pp. 107–128). Bethesda, MD: National Institute on Alcohol Abuse and Alcoholism.

Wills, T. A., Cleary, S. D., & Shinar, O. (1996). *Relationships of coping dimensions over time: Panel analyses in a community sample of adolescents.* Manuscript submitted for publication.

Wills, T. A., DuHamel, K.,& Vaccaro, D. (1995). Activity and mood temperament as predictors of adolescent substance use: Test of a self-regulation mediational model. *Journal of Personality and Social Psychology, 68,* 901–916.

Wills, T. A., & Filer, M. (1996). Stress-coping model of adolescent behavior problems. In T. H. Ollendick & R. J. Prinz (Eds.), *Advances in clinical child psychology* (Vol. 18, pp. 91–132). New York: Plenum Press.

Wills, T. A., & Hirky, A. E. (1996). Coping and substance abuse. In M. Zeidner & N. S. Endler (Eds.), *Handbook of coping: Theory, research, and applications* (pp. 279–302). New York: Wiley.

Wills, T. A., Vaccaro, D., & Benson, G. (1995). Coping and competence in adolescent alcohol and drug use. In J. L. Wallander & L. J. Siegel (Eds.), *Advances in pediatric psychology (Vol. 2): Behavioral perspectives on adolescent health* (pp. 160–178). New York: Guilford.

Wood, J. V. (1989). Theory and research concerning social comparisons and personal attributes. *Psychological Bulletin, 106,* 231–248.

Wood, J. V., Taylor, S. E., & Lichtman, R. R. (1985). Social comparison in adjustment to breast cancer. *Journal of Personality and Social Psychology, 49,* 1169–1183.

# CHAPTER 7

# Social Comparison, Lay Referral, and the Decision to Seek Medical Care

Jerry Suls
René Martin
*University of Iowa*

Howard Leventhal
*Rutgers University*

Pause for a moment and inventory your bodily sensations. Perhaps you will find that all is in order and you are feeling quite well. It is more likely, however, that you will notice a symptom or two. You might have a mild headache, for example, or maybe some discomfort and slight swelling in your left knee. Are you concerned about these symptoms? With whom might you consult if you are uncertain about the meaning of your symptoms? People experience physical signs and symptoms on an ongoing basis. These temporal changes in physical condition must be interpreted, and the individual must decide what response, if any, is appropriate. Actually, different questions tend to be salient at each stage of an unfolding illness episode. As we see here, the number of such questions is considerable, and each tends to elicit a defined set of procedures designed to stimulate specific answers. These questions and procedures are part of the "rules" of self-management, specifically, the rules for the clarification and/or definition of a potential health problem (Leventhal & Diefenbach, 1991; Leventhal, Suls, & Leventhal, 1993).

In this process of interpretation and decision making, individuals may seek to compare their somatic sensations or initial assessment of symptoms with others before seeking expert medical attention (Mechanic, 1972). In fact, social comparison with others may determine whether the person decides the somatic sensations are indicative of illness and whether or not to go for treatment. The network of nonprofessional informational sources comprised of relatives, friends, and acquaintances—what medical sociologists term the "lay referral network" (Friedson, 1961)—provides the context for social comparison and information exchange. This chapter considers the role of social comparison and lay referral in symptom evaluation, focusing on behaviors that occur prior to the delivery of expert medical care, and processes that influence whether medical care is sought.

Although, on first thought, this subject may not traditionally be seen as relevant to the coping process (see Suls, David, & Harvey, 1996), the onset of somatic sensations whose meaning and interpretation are unclear can be as threatening as more commonly studied stressors, such as the death of a relative, or natural disaster. Symptom evaluation, of course, is more straightforward in cases of obvious physical trauma. The person suffering a laceration with copious blood loss, for example, is not likely to experience difficulty deciding whether to seek immediate medical attention. Even traumas are unclear, however; you may not know how deep or extensive the injury.

## BACKGROUND

Leventhal and associates provide a framework within which to consider how social comparison and lay referral processes influence a person's decision to seek medical attention. On the basis of extensive interviews with patients at a clinic, Safer, Tharps, Jackson, and Leventhal (1979) found that the time period that elapses between people's first discovery of a symptom and their entry into medical treatment occurs in three stages. The first stage, *appraisal delay*, reflects the time that passes before the person interprets a symptom as a marker of illness. The time between the recognition that one is ill and the decision to seek medical attention is referred to as *illness delay*. The third and final stage, *utilization delay*, begins when the person decides to seek medical care and ends when that individual actually reports to the physician's office, clinic, or hospital. The social comparison and lay referral processes addressed in the present chapter apply primarily to the appraisal delay and illness delay stages.

Patients have reported in interviews that prior to arrival at the clinic or hospital their attention focused on two critical questions (Safer al al., 1979). First, during the appraisal delay stage, they considered whether or not their symptoms represented an illness (i.e., "Am I sick?"). If the answer to the first question was affirmative, patients then evaluated whether or not their illness warranted professional medical attention (i.e., "Should I go to the doctor?"); this second question characterizes the illness delay stage of Leventhal's model.

A wide range of information and past experience will come into play as the individual addresses the questions, "Am I sick?" and "Should I seek expert care?" For example, a set of symptoms may map onto a known illness schema with a specific diagnostic label, e.g., common cold, a heart attack. When symptoms fit a known pattern, it is easy for the individual to conclude that he or she is ill (Baumann, Cameron, Zimmerman, & Leventhal, 1989; Bishop, 1987). If symptoms are very severe and the person's ability to perform normal responsibilities is impaired he or she may infer that something serious is wrong and in need of medical attention (Apple, 1960; Matthews, Siegel, Kuler, Thompson, & Varat, 1983).

In addition to applying common-sense models and concerns about role impairment to the question of whether or not they are ill, people can draw on prior experiences with symptoms and illnesses (Anderson, Cacioppo, & Roberts, 1995; Cacioppo, Anderson, Turnquist, Petty, 1986). For example, if similar symptoms represented strep throat in the past, the patient is likely to conclude that the present symptoms are also indicative of a strep infection. People may utilize attributional rules in determining whether symptoms might result from external causes or stress. The perceived importance of chest pain, for example, might be discounted after heavy exertion or after an argument with one's boss. Under these circumstances, the individual may infer that muscle strain or stress is producing the symptom. The same chest pain might seem much more alarming, and perhaps even representative of a heart attack, if it occurs at rest. Similarly, Cameron, Leventhal, and Leventhal (1995) found that, when patients experienced ambiguous symptoms during a period of high life stress, they tended to attribute the symptoms to stress rather than illness and delayed seeking medical care.

## SOCIAL COMPARISON THEORY

Comparisons with other people figure prominently among the many types of information that may be used to address the questions "Am I sick?" and "Should I go to the doctor?" Members of the person's lay referral network frequently offer their own interpretations of symptoms before the individual ever seeks medical treatment. Although health care providers may intuitively understand that patients' family members and friends can either facilitate or hinder health care, little theoretical and empirical work has been done on the role of comparison processes in lay referral. This is unfortunate because an understanding of comparison and lay referral may improve our understanding about factors leading to over- and underutilization of health care resources. Some early empirical work suggests that social comparisons with relatives and friends play a significant role in defining symptoms and making decisions about medical care. Suchman (1965) reported that 74% of the respondents in an adult community sample who were experiencing an illness episode talked to at least one layperson regarding symptoms and what to do about them. This person was usually a spouse (53% of the time). Similarly, in a study of patients suffering from head and neck cancer, Miller (1973) reported that 62% of the patients spoke to a layperson about their symptoms and their meaning prior to seeking medical attention. Interestingly, Twaddle (1969) found that if symptoms produced severe pain or disability, respondents sought medical care immediately; for other symptoms the majority of subjects had discussions with nonexperts. The preceding evidence suggests that health care providers are likely to find that a sound theoretical and empirical understanding of lay referral processes will allow them to enhance patient compliance, particularly in the context of chronic illness, by enlisting the aid of members of the lay referral network.

We want to argue that a substantial part of lay referral is most appropriately considered under the rubric of social comparison theory (Festinger, 1954; Latané, 1966; Sanders, 1982; Suls & Miller, 1977). At first glance, the direct role of social comparison in the lay referral network may not be apparent. Social comparison is conceptualized by social psychologists as the process in which one compares one's standing or agreement on an ability or opinion dimension with other peoples' standing on the same dimension in order to gauge capability or correctness; self-evaluation is the purpose of social comparison. (Festinger, 1954; Suls & Martin, 1994). Conferring with members of one's lay referral network does not necessitate comparison, of course; the network may be the context for simple information-seeking. The network also provides a context for obtaining folk wisdom about illness and medical treatment both during illness episodes and at other times (Friedson, 1961). Some uses of the lay referral network, however, involve comparison with others on the so-called illness dimension (e.g., "I have a headache and feel feverish. Have you had those symptoms lately?" to ascertain if the flu is going around). Other instances involve the comparison of opinions about the meaning or severity associated with reported symptoms. "I hurt my arm while lifting a heavy object. Do you think it's probably nothing or should I see my physician?" In the latter situation, members of the network may draw on their general knowledge of physical illness, but they may also make explicit comparisons based on their past or current experiences with similar symptoms.

According to Festinger's (1954) theory of social comparison, people need to possess accurate assessments of their abilities and opinions and they find uncertainty an aversive condition. They prefer physical and objective standards to evaluate themselves, but these are commonly unavailable. Under such circumstances, people compare with others to assess their standing. Although Festinger restricted his model to abilities and opinions, Schachter and Singer (1962) recognized that social comparison may also apply to any situation where people are in a state of uncertainty. They argued that both physiological arousal and the cognitions that label physical sensations combine to create the perception of emotion (and other bodily states). Their experimental studies demonstrated that if people experience visceral arousal for which they have no obvious explanation they engage in a cognitive search to explain the aroused state. The emotions of other people around them may provide the cues, via social comparison, to label their own state. In sum, Schachter and Singer (1962) demonstrated that social comparison also is applicable to the labeling and interpretation of ambiguous physiological arousal as emotional states. Mechanic (1972) extended this argument to situations in which the layperson has no objective criteria to determine whether physical or psychological sensations are indicative of serious illness. Thus, a person experiencing ambiguous somatic sensations may compare with others to determine whether they have or are experiencing the same thing and how they interpret these sensations. Note that the emphasis in these approaches is on self-evaluation; people are intent on obtaining an accurate rendering of their own status and its meaning and significance.

When people choose others, Festinger proposed they prefer others who are similar to them. Subsequent accounts of comparison theory provided more precise descriptions of similarity (Goethals and Darley, 1977). In the evaluation of ability (i.e., "how good am I?"), contemporary social psychologists define similarity in terms of attributes that are related to or predictive of the dimension under evaluation (Goethals & Darley, 1977). If I want to assess how good I am at running, for example, I would compare with someone of the same age, gender, physical shape, and running experience. In contrast, comparing with someone much younger or older would not yield appropriately useful information (Suls, Gastorf, & Lawhon, 1978; Gastorf & Suls, 1978). In ability evaluation, persons should generally choose similar others; they will obtain a greater sense of subjective certainty after comparing with them. (See Wheeler, Martin, & Suls, 1997, for an extension and refinement of ability comparison theory.)

The dynamics of the comparison process in the opinion realm are more complex (Goethals & Darley, 1977). First, following Jones and Gerard's (1965) distinction, there are two kinds of opinions, values and beliefs. Values are opinions that are personally relevant, and there is no "objectively correct" value judgment (Jones & Gerard, 1965). A person making such a judgment is asking, "Is this right or appropriate for me? Will I like it?" Beliefs, in contrast, refer to propositions or statements about the world that are potentially verifiable. According to Goethals and Darley's (1977) attributional recasting of comparison theory, similar others are appropriate sources of information to assist one in making a value judgment. Deciding, for example, whether one would enjoy a particular movie or restaurant may be best answered by comparing with a friend who has similar tastes in movies or food. The opinions of someone with dissimilar attributes, even if they are knowledgeable about food and restaurants, do not necessarily indicate what one will personally like. On this view, similar persons should be preferred as comparison others, and learning that similar others agree or disagree with one's value judgments should have greater impact than agreement or disagreement with someone who does not share similar background attributes.

Beliefs work somewhat differently because they refer to empirically verifiable facts. In their case, the expectation is that the opinions of persons dissimilar on related attributes will be preferred. This somewhat counterintuitive prediction is based on the notion that dissimilar others look at things from a different perspective (because of their different related attributes). Thus, if dissimilar others agree with you about a belief, their agreement has a kind of "triangulation effect," in the same sense that a surveyer gets a better fix on a target by viewing it from different perspectives (Goethals & Nelson, 1973). Similar others share your general perspective and are thus just as likely to be prone to the same biases. Comparison with dissimilar others helps to assure that the same biases are not operating. Consequently, discovering agreement with a dissimilar other should increase your confidence that you are seeing "things" as they really are (Goethals & Nelson, 1973). Of course, if the dissimilar other disagrees, the disagreement can be discounted because of the difference in related attributes. There is empirical evidence that persons prefer to evaluate their beliefs by comparing them with persons who are dissimilar in related atttributes (Gorenflow & Crano, 1989; Reckman & Goethals, 1973). Moreover, confidence in belief judgments is bolstered more by finding agreement with dissimilar others (Goethals & Nelson, 1973).

This brief survey of comparison theory indicates that the dynamics of ability, belief, and value comparisons for self-evaluation all share some basic features. Each type of comparison is set in motion by uncertainty. Uncertainty motivates the individual to compare, to seek information, with relevant others. However, the type of comparison other (similar or dissimilar) sought and the effect of the comparison varies depending on the attribute (ability, belief, value) to be evaluated.

## APPLICATION OF COMPARISON THEORY TO LAY REFERRAL

Elements of social comparison in medical lay referral parallel the distinctions among ability, belief, and value comparisons. In ability comparison, people compare their standing with the standing of others; for example, can they jump higher or run faster or longer? In one form of lay referral for symptom appraisal that is akin to ability comparison ("context-induced comparison," described in detail later), to ascertain whether he or she is ill, an individual judges whether his or her symptoms are the same as or more or less severe than those of another person or persons. In this case, the comparison is with others on the dimension or attribute (i.e., symptoms) under evaluation.

Other forms of comparison in lay referral involve the evaluation of opinions about the meaning of symptoms. The belief–value distinction, described earlier, has parallels in symptom evaluation. Discerning the meaning of symptoms can be considered a form of belief evaluation because, at one level, symptom interpretation involves the verification of an actual entity. For example, are chest heaviness, shortness of breath, and fatigue symptoms of coronary heart disease? In this case, agreement from someone with a dissimilar perspective may increase certainty that one should seek medical attention by virtue of the triangulation process we referred to earlier (cf. Goethals & Nelson, 1973). (Of course, if a dissimilar other disagrees, the disagreement may be discounted because of their different background.) Medical experts may be even more useful. Not only do they have a different perspective but as experts, they may be perceived to provide "objective criteria." Recall that social comparison theory posits that objective or physical standards are preferred to social comparison. In the medical arena, experts probably are treated as objective referents. There may also be members of the lay network who also have "expert status" conferred upon them even if it is not justified (Suls & Goodkin, 1994). In such cases, the dynamics described above regarding similarity and dissimilarity may be "short-circuited."

The interpretation of symptoms can also be treated as a value question because some illnesses manifest themselves differently in different people and affect them in unique ways. Just as someone with similar taste and background may be seen as a good source of information about what restaurant or movie we would enjoy, so too, someone with a similar background or experience may be viewed as a more appropriate standard to compare with to decide whether somatic sensations are indicative of illness. (Unless the dissimilar other is a medical expert who, as noted above, may be treated as an objective standard rather than a social referent.) For example,the level of pain reported by an elderly person is unlikely to be perceived as an appropriate standard for assessing the significance of pain experienced by a younger person. Because symptom interpretation has elements that resemble both beliefs and values, the choice of social comparison referents in lay referral may involve a blend of similar and dissimilar others.

It is worth noting that our analysis represents an extension of Heider's (1958) and Kelley's (1967) notion that people attempt to understand the behavior of others just as scientists would. They initially collect data and then, by examining that data, make a rational judgment about the causes of events. In other words, people operate as "intuitive scientists" in explaining behavior or events. Analogously, when people experience new bodily sensations or signs, they operate as "intuitive physicians" to decide whether they need to be concerned, take some action, or seek a medical professional. This is not a disinterested process, however. People may want an accurate evaluation, but they may also want to be reassured if the outcome of initial consultation suggests an unfavorable diagnosis. Thus, various defensive processes may be engaged subsequent to the first encounters with members of the lay network (Taylor, Buunk, & Aspinwall, 1990; VanderZee, Buunk, & Sanderman,1995; Wills, 1981). Once one obtains information, especially if the outcome is negative, one may be motivated to minimize or reconstrue its implications in a more positive light. Recent research on comparison has emphasized the use of upward and downward comparisons to reduce the impact of information threatening to the self (Buunk, Collins, Taylor, VanYperen, & Dakof, 1990; Wheeler & Miyake, 1992; Wills, 1981). We elaborate on the role of defensive comparisons later in the chapter.

In the sections that follow, we develop the role of social comparison in lay referral in three scenarios. Each scenario describes different circumstances that might prompt the individual to question, "Am I ill?" It is apparent in these scenarios that social comparison as used to appraise physical symptoms resembles ability, belief, and value comparison. As we consider possible symptom scenarios, we comment on how the process approximates ability, value, and belief comparison and on the different roles of similar, dissimilar, and expert sources of referral. After considering social comparison processes in the appraisal delay stage, we describe the processes evoked during the illness delay stage by the question, "Should I go to the doctor?"

### Scenario 1: Symptom-Induced Social Comparison

A middle-aged man experiences pain on the left side of his chest, which later spreads to his left arm. Chest pain might seem similar to "heartburn" from eating a spicy meal; on the other hand, pain extending to the left arm might elicit concerns about angina. Each experience of changes in bodily sensations may prompt a state of uncertainty. What do these symptoms mean? Are they indicative of illness?

By seeking information from others in the immediate social context, people experiencing unexplainable somatic sensations can attempt to evaluate whether their assessment and interpretation of their experience is appropriate. In most cases, people form a tentative opinion for themselves; finding validation from others reduces residual uncertainty. In essence, this situation involves social comparison for opinion evaluation. The individual in this scenario describes the sensations to a friend or relative and then asks the listener for his or her opinion. If the listener agrees with the individual's initial assessment, then the latter probably gains confidence in that assessment. If the listener disagrees, people perceiving the symptom will experience even greater ambiguity and may continue to seek information regarding the symptoms' meaning.

Although people act as an "intuitive physicians," they are not guided completely by logical considerations. Fiske and Taylor's (1991) review of the empirical literature on cognitive processes suggests that the individual may best be characterized as a "motivated tactician." By this they mean that the individual is a "fully engaged thinker who has multiple cognitive strategies available and chooses among them based on goals, motives, and needs. Sometimes the motivated tactician chooses wisely, in the interests of adaptability and accuracy, and sometimes the motivated tactician chooses defensively, in the interests of speed or self-esteem" (p. 13). Given the potential costs of underestimating the significance of physical symptoms, the individual will frequently be caught between the "intuitive physician" and "tactician" roles. It is, therefore, scarcely surprising that ambiguous symptoms can evoke so much distress and anxiety.

Of course, the individual probably would prefer to hear the most positive interpretation of the symptoms. In fact, there is empirical evidence that people try to minimize the threat value of symptoms (Ditto, Jemmott, & Darley, 1988). Consequently, people may delay for a time before seeking consultation with a relative or friend. If the symptoms persist, however, the individual will probably seek advice. The result of initial consultation and comparison with members of the lay network may lead to labeling the symptoms as benign and not meriting medical attention. On the other hand, laypersons may suggest that formal medical treatment should be sought. In the case of an unfavorable "diagnosis" by friends and relatives, which may constitute a threat to the self, the individual may seek other lay consultations. Ditto and Lopez (1992) found that people given an unfavorable medical opinion from experts were more likely to distrust the result, cited more life irregularities that affected accuracy of the assessment, and were more likely to seek another assessment than were people receiving a favorable diagnosis. If people distrust unfavorable diagnoses from experts, one would expect them to be even more rejecting of the medical opinions of laypeople. This suggests that people may seek a second opinion about bad news. Defensive processes may prompt the individual to "shop around." However, if several members of the lay network judge a pattern of somatic sensations or bodily signs as serious, one may expect the person to seek formal medical attention.

***Selection of Comparison Other.*** As noted above, the selection and effect of an appropriate comparison on opinion evaluation depends on whether the opinion under consideration reflects a belief or a value. Social comparison prompted by the perception of symptoms incorporates aspects of both belief and value comparison. The desired information (i.e., whether one has some definable medical condition) represents a potentially verifiable belief that might be best addressed by a dissimilar comparison other by means of the triangulation process described earlier.

There is good reason to think, however, that people with medical or health expertise should provide the most informative feedback. Not only will such persons have a dissimilar perspective, but they may also possess expert information that may be considered objective. As noted earlier, we can expect people to prefer objective information to social comparison information. Absent a physician or other health care professional, a lay expert may offer a useful opinion that will provide a more learned perspective. For example, the neighbor who works part time as a nursing assistant might provide especially useful comparison information.

Whereas symptom-induced social comparison has elements of belief evaluation, value comparison is also relevant to the question of whether one is ill. Illnesses manifest themselves differently in different people. A physican or the opinion leader in the lay referral network may be very knowledgeable about illness but may be different in age, experience, and perceived susceptibility from oneself. Many questions about illness are not answered by "objective" physical tests or expert diagnosis, but rather with reference to a particular person's situation and life responsibilities. Someone with a similar physical constitution and background may provide a more appropriate benchmark for interpreting one's symptoms. For example, increasing aches and pains usually are "part and parcel" of aging. Someone who is going through the same thing may be perceived to be a better guide for determining whether there is something to be concerned about and what it means for someone like me.

According to this reasoning, symptom-induced comparison has aspects both forms of evaluation–belief (are these symptoms indicative of a disease?) and value (e.g., am I the kind of person who contracts this disorder? how will these symptoms affect my lifestyle?). Even if lay experts have never experienced the precise symptoms themselves, they may provide knowledgeable opinions about symptoms, disease, and appropriate medical care. Peers or similar comparison others may have the attributes and experience necessary to suggest whether the symptoms are indicative of illness and how the illness will be manifested in people like themselves (see Kulik & Mahler, chapter 8, this volume). Symptom-induced comparison consequently may occur both with dissimilar others and similar others. Dissimilar experts may, however, play a special role because they have the additional virtue of providing objective criteria. According to this perspective, people should be ambivalent about whether similar or lay experts are better sources of feedback about their symptoms. In the best of all possible situations, the "expert" would be someone of similar age and physical history, thereby satisfying both value and belief concerns. See Table 7.1 for a summary of the comparison processes operating in the "symptom-induced" scenario.

***If Experts Are Best, Why Lay Referral?*** If, in light of their expert knowledge, health care professionals are generally believed to have the most useful information, the reader may ask why the lay referral network is consulted at all. In other words, why not seek medical attention immediately at the onset of symptoms? One reason is that, by definition, the lay referral network is nearby, convenient, and easily accessible. The health care establishment is distant. By the principle of least effort, the informal community of friends and relatives is psychologically and physically closest to the patient (Sanders, 1982). Financial cost is another obvious reason why people carefully consider the significance of their symptoms before seeking formal medical attention.

There are a variety of additional reasons that the lay referral network

TABLE 7.1
Comparison Processes Operating in Three Lay Referral Scenarios

| | *Symptom-Induced* | *Context-Induced* | *Mass Psychogenic* |
|---|---|---|---|
| Comparison trigger | Personal symptoms | Relevant other with objective disease and possibility of contagion or shared exposure | Relevant other with subjective complaints and possibility of contagion or shared exposure |
| Evaluation dimension | Opinion evaluation including aspects of value and belief | Ability evaluation | Ability evaluation |
| Similarity of comparison other | Values: similar on related attributes Beliefs: dissimilar on related attributes; expert provides dissimilar perspective and objective reality | Similar other on related attributes | Similar other on related attributes |

is utilized prior to, or even instead of, professional health care. People tend to believe that the source of their symptoms is transient and likely to improve, rather than persistent and increasingly severe (Cacioppo et al., 1986). This propensity is supported by empirical findings (Fries & Frey, 1980; Higgins, Rhodewalt, & Zanna, 1979) and anecdotal accounts of heart attack survivors (Hackett & Cassem, 1969). The bias toward perceiving symptoms as transient and benign is also consistent with the well documented tendency for people to think of themselves as relatively invulnerable to disease and negative events (Weinstein, 1980; see also Klein & Weinstein, chapter 2, this volume) and in better health than others (Suls, Marco, & Tobin, 1991; Taylor & Brown, 1988). Medical experts may also be avoided if the individual fears hearing a threatening or dismal diagnosis. Compared to the pronouncement of a physician, it is relatively easy to discount or derogate pessimistic information provided by a relative or friend (Sanders, 1982). These results are suggestive of the "motivated tactician" described earlier.

Another reason favoring the use of lay referral information is the potential embarrassment associated with health care visits. The individual who makes a doctor's appointment or rushes to the local emergency room for a symptom that turns out to be benign or trivial is likely to be embarrassed. He or she may even be criticized for overreacting and using medical resources inappropriately. Although disclosing certain kinds of symptoms to one's friends can also provoke embarrassment, many symptoms do not have this quality. A chat over coffee with a friend or relative does not involve the same costs as making a medical appointment and taking up a medical professional's time with what might be a trivial condition. There is at least anecdotal evidence that patients do not like to be labeled as hypochondriacs or hysterics by their physicians.

***Empirical Data on Symptom-Induced Comparison.*** As a preliminary examination of the analysis of comparison in the symptom-induced scenario, we asked a sample of 106 college students to report on the last time they made an unscheduled visit to a physician, medical clinic, or hospital for some symptom or injury. Questions concerned whether they talked to anyone prior to going for medical consultation, whom they talked to, and why. The first notable feature of the responses was that approximately 94% of the participants mentioned wanting to talk to someone else. Clearly, consultation with friends and relatives about physical symptoms is very common. Table 7.2 provides a breakdown of the reasons these students gave for talking to others. As can be seen, seeking information was a major reason reported. About 80% of the respondents said they talked to someone else about their symptoms to find out what they thought the problem was; 75% talked to others to get advice about what should be done. In a study with middle-aged and older adults seeking medical care, Cameron, Leventhal, and Leventhal (1993) reported that wanting to find out what the symptoms might mean and what should be done also were mentioned frequently (33% and 38%) as reasons for talking to friends and family. The fact that young adults mentioned these reasons more often than did the older persons in this study might reflect young adults' lack of experience and their consequent greater uncertainty with regard to symptoms and illness. It is also noteworthy that 61% of Cameron et al.'s respondents spoke to someone else about their symptoms compared to 94% of the young adult sample. Again, although older subjects also appear to have a need

TABLE 7.2
Reasons Provided for Seeking Lay Referral

| *Reasons* | *Percent* |
|---|---|
| Wanted to know what others thought the symptoms or injury could be | 82 |
| Sought advice on what to do about the problem | 75 |
| Wanted to know if the other person had similar symptoms | 24 |
| Wondered if others would worry if they had similar symptoms | 24 |
| Just wanted to talk about it | 35 |

to talk to others about signs and symptoms, the need to communicate is not quite as great, perhaps because the elderly have more experience and knowledge about interpreting the meaning of symptoms. It is also possible that because the elderly have more health problems and concerns, they are more likely to take their concerns to their physician without first conferring with friends or family. The more critical point about both samples is that a majority of people appear to act like "intuitive physicians," by trying to learn what they can from other people prior to seeking medical attention.

For the young adult sample, we asked with whom the person communicated. As indicated in Table 7.3, parents and friends were frequent choices. Friends can be considered as similar others. Parents are also similar in some ways (shared heredity and family background, of course), but dissimilar by virtue of age and level of experience. The latter features are likely to provide parents with more relevant medical knowledge. These results are broadly consistent with our analysis that both similar others and dissimilar others who have more expertise are likely to be chosen to obtain useful comparison information.

The survey also asked respondents whether the person they spoke to had any medical expertise. Thirty-seven percent mentioned communicating with a friend, acquaintance, or relative who was involved in medical care (e.g., physician, dentist, registered nurse) prior to seeking formal medical attention. We examined whether the reasons given for talking to someone else about their symptoms differed depending on whether the other had some medical expertise or not. As shown in Table 7.4, people tended to ask the same questions of others regardless of whether the other had medical expertise. There were two notable exceptions. About 32% of the respondents mentioned talking with others to see if they had had similar symptoms when the others did not have medical expertise; when the people consulted had medical expertise; only 16% of respondents mentioned wanting to know if their referents had had similar symptoms. Also, 30% of the sample mentioned talking to someone about whether they would be worried if they had the same symptoms when the other had no medical expertise; less

TABLE 7.3
Choices of Referents for Health-Related Information and Advice

| *Referents* | *Percent* |
|---|---|
| Parents | 58 |
| Friends | 36 |
| Other relatives | 3 |
| Acquaintances | 2 |
| Strangers | 1 |

TABLE 7.4
Reasons for Seeking Lay Referral of Referents With and Without Medical Expertise

| *Reason* | *Referent With Medical Expertise* | *Referent Without Medical Expertise* |
|---|---|---|
| Wanted to know what others thought the symptoms or injury could be | 89.2% | 77.8% |
| Sought advice on what to do about it | 81.0% | 73.0% |
| Wanted to know if the other person had similar symptoms | 16.2% | 31.8% |
| Wanted to know if others would worry if they had similar symptoms | 18.9% | 30.2% |
| Just wanted to talk about it | 35.1% | 36.5% |

than twenty percent mentioned wanting to know if the other would worry when they had medical expertise. These data suggest that persons perceived to have medical expertise function as knowledgeable dissimilar others who need not experience the same illness to be a useful source of information, but these "experts" appear to answer questions relating to the nature of the symptoms and what course of action should be taken. These results are reminiscent of belief concerns. However, similar (nonexperts) are more useful when the issue is whether the other person has the same symptoms or would worry with the same symptoms. These issues are reminiscent of value concerns: is this appropriate for me?

### Scenario 2: Context-Induced Social Comparison

Imagine that your spouse has been diagnosed with infectious mononucleosis. Though you are feeling well, you nevertheless begin to monitor yourself closely. Pennebaker (1982) found that manifestation of symptoms by others tends to increase self-symptom monitoring. Perhaps your fatigue after a long day at work or the slight tickle in your throat represent the early stages of mononucleosis. You consult your spouse: did his or her symptoms also begin with fatigue and a tickle in the throat? After considering your spouse's condition, you may go so far as to measure your own temperature and palpate your neck for enlarged lymph nodes. You are seeking context-induced social comparison information.

Context-induced social comparison probably occurs most frequently when a member of the social network is verifiably ill with some contagious disorder, or when parties share exposure situations, such as food poisoning or environmental toxins. The awareness of exposure to contagious elements induces symptom vigilance. The individual observes his or her physical condition and attempts to match the signs and symptoms experienced with those presented by the contagious other. If the symptoms match, then the target will infer that he too is ill. In this second scenario, social comparison is prompted by the presence of another person who is ill, rather than the initial manifestation of symptoms per se as described in the first scenario.

When considered in light of social comparison theory, the context-induced scenario most closely resembles the evaluation of abilities. In this case, when we learn that someone who is physically close or similar to us is ill we are prompted to make a comparison between ourselves and that person. Because of our knowledge that some illnesses are contagious, we may become vigilant about our own physical health. In the context-induced scenario, there may be no discussion and exchange of opinions about the significance of symptoms, as there is in the symptom-induced situation. Merely being exposed to someone who is physically ill may prompt a self-evaluation and monitoring of relevant symptoms, in much the same way that exposure to a higher ability or high-status other induces a social comparison and consequent self-assessment (Gilbert, Geisler, & Morris, 1995; Morse & Gergen, 1970; Tesser, 1991). In ability evaluation, the comparer considers whether he or she can accomplish a particular task—climb a mountain, for example, or earn a high score on an academic achievement examination. In context-induced evaluations of illness, the comparer ponders whether he or she exhibits a particular set of physical symptoms, the meaning of which is provided by the proximity of a contagious other.

Who are we likely to chose as a similar comparison other in context-induced illness evaluations? In the case of many common contagious illnesses, such as colds and the flu, any other person with whom one has had contact or with whom one shares exposure is considered a relevant and similar comparison other. This is because attributes related to or predictive of having these illnesses are considered "universal." That is, human beings share attributes that render them vulnerable to a great number of diseases or toxins so that merely having physical contact or sharing the same space or being exposed similarly may be sufficient to become ill. There are also instances, however, when similarity is defined by factors beyond physical contact. For example, if your child comes down with the chicken pox, this should only induce symptom vigilance and matching if you have never had the chicken pox. If you have had the chicken pox previously, you know you will be immune to future episodes and you will not attempt to match any symptoms you begin to experience to those of your child's illness.

Other physical disorders involve more complicated and subtle types of comparisons, extending the role of context-induced illness comparisons beyond the realm of contagious diseases. Let us suppose that you and a friend are both employed in the same factory doing the same kind of work. If this friend is diagnosed with cancer, you might become highly vigilant about bruises, weight loss, and fatigue because there are common-sense beliefs and some solid scientific evidence linking environmental exposure to certain toxins and the risk of cancer. Here, work-site similarity becomes a relevant dimension.

Shared characteristics as general as age and gender may even prompt symptom vigilance. Suppose a neighbor who is the same age and who shares your lifestyle and habits (e.g., smokes two packs of cigarettes per day) is struck by a heart attack. This may prompt you to be more vigilant about chest pain, fatigue, and other symptoms of heart disease. The main point in context-induced illness comparisons is that people become vigilant about their own symptoms as a result of sharing contact or exposure with others who are ill. If the person detects symptoms they are probably labeled in a manner consistent with the disorder of their similar friend, relative, or acquaintance. Similarity becomes important to the extent the physical disorder is seen to be related to personal attributes.

Although we conceive this process as analogous to the way in which people construe their abilities, there is at least one notable difference. In ability social comparison, the process begins when people are uncertain about their standing, usually because they lack an objective standard. In context-induced social comparison, the illness of another person with whom one has shared contact or exposure creates the uncertainty about one's standing on the illness dimension. That is, the context (a similar other becoming ill) is the social comparison (see Table 7.1).

Context-induced evaluations of symptoms may engender both positive and negative outcomes. The symptom vigilance induced by the presence of a similar other who is ill may lead to the early awareness of important symptoms, encouraging the comparer to receive early medical diagnosis and intervention. However, the same context-induced symptom vigilance may cause the individual to become overconcerned with ambiguous physical sensations, producing unwarranted concern and unnecessary health care visits.

## Scenario 3: Mass Psychogenic Illness

A third scenario involves instances of mass psychogenic illness, or widespread symptom perception among a large group of individuals working or living close to one another even though there is no objective evidence of illness (based on medical tests) or of environmental pollution (based on tests of water, air, etc.) (Colligan, Pennebaker, &

Murphy, 1982). Characteristic features of these cases are that symptoms tend to occur during periods of extreme stress and show rapid onset and resolution. Generally the "illness" spreads among people one works closely with or knows personally.

The classic and perhaps best documented case is the so-called "June Bug" episode studied by Kerckhoff and Back (1968). During an especially busy time of the year, an industrial plant was closed down because of a mysterious illness afflicting about one quarter of the plant's 200 employees. Reported symptoms included nausea and feverishness that sent several workers to their physicians and a few to the hospital, although no objective evidence of illness was found. In interviews, several stricken workers reported seeing or being bitten by an insect at the plant sometime prior to the onset of their symptoms. Careful inspection failed, however, to find evidence of insect bites or strange insects. Examiners from the Center for Disease Control concluded after a complete examination of the plant and the victims, that the afflicted were "victims of nothing more than extreme anxiety" (Kerckhoff & Back, 1968, p. 7). The conclusion was that the people who became "ill" showed a classic pattern of hysterical contagion in which the symptoms were mislabeled as physical illness.

In cases of mass psychogenic illness, members of one's social context present ambiguous symptoms—that is, symptoms that might or might not be indicative of illness. These symptoms "spread" to others living or working nearby. Consistent with this interpretation, the vast majority of cases in the "June Bug" epidemic occurred on two consecutive days after the news media publicized earlier incidents. Second, most of those afflicted worked at the same time and same place in the plant. Third, most of the ill were women who were married and had children; they were accordingly trying to combine job and motherhood, often an exhausting arrangement. It is also of interest that the "epidemic" occurred at a busy time in the plant during which there were incentives for employees to put in overtime and to work at a fast pace. Job anxieties coupled with physical manifestations of fatigue created a set of circumstances that could be labeled as illness.

This is a scenario for mass psychogenic illness. Like Scenario 2, a social comparison process induced by the social context was operating, but here the symptoms were not really indicative of physical disease. There was no "real" disease being transmitted between the workers. In other words, the social reality was not veridical. Nonetheless, if the individual learns of others' symptoms and is already fatigued and anxious, then the person may be particularly likely to label ambiguous, everyday symptoms, such as fatigue and headache, as signs of illness. We assume that under these conditions there is some arousal, boredom, or anxiety that contributes to the situation. In addition, there probably is some incentive for playing the sick role, such as a brief respite from a hectic work schedule. In a related vein, Buunk and Ybema (chapter 12, this volume) discuss the way social comparison may induce burnout as well as absenteeism among individuals faced with more or less ambiguous stress at work.

There is a parallel in the work of Schachter and Singer (1962) on emotion, described earlier, in which people labeled unexplained arousal consistently with the emotions exhibited by other people in the same situation. In mass psychogenic illness, people have vague, ambiguous symptoms and adopt the same label and explanation for these symptoms as do other people. The difference between Schachter and Singer's analysis and mass psychogenic illness is that in the latter, the ambiguous physical state is labeled as an illness rather than as an emotional state. Typically, in psychogenic episodes, people are fatigued, anxious, and experience symptoms which frequently are ambiguous. If others claim to have been bitten by a strange bug or contracted the flu, this becomes a plausible label for one's own state.

As in cases of context-induced comparison, the information sought in mass psychogenic illness most closely resembles ability evaluation in the initial detection of symptoms (see Table 7.1). People are prompted by others' reports of illness to monitor their own symptoms vigilantly and to compare them with the ones reported by others. We suspect that similarity of environment and exposure are critical to the selection of a comparison other in mass psychogenic illness. Someone with similar constitutional attributes (such as gender, age, general level of vigor) who becomes ill may facilitate self-attribution of illness because similarity may suggest similar levels of vulnerability. Also, if stress and anxiety play a role, hysterical contagion is more likely in individuals who are also feeling anxious and distressed. Note in the latter case that although information that a similar other is ill faciliates contagion, it is not because the other is a more appropriate comparison other but because the target person has existing feelings that also are congruent with the notion of some infectious or pathogenic agent in the immediate environment (see Table 7.1).

Studies on mass psychogenic illness have not systematically assessed similarity of those who are "stricken" by the illness versus those who are not. However, Wrightsman (1960) found that similarity was important in the related phenomenon of emotional contagion. Recently, Sullins (1991) also reported results of two experimental studies showing that the emotions of two previously unacquainted individuals became more alike when they expected to undergo the same experience, but not when they were in different circumstances. More directly relevant to mass psychogenic episodes, Kerckhoff and Back (1968) found that those affected at the plant were more likely to be linked together by bonds of friendship and work-related associations. Similarly, Stahl and Lebedun (1974) found that workers who exhibited the most severe symptoms to a "mystery gas" at a Data Center were more likely to be friends. Stahl and Lebedun also found no ecological (physical) clustering of symptomatology: "instead similarities in symptomatology were better defined by interpersonal networks of friendship patterns" (p. 48). Commonly, such individuals also share other attributes.

## Lay Referral in the Illness Delay Stage

If the symptom perceiver in any of the three scenarios concludes that he or she is ill, attention then turns to the question of whether expert medical care should be sought. Zola (1973) described a number of "triggers" that prompt an individual to seek treatment. These included degree to which the symptoms create distress and whether a symptom (such as reporting always being in pain or tired) threatens a relationship between the individual and some other person. As in the appraisal phase, common sense models and prior experience influence whether people decide to seek formal care and how long they delay before entering the health care delivery system (Leventhal et al., 1980). If beliefs about an illness suggest that the condition will spontaneously resolve in a short time, then a doctor may not be consulted even though the symptom perceiver considers himself or herself ill. The symptom perceiver also may elect to simply observe the course of the illness without medical intervention if previous experience indicates that the symptomatic period will be brief or mild.

Safer et al. (1986) also reported that patients with longterm, chronic symptoms and those who imagined possibly, severe consequences of their illnesses took longer than others to seek medical attention. It appears that people see some kinds of ongoing symptoms as indicative of illnesses that will go away on their own. (Perhaps they also come to recognize chronic symptoms as ordinary and therefore of little concern. They may also anticipate that little can be done to correct ongoing chronic symptoms.) It seems counterintuitive that those persons who imagine grim consequences of their symptoms apparently are the ones to delay before seeking medical attention. This tendency probably reflects fears about the prospect of receiving a serious diagnosis, the discomfort people associate with medical procedures, and a focus on the short-term rather than the long-term consequences of the symptoms. Here, again, the person may act more as the "motivated tactician" than the "intuitive physician." However, if symptoms interfere with role performance, such as work or family responsibilities, then people are likely to seek medical attention promptly (Apple, 1960).

In addition to common sense models, symptom novelty, and prior experience, people also rely on their lay referral network for information regarding the importance of seeking medical care. For example, there is evidence that people are more likely to seek medical attention if there is a history of a similar problem in the family or if a relative had a similar problem (Turk, Litt, Salovey, & Walker, 1985). In some cases, family, friends, or employers may pressure the patient to seek treatment; what Zola (1973) refers to as "social sanctioning."

Conferring with family and friends in this domain also involves the social comparison of opinions, focusing on the question "Should I go to the doctor?" As in symptom appraisal, evaluation of this question incorporates elements of both belief and value comparison. Whether medical attention is needed is a potentially verifiable proposition. Receiving validation from a party with a different perspective should add confidence to one's own assessment, especially if the comparison other has some expertise. Note also that if the layperson is viewed as having expertise, his or her assessment may also be considered indicative of objective criteria. But deciding to go to a physican also has aspects of a value decision. The ill person must determine whether it is appropriate for him or her to go to a physician. "Should I seek medical attention and obtain medication or should I endure the pain?" Obviously, in cases of extreme symptoms, there is little ambiguity; in these instances, information from the lay referral network is unlikely to be sought at all. In more ambiguous cases, the individual needs to decide whether his or her illness requires professional attention given other aspects of his or her physical or psychological constitution. Lay referral may be most pertinent to considerations about whether to use medical resources or treat him or herself; whether seeking medical care will threaten a relationship, or tax financial resources. Here, a similar other may provide needed information, just as similar others seem to be more helpful in evaluating subjective values and personally relevant issues.

There is some empirical evidence relevant to the notion that similar and dissimilar expert comparison others are influential in making decisions about seeking health care, though research in this domain is limited. Oberlander, Pless, and Dougherty (1993) interviewed a sample of approximately 500 parents who visited a pediatric emergency department. Parents were asked whether they had previously sought advice from family, friends or a physician. The researchers also had coders evaluate whether the emergency room visit was appropriate, based on the child's age, time of visit, clinical state, and problem at presentation. The results indicated that the proportion of visits deemed appropriate was higher (47%) when a parent had spoken to both a nonphysician and a physician prior to visiting the emergency room, than when no advice was sought (27%). When a parent spoke to a nonphysician, the greatest likelihood of an appropriate visit occurred when that person was a nurse (71%) and the least when the person was a family member (32%). Not surprisingly, the advice of other medical professionals led to a higher frequency of appropriate visits. Nonetheless, seeking the council of other family members also led to slightly more appropriate visits than not seeking others' advice at all. Thus, there is at least some support for the idea that both dissimilar experts and similar family members may provide useful information. Most importantly, it appears that family members, regardless of expertise, are a major trigger in getting a person to seek formal medical attention (Zola, 1973)

## LAY REFERRAL: DELAY OR ENCOURAGEMENT?

Does lay referral encourage or delay seeking medical attention? Sanders (1982) review of the literature suggested that lay consultants' opinions are heavily loaded in favor of obtaining professional advice. In a longitudinal study of medical care seekers who were between the ages of 45 and 80 (mean age 60.9 years) and who belonged to a health maintenance organization (HMO), described earlier, Cameron et al. (1993) found that 50% of their sample had been advised by family or friends to seek medical care. However, in our view, the complexity of medical disorders and contemporary practices and the rapidity with which the biomedical sciences are advancing should render most laypeople rather confused and prone to misinformation. It is unclear whether such misinformation would lead to overadvising or underadvising when it comes to the decision about seeking a doctor's care. This may also explain why Cameron et al. (1993) found that patients were advised to see a physican only about half of the time.

Sanders (1981) investigated the effects of objective information and (lay referral) comparison information on the decision to go to a physician. Subjects were asked to imagine that they were experiencing various symptoms and then were given social comparison information (from friends) suggesting they either should or should not seek medical attention. The receipt of objective information, in the form of a simple physical test, was also manipulated to suggest either that the symptoms did or did not require professional attention. After receiving the information, participants were asked to indicate how likely they were to consult a doctor. Sanders found that in the absence of objective information, subjects' decisions were strongly swayed by friends' opinions. When there was objective information indicating that the subject should seek medical assistance, comparison had little additional impact. However, when objective information suggested the symptoms were harmless (i.e., a negative test), the impact of social comparison was still substantial! In other words, even if the physical test suggested that the symptoms were trivial, subjects reported they would still go to the doctor if their friends advised that they should. The reason for this may lie, according to Sanders, in the major function of the lay referral system which is to validate the sick role (see also Suchman, 1965). If significant others are willing to let one forgo responsibilities, then objective criteria become less important. In addition, it is well-documented that negative instances are less informative than positive instances (Wason, 1961), hence, "go" social comparison information may offset "don't go" objective information.

Jemmott, Ditto, and Croyle (1986) provide additional empirical evidence that has bearing on when lay consultation delays medical care-seeking. College students were recruited to undergo some medical tests, one of which fictitiously assessed an enzyme deficiency, called thioamine acetylase deficiency (TAA), that could lead to a disorder of the pancreas (also fictitious). Each subject was given bogus feedback, indicating that he or she had or did not have the enzyme deficiency; participants were then told either that the deficiency was rare or that it was prevalent. The subjects were then asked to complete a questionnaire which included items about the seriousness of various disorders, including TAA. Participants led to believe that TAA was rare rated the disorder as more serious than those told TAA was prevalent. (Needless to say, subjects were debriefed at the conclusion of the study.) Apparently common maladies are considered less problematic and threatening than infrequent disorders. Other evidence indicates that people with a history of a medical condition estimate its prevalence to be greater and regard it as less life-threatening than people with no history of the condition (Jemmott, Croyle, & Ditto, 1988). Extrapolating from these data, it would be expected that illnesses or symptoms that are prevalent among members of one's network would be perceived as minor and less deserving of medical attention. Consequently, the network may prompt the individual to underestimate the need for medical attention.

The role of illness prevalence among members of one's social network is also nicely demonstrated in Clark's (1959) study of Mexican-American migrant workers. Clark found that migrant workers had all sorts of symptoms that medical professionals regard as serious but that the workers did not feel were serious or requiring medical attention, apparently because the symptoms were so prevalent and no one had died.

So although members of the lay referral network often encourage their ill member to seek professional health care, lay consultation potentially can also contribute to illness delay. Family and friends may help the symptom perceiver make a positive appraisal about whether the physical signs are indicative of illness, but they may not necessarily agree that medical attention is warranted. Relatives and friends, lacking expert training, may "misdiagnose" the source and seriousness of the ill person's problems, leading to inappropriate advice. Members of the lay referral network who distrust health care providers or who have had unpleasant health care experiences may persuade the ill target to delay or avoid professional consultation (Suls & Goodkin, 1994). The act of communicating with relatives and friends regarding symptoms requires time; prolonged illness delay may result if multiple sources are consulted or if members of the network offer conflicting interpretations. Finally, the illness delay stage may become extended if the lay network becomes involved in lengthy discussions of which physician or clinic is most appropriate, least expensive, or easily accessible.

Medical sociologists have presented evidence that people with strong social support networks tend to delay in seeking medical care. Granovetter (1978) and Liu and Duff (1972) reported that persons who have so-called "strong tie" networks, characterized by involving consultation with a few persons, tended to delay longer before seeking medical attention than people with weak ties (i.e., more diffuse contacts). These researchers suggested that diffuse networks may provide confusing and disparate information that causes people to seek professional advice sooner. Berkanovic, Telesky, and Reeder (1981) also found that people who had more contact with their social network were less likely to see a physician. The greater the physical distance between the individual and his or her network, the more likely formal medical attention was sought. Granovetter proposed that the network effects resulted because strong networks encouraged the individual to stay well (or perhaps discourage the sick role). It is just as plausible that persons who are isolated experience greater feelings of anxiety and uncertainty. In the absence of close informal support, they resort to the more formal medical attention. In any case, the nature of these (retrospective) data makes it difficult to judge whether this sort of delay is appropriate or not.

In our view, the critical factor in illness delay is not whether one's network is large or small, but the nature of interactions between members of the network and whether people feel comfortable soliciting opinions about the significance of their symptoms or actively engaging in social comparisons. Of course, obvious physical indicators of disease or disability permit the opportunity for comparison simply because they are public. However, other symptoms are more subtle and private. If an individual says he is not feeling well or has certain symptoms in a large group such as a party or large family get-together, a kind of pluralistic ignorance may be operating which discourages the group from offering the interpretation that the symptoms are serious and in need of attention. Pluralistic ignorance is characterized by the belief that one's private thoughts, feelings, and behaviors are different from those of others, even though one's public behavior is identical (Katz & Allport, 1928; Miller & McFarland, 1987).

The concept of pluralistic ignorance has been linked to the hesitancy of bystanders to intervene in emergencies (Latané & Darley, 1970). Bystanders who are unsure about the seriousness of the situation often assume that other bystanders, despite acting similarly to themselves, are confident that the situation is not an emergency. The more bystanders present, the more powerful the effect, resulting in a lower probability that any given individual will label the situation an emergency and intervene. Analogously, a person may share information about her symptoms, but because family and friends are looking to each other for a response, no one explicitly reacts and the person's physical condition is minimized or ignored. The problem here is that no one is willing to be candid. This may seem surprising among friends and family, but we suspect that in groups even close acquaintances are unlikely to come forward. On the other hand, if the individual shares information about her symptoms with a single member of the family or a friend, then pluralistic ignorance is less apt to operate. That lone member of the lay referral network is more likely to take an active role in offering an interpretation of the symptoms and suggesting that a physician be consulted. According to this account, being a member of large network is not so critical as the opportunity to consult privately with individual members of the network.

In summary, the lay referral network can have both a positive and negative influence in terms of prompting the individual to seek medical attention. The empirical literature is inconsistent about whether the lay referral facilitates or impedes seeking medical attention because social comparison (and other) processes have both facilitatory and inhibitory elements.

## CONCLUDING COMMENTS

***Social Comparison, Lay Referral, and the Inappropriate Use of Health Resources.*** The preceding discussion of the role of social comparison processes in the lay referral system may clarify a puzzling set of empirical findings. Estimates suggest that only about one third of people with physical symptoms actually refer themselves for medical consultation (Scambler, Scambler, & Craig, 1981). This would not be problematic, of course, if the untreated symptoms were mild or did not indicate of any disease. However, there is evidence to suggest that persons experiencing significant symptoms often fail to refer themselves for professional attention. Ingham and Miller (1979) used a mobile health clinic to administer an extensive battery of medical screening tests to virtually all of the citizens of a borough in the United Kingdom. They found that 57% of the 3,160 participants had symptoms necessitating treatment that they had never sought. The large proportion of unreported, untreated symptoms led Scambler and Scambler (1985) to refer to this phenomenon as the "illness iceberg."

Although consequential symptoms often go untreated, there is surprising evidence that a large proportion of the people who do report symptoms to their physicians have no demonstrable disease. For example, some studies estimate that 20% to 40% of all patients seeking primary care have no major medical illness and 30% to 60% of all visits to primary care physicians involve symptoms for which no serious underlying medical cause can be detected (Backett, Heady, & Evans, 1954; Barsky, 1981).

Putting all of these findings together, we are led to the conclusion that many people visit their physicians when they are not actually ill, while others who are suffering from consequential symptoms fail to seek health care. Advice and other forms of information from family members and friends regarding the interpretation of physical symptoms (i.e., social comparison processes operating in the lay referral network) may be among the factors that lead to inappropriate use of health care resources, including both overuse and underuse.

***The Importance of the Lay Referral Network after Medical Consultation.*** Although the current chapter has focused on the operation of social comparison prior to entry into the health care delivery system, social comparison persists as a powerful agent of social influence even after the patient consults his physician. Many illnesses are chronic rather than curable. The patient receives a treatment regimen, often including medications, and is asked to monitor his ongoing condition carefuly. Although the patient has had some experience with the symptoms, flare-ups may present as much ambiguity as the first episodes. For example, suppose that a person with asthma experiences increased chest tightness and wheezing in April. Should the increase in these familiar symptoms occasion a visit to the internist, or should the patient simply attribute the increased symptoms to the presense of mold spores and pollen common in the spring? The familiarity of the symptoms may encourage the patient to treat herself by increasing the dosage of prescription drugs without first conferring with a health care provider, a practice prone to untoward consequences.

In the context of chronic illness, consultation with family and friends operates very much as it did in the initial episodes described above. However, the health care provider has the unique opportunity under these circumstances to capitalize on the power of the lay referral network. Nurses and physicians should identify important members of lay referral network for their chronically ill clients. Relatives and close friends should be included in educational discussions of symptoms that serve as warning markers of impending exacerbations. Such efforts would alert members of the network to relevant symptoms and assist them in offering accurate interpretations and advice. Finally, the contribution and effectiveness of lay consultation should be evaluated on an ongoing basis over the course of the patient's chronic illness, with educational interventions made as necessary.

***Implications for Future Research.*** This chapter distinguished among three scenarios, symptom-induced comparison, context-induced comparison, and mass psychogenic illness, and linked them to traditional aspects of social comparison theory. As such, our discussion seeks to be informative about the role of comparison processes in lay medical decision making. Interpersonal comparison processes were initially applied by Festinger to opinions and abilities and then later extended by Schachter and Singer to emotional states and to physical symptoms by David Mechanic (1972).The chapter extends previous analyses by presenting three different scenarios in which social comparisons operate, and by elaborating on the usefulness of the belief and value distinction developed in contemporary comparison theory for the interpretation of physical symptoms. Examination of comparison processes in symptom interpretation may, as noted previously, be helpful in implementing medical treatments and compliance and also in understanding why people sometimes go for treatment when it is not needed and at other times don't seek medical attention or delay in doing so.

More research is clearly needed. The study of comparison processes in lay referral is still in its early stages; we know little, for example, about what confers an aura of medical expertise on some members of the social network. The chapter treated the referral network as a single group of people, but more likely individuals have multiple referral groups. Which groups are sought, and how people reconcile disparate opinions or comparisons is not well understood. We have treated people as if they all operate in the same ways, but it seems more likely that individual predispositions play a role. Research on individual differences in social comparison of lay referral would be desirable. Persons high in extraversion are more likely to more extensive social networks and social contacts. Does this mean they confer with other laypeople prior to seeking expert medical attention more than introverts do? According to Watson and Pennebaker (1989), persons high in *negative affectivity* (chronic feelings of dissatisfaction and life stress) are more likely to interpret benign bodily sensations as potential signs of physical illness. Are such persons less likely to confer with network members and more likely to seek formal medical attention? Finally, our emphasis has been on the "intuitive physician" model, which emphasizes an accurate rendering of symptoms and their meaning, but there is evidence available that people under certain circumstances operate more like "motivated tacticians" to protect self-esteem and maintain positive emotions. Understanding how people balance these distinct motivations is important if we are to understand and facilitate timely and appropriate medical care-seeking.

***Further Extensions of Comparison Theory.*** The application of comparison theory to lay referral may also be of benefit to the development and refinement of comparison theory. As noted by Wills and Suls (1991), the lack of attention to the social comparison of opinions has been conspicuous in recent years; ability and trait evaluation has tended to take center stage for theorists and researchers. Analysis of medical lay referral reinforces the need to look more carefully at opinion comparison especially as it relates to beliefs and values. Contemporary accounts of comparison theory (Goethals & Darley, 1977) have treated belief and value comparison as distinct; however, we have described how some comparison instances involve blends of the two (see also Suls, 1986). The medical domain may be an appropriate place to examine the subtleties of opinion evaluation.

One of the comparison scenarios, context-induced comparison, suggests that uncertainty need not be the instigator of comparison processes, contrary to the general thesis of Festinger's theory. In the usual process, the person is uncertain about his or her standing or correctness, lacks an objective standard, and consequently compares with others. In the context-induced scenario, however, the illness of others creates a comparison with self, which, in turn, induces self-monitoring and information search. In this case, the comparison induces uncertainty rather than uncertainty inducing comparison. This kind of situation may not be unusual in other domains and suggests some emendation of social comparison theory.

In conclusion, the study of social comparison and medical lay referral provides the opportunity to contribute to the understanding of lay medical decision-making as well as to refine and advance the basic theory of interpersonal comparisons. We are reminded of Kurt Lewin's dictum, "That there is nothing so practical as a good theory." And we would add that there is nothing so good for theory as a practical proving ground.

## ACKNOWLEDGMENTS

Work on this chapter was partially supported by NIH grant 46448. The authors wish to thank James Kulik, Lisa Aspinwall, and the editors for their helpful comments on earlier versions of this chapter.

## REFERENCES

Anderson, B., Cacioppo, J. T., & Roberts, D. C. (1995). Delay in seeking a cancer diagnosis: Delay stages and psychophysiological comparison processes. *British Journal of Social Psychology, 34,* 33–52.

Apple, D. (1960). How laymen define illness. *Journal of Health and Social Behavior, 13,* 219–228.

Barsky, A. (1981). Hidden reasons some patients visit doctors. *Annals of Internal Medicine, 94,* 492–497.

Backett, E. M., Heady, J. A., & Evans, J. C. (1954). Studies of a general practice. II The doctor's job in an urban area. *British Medical Journal, 1,* 109–123.

Baumann, L., Cameron, L., Zimmerman, R., & Leventhal, H. (1989). Illness representations and matching labels with symptoms. *Health Psychology, 8,* 449–470.

Berkanovic, E., Telesky, C., & Reeder, S. (1981). Structural and social psychological factors in the decision to seek medical care for symptoms. *Medical Care, 19,* 693–709.

Bishop, G. D. (1987). Lay conceptions of physical symptoms. *Journal of Applied Social Psychology, 17,* 127–146.

Buunk, B. P., Collins, R. L., Taylor, S. E., Van YPeren, N., & Dakof, G. A. (1990). The affective consequences of social comparison: Either direction has its ups and downs. *Journal of Personality and Social Psychology, 59,* 1238–1249.

Cacioppo, J. T., Anderson, B. L., Turnquist, D. C., & Petty, R. E. (1986). Psychphysiological comparison processes: Interpreting cancer symptoms. In B. L. Anderson (Ed.), *Women with cancer: Psychological perspectives* (pp.141–171). New York: Springer-Verlag.

Cameron, L., Leventhal, E. A., & Leventhal, H. (1993). Symptom representation and affect as determinants of care seeking in a community-dwelling, adult sample population. *Health Psychology, 12,* 171–179.

Cameron, L., Leventhal, E. A., & Leventhal, H. (1995). Seeking medical care in response to symptoms and life stress. *Psychosomatic Medicine, 57,* 37–47.

Clark, M. (1959). *Health in the Mexican-American culture.* Berkeley: U. Cal. Press.

Colligan, M., Pennebaker, J., & Murphy, L. (Eds.). (1982). *Mass psychogenic illess: A social psychological analysis.* Hillsdale, NJ: Lawrence Erlbaum Associates.

Ditto, P. H., Jemmott, J. B. III., & Darley, J. M. (1988). Appraising the threat of illness: A mental representational approach. *Health Psychology,7,* 183–200.

Ditto, P. H., & Lopez, D. F. (1992). Motivated skepticism: Use of differential criteria for preferred and nonpreferred conclusions. *Journal of Personality and Social Psychology, 63,* 568–584.

Festinger, L. (1954). A theory of social comparison processes. *Human Relations, 1,* 117–140.

Fiske, S., & Taylor, S. (1991). *Social cognition* (2nd ed.). Reading, MA: Addison-Wesley.

Freidson, E. (1961). *Patients' views of medical practice.* New York: Russell Sage.

Fries, A., & Frey, D. (1980). Misattribution of arousal and the effects of self-threatening information. *Journal of Experimental Social Psychology, 16,* 405–416.

Gastorf, J. W., & Suls, J. (1978). Performance evaluation via social comparison: Performance similarity versus related attribute similarity. *Social Psychology, 41,* 328–340.

Gilbert, D. T., Giesler, R. B., & Morris, K. A. (1995). When comparisons arise. *Journal of Personality and Social Psychology, 69,* 227–236.

Goethals, G. R., & Darley, J. (1977). Social comparison theory: An attributional approach. In J. Suls & R. L. Miller (Eds.) *Social comparison processes: Theoretical and empirical perspectives* (pp. 259–278). Washington, DC: Hemisphere.

Goethals, G. R., & Nelson, R. E. (1973). Similarity in the influence process: The belief-value distinction. *Journal of Personality and Social Psychology, 25,* 117–122.

Gorenflo, D. W., & Crano, W. D. (1989). Judgmental subjectivity/objectivity and locus of choice in social comparison. *Journal of Personality and Social Psychology, 57,* 605–614.

Granovetter, M. S. (1978). The strength of weak ties. *American Journal of Sociology, 31,* 1360–1369.

Hackett, T. P., & Cassem, N. H. (1969). Factors contributing to delay in responding to the signs and symptoms of acute myocardial infarction. *American Journal of Cardiology, 24,* 651–658.

Heider, F. (1958). *The psychology of interpersonal relations.* New York: Wiley.

Higgins, E. T., Rhodewalt, F., & Zanna, M. P. (1979). Dissonnace motivation: Its nature, persistance, and reinstatement. *Journal of Experimental Social Psychology, 15,* 16–34.

Ingham, I., & Miller, P. (1979). Symptom prevalence and severity in a general practice. *Journal of Epidemiology and Community Health, 33,* 191–198.

Jemmott, J. B., III, Croyle, R. H., & Ditto, P. H. (1988). Commonsense epidemiology: Self-based judgments from laypersons and physicians. *Health Psychology, 7,* 55–73.

Jemmott, J. B., III, Ditto, P. H., & Croyle, R. T. (1986). Judging health status: Effects of perceived prevalence and personal relevance. *Journal of Personality and Social Psychology, 50,* 899–905.

Jones, E. E., & Gerard, H. B. (1965). *Foundations of social psychology.* New York: Wiley.

Katz, D., & Allport, F. H. (1928). *Student attitudes: A report of the Syracuse University research study.* Syracuse, NY: Craftsman Press.

Kelley, H. (1967). Attribution theory in social psychology. In D. L. Levine (Ed.), *Nebraska symposium on motivation* (pp. 192–241). Lincoln: University of Nebraska Press.

Kerckhoff, A. C., & Back, K. W. (1968). *The June Bug: A study of hysterical contagion.* New York: Appleton-Century-Crofts.

Latané, B. (Ed.). (1966). Studies in social comparison. *Journal of Experimental Social Psychology,* Supplement 1.

Latané, B., & Darley, J. (1970). *The unresponsive bystander: Why doesn't he help?* New York:Appleton-Century-Crofts.

Leventhal, H., & Diefenbach, M. (1991). The active side of illness cognition. In A. Skelton & R. T. Croyle (Eds.), *Mental representations in health and illness* (pp. 247–272). New York: Springer-Verlag.

Leventhal, E., Suls, J., & Leventhal, H. (1993). Hierarchical analysis of coping: Evidence from life-span studies. In H. Krohne (Ed.). *Attention and avoidance* (pp. 71–100). Seattle, WA: Hogrefe & Huber.

Leventhal, H., Meyer, D., & Nerenz, D. (1980). The common sense representation of illness danger. In S. Rachman (Ed.), *Contributions to medical psychology* (Vol. 2, pp. 7–30).

New York: Pergamon.

Liu, W. T., & Duff, R. W. (1972). The strength in weak ties. *Public Opinion Quarterly, 42,* 361–367.

Matthews, K. A., Siegel, J. M., Kuler, L. H., Thompson, M., & Varat, M. (1983). Determinants of decisions to seek medical treatment by patients with myocardial infarction symptoms. *Journal of Personality and Social Psychology, 44,* 1144–1156.

Mechanic, D. (1972). Social psychological factors affecting the presentation of bodily complaints. *New England Journal of Medicine, 286,* 1132–1139.

Miller, D. T., & McFarland, C. (1987). Pluralistic ignorance: When similarity is interpreted as dissimilarity. *Journal of Personality and Social Psychology, 53,* 298–305.

Miller, M. H. (1973). Seeking advice for cancer symptoms. *American Journal of Public Health, 63,* 955–961.

Morse, S., & Gergen, K. J. (1970). Social comparison, self-consistency, and the concept of the self. *Journal of Personality and Social Psychology, 40,* 624–634.

Oberlander, T. F., Pless, I. B., & Dougherty, G. E. (1993). Advice seeking and appropriate use of a pediatric emergency department. *American Journal of Developmental Care, 147,* 863–867.

Pennebaker, J. W. (1982). *The psychology of physical symptoms.* New York: Springer-Verlag.

Reckman, R. F., & Goethals, G. R. (1973). Deviancy and group-orientation as determinants of group composition preferences, *Sociometry, 36,* 419–423.

Safer, M., Tharps, Q., Jackson, T., & Leventhal, H. (1979). Determinanta of three stages of delay in seeking care at a medical care clinic. *Medical Care, 17,* 11–29.

Sanders, G. S. (1981). The interactive effect of social comparison and objective information on the decision to see a doctor. *Journal of Applied Social Psychology, 11,* 390–400.

Sanders, G. S. (1982). Social comparison and perceptions of health and illness. In G. S. Sanders & J. Suls (Eds.), *Social psychology of health and illness* (pp. 129–157). Hillsdale NJ: Lawrence Erlbaum Associates.

Scambler, A., Scambler, G., & Craig, D. (1981). Kinship and friendship networks and women's demand for primary care. *Journal of the Royal College of General Practitioners, 26,* 746–750.

Scambler, G., & Scambler, A. (1985). The illness iceberg and aspects of consulting behavior. In R. Fitzpatrick & J. Hinton (Eds.), *The experience of illness* (pp. 32–50). London: Tavistock.

Schachter, S., & Singer, J. E. (1962). Cognitive, social, and physiological determinants of emotional state. *Psychological Review, 69,* 379–399.

Stahl, S. M., & Lebedun, M. (1974). Mystery gas: An analysis of mass hysteria. *Journal of Health and Social Behavior, 15,* 44–50.

Suchman, E. A. (1965). States of illness and medical care. *Journal of Health and Social Behavior, 6,* 114–128.

Sullins, E. S. (1991). Emotional contagion revisited: Effects of social comparison and expressive style on mood convergence. *Personality and Social Psychology Bulletin, 17,* 166–174.

Suls, J. (1986). Notes on the occasion of social comparison theory's thirtieth birthday. *Personality and Social Psycholgy Bulletin, 12,* 289–296.

Suls, J., David, J. P., & Harvey, J. H. (1996). Personality and coping: Three generations of research. *Journal of Personality, 64,* 711–736.

Suls, J., Gastorf, J., & Lawhon, J. (1978). Social comparison choices for evaluating a sex- and age-related ability. *Personality and Social Psychology Bulletin, 4,* 102–105.

Suls, J., & Goodkin, F. (1994). Medical gossip and rumor: Their role in the lay referral system. In R. F. Goodman & A. Ben-Ze ev (Eds.), *Good gossip* (pp. 169–179). Lawrence: University Press of Kansas.

Suls, J., Marco, C., & Tobin, S. (1991). The role of temporal comparison, social comparison, and direct appraisal in the elderly's self-evaluations of health. *Journal of Applied Social Psychology, 21,* 1125–1144.

Suls, J., & Martin, R. (1994). Social comparison. In A. Manstead & M. Hewstone (Eds.), *Blackwell encyclopedia of social psychology.* Oxford: Blackwell.

Suls, J., & Martin, R. (1995). *A study of reasons given for lay referral in cases of physical symptoms and injury in young adults.* Unpublished manuscript, University of Iowa.

Suls, J., & Miller, R. L. (Eds.). (1977). *Social comparison processes: Theoretical and empirical perspectives.* Washington, DC: Hemisphere.

Taylor, S. E., & Brown, J. D. (1988). Illusion and mental health: A social psychological perspective. *Psychological Bulletin, 103,* 193–210.

Taylor, S. E., Buunk, B., & Aspinwall, L. (1990). Social comparison, stress, and coping. *Personality and Social Psychology Bulletin, 16,* 74–89.

Tesser, A. (1991). Emotion in social comparison and reflection processes. In J. Suls & T. A. Wills (Eds.), *Social comparison: Contemporary theory and research* (pp. 117–148). Hillsdale, NJ: Lawrence Erlbaum Associates.

Turk, D. C., Litt, M. D., Salovey, P., & Walker, J. (1985). Seeking urgent pediatric treatment: Factors contributing to frequency, delay, and appropriateness. *Health Psychology, 4,* 43–59.

Twaddle, A. C. (1969). Health decisions and sick role variations: An exploration. *Journal of Health and Social Behavior, 10,* 105–114.

VanderZee, K., Buunk, B., & Sanderman, R. (1995). Social comparison as a mediator between health problems and subjective health evaluations. *British Journal of Social Psychology, 34,* 53–65.

Wason, P. C. (1960). On the failure to eliminate hypotheses in a conceptual task. *Quarterly Journal of Experimental Psychology, 12,* 129–140.

Watson, D., & Pennebaker, J. W. (1989). Health complaints, stress, and distress: Exploring the central role of negative affectivity. *Psychological Review, 96,* 465–490.

Weinstein, N. (1980). Unrealistic optimism about future life events. *Journal of Personality and Social Psychology, 39,* 809–820.

Wheeler, L., Martin, R., & Suls, J. (1997). The proxy social comparison model for self-assessment of ability. *Personality and Social Psychology Review, 1,* 54–61.

Wheeler, L., & Miyake, M. (1992). Social comparison in everyday life. *Journal of Personality and Social Psychology, 62,* 760–773.

Wills, T. A. (1981). Downward comparison principles in social psychology. *Psychological Bulletin, 90,* 245–271.

Wills, T. A., & Suls, J. (1991). Commentary: Neo-social comparison theory and beyond. In J. Suls & J. A. Wills (Eds.), *Social comparison: Contemporary theory and research* (pp. 395–411). Hillsdale, NJ: Lawrence Erlbaum Associates.

Wrightsman, L. (1960). Effects of waiting with others on changes in level of anxiety. *Journal of Abnormal and Social Psychology, 61,* 216–222.

Zola, I. (1973). Pathways to the doctor: From person to patient. *Social Science and Medicine, 7,* 677–689.

# CHAPTER 8

# Social Comparison, Affiliation, and Coping With Acute Medical Threats

James A. Kulik
*University of California, San Diego*

Heike I. M. Mahler
*California State University, San Marcos, and University of California, San Diego*

> *I would try to find out as much as I possibly could . . . . Maybe, well, I could see and ask him what he's doing so I can do the same thing.*
>
> —Kulik and Mahler (1989)

The foregoing statement was made by a man faced with the imminent prospect of coronary-bypass surgery. He was explaining why he would prefer to be assigned a hospital roommate who was recovering from such surgery rather than a roommate who was awaiting it. The remark demonstrates the patient's belief that affiliation with other patients who have been through the same thing may help him cope with his situation. For almost 10 years, we have been interested in the affiliation patterns of people who face acute medical threats such as surgery and in how those affiliations might affect their ability to cope with such situations. In this research, we have been interested in a number of practical questions related to the assignment of surgical patients to hospital roommates: For example, is it better to assign patients who are awaiting surgery to roommates who have similar medical problems or different ones? Should one assign patients awaiting surgery to roommates who also await surgery or roommates who have already undergone surgery? Does an anxious roommate make a preoperative patient more anxious? While pursuing answers to these and other everyday issues of patient management, we have also found it useful to work from a social comparison theory framework (Festinger, 1954) to guide the design of both laboratory and field studies. Like Lewin (1948), we believe that an interplay between laboratory and field research is essential both for establishing the validity and parameters of a theory and for achieving results of practical value (cf. Kulik & Mahler, 1990).

To provide some theoretical and historical background to the primary focus of the chapter, we begin by reviewing some of the classic laboratory studies of affiliation choices in the face of acute threat. In doing so, we focus on several of the central concepts presented in Schachter's (1959) seminal work that extended social comparison theory to the domain of emotion and affiliation. Of particular interest are conclusions about the role that the desires to compare emotional response and to achieve cognitive clarity play in affiliation preferences, for we apply these concepts to our primary concern—our discussion of what is known about the actual affiliative behaviors of individuals under threat and their possible implications for health outcomes. We consider in some detail the handful of studies that have gone beyond traditional fear and affiliate-choice paradigms to consider the extent to which social comparison principles account for how people actually affiliate with others in the face of acute physical threats. We then consider the existing evidence that patient affiliations prior to aversive medical procedures actually affect the patient's ability to cope both emotionally and physically with the threat.

## CLASSIC SOCIAL COMPARISON STUDIES OF AFFILIATION AND THREAT

Social psychologists have long been interested in the affiliation preferences of people who are faced with a novel, physical-threat situation. As noted by Buunk, Gibbons, and Reis-Bergan (chapter 1, this volume), the theoretical cornerstone of this fear and affiliation research was laid by Festinger's (1954) social comparison theory. Festinger argued that people have a basic need for accurate appraisals of their opinions and abilities and that lacking an objective standard for a reference, individuals will evaluate their opinions and abilities by comparing themselves with other people. Festinger proposed further in his so-called similarity hypothesis that people prefer particularly to compare themselves to others of relatively similar ability or opinion. It was Festinger's belief that similar others provide a more accurate and stable gauge for evaluating one's relative standing than do people of very different ability or opinion.

As Taylor, Buunk, and Aspinwall (1990) have noted, implicit in

Festinger's original formulation was the potential relevance of social comparison processes for efforts to cope with stressful situations. That is, when confronting novel, threatening, or challenging situations, people generally need to evaluate the nature of the situation, their resources, and their emotional reactions. It was Schachter (1959), however, who explicitly extended social comparison theory to the domain of stress and emotion by proposing that people facing novel threats will experience an increased desire to affiliate with others, particularly with others who are currently facing the same threat. Consistent with this prediction, several early laboratory experiments found that when given the choice, individuals made fearful by the threat of imminent electric shock generally preferred to wait with similarly threatened others rather than alone or with others not facing the threat (e.g., Darley, 1966; Firestone, Kaplan, & Russell, 1973; Schachter, 1959, Experiments 1 and 2). As Schachter (1959) phrased it, "misery doesn't love just any kind of company, it loves only miserable company" (p. 24).

Considerable theoretical interest has focused on the question of why individuals under threat might experience an increased desire to affiliate with similarly threatened others. Schachter (1959) considered various possibilities but, in an extension of basic social comparison theory, clearly favored a self-evaluation explanation. According to this view, people experiencing physiological arousal that they have difficulty labeling because it accompanies an unfamiliar event or situation. They are motivated to affiliate with similarly threatened others, Schachter proposed, because such individuals are thought to provide the best gauge for evaluating the intensity, nature, or appropriateness of their emotional state. Thus Schachter proposed an "emotional similarity hypothesis," wherein needs for emotional self-evaluation are induced by novel threat and are met through social comparison or, more specifically, through comparing one's own emotional state with that of similarly threatened others.

Schachter also considered the possibility that a desire to increase "cognitive clarity" about the impending threat, that is, to reduce uncertainty regarding the nature and dangerousness of the situation, might motivate affiliation with similarly threatened others. In doing so, he acknowledged that comparisons of emotions can be viewed as a special case of cognitive clarity efforts (that is, part of reducing uncertainty about a novel threat situation may involve reducing uncertainty about how one should respond emotionally). Schachter, however, preferred to differentiate cognitive clarity, which he viewed in relatively nonsocial terms of threat-relevant information gathering, from emotion comparison processes, which he argued were inherently interpersonal and intended to evaluate one's feelings. Thus defined, he argued against cognitive clarity as an important determinant of affiliation. His argument was based largely on a laboratory experiment in which subjects who faced either high or low threat were asked to make their affiliation choice (to wait with fellow subjects or wait alone) either under conditions in which all verbal affiliation would be prohibited (no-talk condition) or verbal affiliation would be permitted for threat-irrelevant topics only (irrelevant-talk condition) (Schachter, 1959, Experiment 3). Schachter reasoned that talking with an affiliate about the threat is not essential to compare one's emotional response but is essential to gain cognitive clarity about the situation. He therefore expected to find that high threat individuals would exhibit more desire to affiliate than low threat subjects, whether in no-talk or in irrelevant-talk conditions. The results, however, showed that subjects in the high threat condition did not choose more than low threat subjects to wait with the similar others in either talk condition (pp. 34, 37). Despite this disconfirmation, Schachter concluded on the basis of subsequent internal analyses that desire for cognitive clarity had been ruled out "as any sort of potent motive" for affiliation under threat (p. 39), and that the emotional similarity hypothesis had been supported (i.e., that threat leads to an increased desire to be with similarly threatened others for purposes of emotional comparison).

This rather weak evidence was followed by other laboratory experiments that found only qualified support for the emotional similarity hypothesis (e.g., Darley & Aronson, 1966; Gerard, 1963; Gerard & Rabbie, 1961). Particularly pertinent, Zimbardo and Formica (1963) found that under high compared to low threat (of electric shock), individuals indicated a greater preference for awaiting the threat in the presence of someone likewise facing the same threat (similar emotional state) than with someone who had already experienced the threat (dissimilar emotional state). On the surface, this finding would seem to suggest that affiliation choices were more likely motivated by desires to compare one's emotions than to achieve cognitive clarity, if one assumes that someone who has already experienced a particular threat would be better able to provide cognitive clarity than someone who is awaiting the threat. By extrapolation, the Zimbardo and Formica result also would seem to predict that if patients were given a choice prior to surgery, they should be more apt to want a roommate who was awaiting the same surgery than a roommate recovering from the same surgery. Such a prediction would be tenuous, however, for several reasons. Most obvious, results based on relatively low-level, simple laboratory threats may not generalize to real-world medical threat situations. More subtle, but we believe at least as important, a critical procedural point in the Zimbardo and Formica experiment is that subjects' affiliation choices were made with the proviso that subjects could not discuss the experiment with the potential affiliate. This prohibition was imposed in an effort to rule out cognitive clarity a priori as an explanation for the observed tendency for subjects to want to affiliate more with others awaiting the same threat. As noted elsewhere, however (Kulik & Mahler, 1990), eliciting an affiliate-choice preference, while experimentally removing any chance for one's desire for cognitive clarity to operate, does not rule out the possibility that a desire for cognitive clarity normally is a significant motivator of affiliation under threat (cf. Kirkpatrick & Shaver, 1988; Rofe, 1984). Thus what the Zimbardo and Formica results actually suggest is that when the motivation for cognitive clarity is presumably blocked, affiliation choices in the face of threat may be determined by the desire to compare one's emotional response with that of others. This clearly is not the same as saying affiliation choices under threat are motivated principally or generally by desires for emotion comparison, particularly when one considers how unlikely it is that threat-relevant affiliation is prohibited in real world contexts.

Indeed, when we examined the affiliation choices of patients who faced the imminent prospect of coronary bypass surgery—and imposed no constraints on talking with affiliates—we found a very different pattern of affiliation, one that suggests a more prominent role for cognitive clarity as a motivator (Kulik & Mahler, 1989). Specifically, the night before surgery, we asked men hospitalized for coronary bypass procedures whether they would prefer assignment to a roommate who was awaiting bypass surgery, whether they would prefer a roommate who was back on the main ward recovering from bypass surgery, or whether they had no preference. The results indicated that patients most often preferred assignment to a roommate who was already recovering from bypass surgery. Even though a preoperative roommate is apt to be more similar in emotional status and therefore presumably a better referent for emotion comparison, a postoperative roommate was perceived as having greater information value, that is, as having more potential for providing cognitive clarity or reduction of uncertainty about what was to come. As one patient explained, "It's more helpful for me to talk to someone who's already had it, because the guy that's waiting doesn't know anything about it, only what he's been told." Another noted, "I could see how fast he [a recovering roommate] recovers, how they treat him after he's been operated on, you know, what to expect." Another noted that a recovering roommate should have information not even available to physicians; for example, "I'm not saying the doctors are liars. I'm not saying that. But you'd rather talk to a guy that's been through it . . . the doctors know the technicalities but they've never felt the pain." Still others, like the patient who opened this chapter, focused on the potential ability of the recovering roommate to provide specific coping strategies. Another patient explained similarly, "if you go out and get the information and you understand it and talk to the guy that already had it done and all . . . then take it from there . . . ask them [postoperative patients] a few questions, what'd they do here and what they'd do there."

***Summary.*** From the foregoing brief review, we are left with the conclusion that the early fear and affiliate-choice research appears to have underemphasized desires for cognitive clarity in favor of desires for emotion comparison as determinants of affiliation choices made under acute threat. More comprehensive reviews of this early literature appear at least implicitly to reach the same conclusions (see Cottrell & Epley, 1977; Shaver & Klinnert, 1982; Suls, 1977). Rofe (1984) is perhaps most explicit, arguing that when a person faces threat, the desirability of a potential affiliate will depend on the perceived ability of that individual to eliminate or reduce the stressfulness or uncertainty of the situation, not on the emotion-comparison potential of the affiliate per se. This conclusion makes sense when considered in relation to current conceptualizations of stress and coping that emphasize the importance of cognitive appraisal processes (e.g., Cohen & Lazarus, 1983; Lazarus & Folkman, 1984). According to these models, when we encounter a novel situation we engage in a primary appraisal process whose goal is to assess the likelihood that the situation will cause us harm. Efforts to obtain cognitive clarity can be viewed as central to primary appraisal efforts. Seeking information about the situation is believed also to play a role in subsequent problem-focused coping efforts, aimed at reducing the demands of the situation, or emotion-focused coping efforts, aimed at controlling the emotional response to the situation (Cohen & Lazarus, 1979). Thus when we are faced with a novel threat, as a part of coping, we may experience an increased desire for information relevant to the threat, and want to affiliate according to the ability of the other to provide such information (see also Suls, Martin, & Leventhal, chapter 7, this volume).

The role that one's desire for cognitive clarity plays in motivating affiliation in the face of threat is also interesting to consider in the light of recent theoretical expansions of social comparison theory. It is now generally believed, for example, that people engage in social comparison processes for a number of reasons, including self-evaluation (Festinger, 1954); self-enhancement, that is, to feel better about themselves (e.g., Hakmiller, 1966; Thornton & Arrowood, 1966; Wills, 1981); and self-improvement (cf. Brickman & Bulman, 1977; Festinger, 1954; Wood, 1989; Wood & Taylor, 1991; Wood & VanderZee, chapter 10, this volume; see also Helgeson & Mickelson, 1995, for other possible motives). According to Wills (1981), situations that decrease one's sense of well-being should lead to a desire for self-enhancement and, therefore, generally should lead individuals to prefer to compare with others who are worse off (i.e., to make downward comparisons). In an important refinement, Taylor and Lobel (1989) proposed that although threat may generally lead people to prefer to compare themselves cognitively to others worse off for purposes of self-enhancement, threat also may lead people to seek upward comparison information and affiliation (i.e., information or contact with others who are better off) for purposes of self-improvement, that is, in order to gain information that will enable them to improve their situation (cf. Helgeson & Taylor, 1993; Molleman, Pruyn, & van Knippenberg, 1986). Social comparison for self-improvement can be viewed as a close cousin, if not a direct descendant, of the original concept of cognitive clarity in that at issue fundamentally is seeking of threat-relevant information. Note also that upward comparisons theoretically can be made along at least two orthogonal dimensions, namely, the severity of the problem (the other person has a less severe problem than me) and coping adequacy (the other person is coping better than I am) (see Buunk, 1995; Gibbons & Gerrard, 1991). It has been suggested that individuals under stress may be more inclined to prefer upward affiliation on the coping dimension than on the problem severity dimension. Someone who faces a similar problem but who is coping better may be a particularly desirable affiliate, because such an individual is likely to have relevant information that can enhance cognitive clarity and benefit problem-focused coping. In contrast, affiliation with others who face a less serious problem appears to afford relatively little potential for cognitive clarity or problem-solving information and may more likely engender envy (Buunk, 1995).

Viewed from the perspective of upward and downward comparisons, it may be that the preoperative bypass patients in our study (Kulik & Mahler, 1989) were in effect expressing a desire for upward comparisons on a coping dimension when they indicated a preference for a roommate who had already undergone bypass surgery. Although we did not attempt to manipulate our respondents' perceptions of their roommates' relative coping skills, respondents clearly perceived the prospective roommate who was already recovering as having greater cognitive clarity and instrumental information for the situation than they themselves did or than other preoperative bypass patients might have; that is, as having more information that might reduce uncertainty and benefit their coping efforts. In addition, the fact that the postoperative roommate was described as having already had bypass surgery, and as back on the main ward, implies some degree of coping success. It is entirely possible, if not probable, that a prospective roommate who had just had bypass surgery only a few hours prior would not be nearly so desirable. Such an individual would likely be perceived (correctly) as less informative and perhaps additionally as frightening (by virtue of being attached to a ventilator and myriad tubes). It is likewise probable that a potential postoperative bypass roommate who is back on the main ward, but who is described explicitly as having had a difficult time coping with recovery, would not be as desirable as one described (or assumed) to be coping well. Much more empirical work is needed, but we believe therefore that it is not the postoperative status of the other per se that invites the preoperative patient to want contact, but rather the extent to which the prospective roommate is believed able to provide cognitive clarity, inspiration, and relevant coping information (cf. Rofe, 1984).

Although certainly interesting, none of the work on fear and affiliation choice, nor more recent extensions of this work that suggest with whom individuals generally affiliate or about whom they want information (see reviews by Buunk, 1994; Taylor, Buunk, Collins, & Reed, 1992), tells us specifically the extent to which social comparison processes determine actual affiliative behaviors in an acute threat situation. It should be obvious that what determines initial affiliation desires or choices in the face of threat is not necessarily what determines how people affiliate in an actual threat situation. It is well known that attitudes and behavior toward an object are often divergent (Ajzen & Fishbein, 1977; Wicker, 1969), and the correspondence between stated desire to be in the presence of another person, which is essentially an attitude, may not necessarily predict the nature or amount of actual affiliation with that person. Buunk (1994, 1995) has further noted that individuals under stress appear more interested in obtaining information about how others are doing than in having direct contact in which they share their experiences. Thus, in considering threat and affiliation relationships from a social comparison perspective, distinctions should be made among desires for information about others, desires for affiliation with others, and actual affiliation with others (cf. Buunk, 1994). We now turn to a consideration of the evidence that social comparison processes are relevant to actual affiliation with others.

## NONVERBAL AFFILIATION IN THE FACE OF ACUTE THREAT

Affiliative behavior comes in two general forms, nonverbal and verbal. Facial gaze has been used previously by social interaction researchers as a primary indicator of nonverbal affiliation (e.g., Argyle & Dean, 1965). Unfortunately, there are at this time only a few studies that have examined visual affiliation in an acute threat situation. Almost all have done so under conditions in which subjects were prohibited from engaging in verbal affiliation. Buck and Parke (1972), for example, compared visual affiliation of subjects faced with either threat of shock or threat of embarrassment (sucking on infantile oral objects). Threatened subjects waited alone or in the presence of a confederate who ostensibly was in the control condition and therefore was not faced with the same situation. The confederate acted either nonsupportively (said nothing) or supportively (made a supportive remark before "remembering" the prohibition against talking). The results of primary interest indicated that subjects made fearful by threat of shock increased their looking to both supportive and nonsupportive confederates, whereas subjects faced with embarrassment appeared to increase their looking only when the confederate appeared explicitly supportive.

These results are consistent with the affiliate-choice results of Sarnoff and Zimbardo (1961), which suggested that desire for affiliation with similar others is greater when fearful than when embarrassed. However, particularly given that the (confederate) affiliate in the Buck and Parke (1972) study was not a fellow sufferer, it is not clear that these results involve social comparison processes per se. Rather the results suggest more simply that support received from the affiliate is one determinant of how much visual affiliation occurs under threat (whether physical threat or embarrassment). Given that there was not a low or no-threat condition, there is no evidence that support from others is a determinant of affiliations specifically under threat.

A recently completed laboratory study by Gump and Kulik (in press) was designed more specifically to test the emotional similarity hypothesis in the context of visual affiliation. Subject pairs listened over headphones to audiotaped instructions in which an ischemia task that they were to perform was described as either innocuous (low threat condition) or as likely to be quite painful (high threat condition). Of immediate interest were the visual affiliation patterns of pairs in which both participants were either under high or low threat. Independent of threat level, subjects also were led to believe through instructions and various props either that their "partner" would be performing the same task or a completely different task. According to the emotional similarity hypothesis, emotional comparison needs should be greater under high than under low threat and served principally by affiliation with someone facing the *same* high threat situation.

Probe items supported the validity of both manipulations; subjects believed either that their partner was in the same or a different experiment, as intended, and high threat subjects indicated that they were more anxious and fearful than low threat subjects. Beyond this, videotaped recordings that were made while subjects listened to the audiotape indicated that high threat pairs demonstrated significantly greater visual affiliation than low threat pairs ($p < .01$). Independent of this threat effect, pairs facing the same situation also spent more time looking at each other than pairs facing dissimilar situations ($p < .05$). Finally, and most interesting, further analyses revealed that low threat (calm) subjects looked at their partner about the same regardless of whether or not the partner was facing the same situation (*M*s = 5.83 vs. 5.16 s, *ns*), whereas high threat (fearful) subjects looked significantly more at the partner they believed faced a similar compared to a dissimilar situation (*M*s = 12.88 vs. 5.90 s, $p < .05$). As far as we know, this is the strongest evidence to date suggesting that threat increases visual affiliation specifically toward others facing the same situation.[1] This pattern is consistent with the emotional similarity hypothesis, although more direct evidence that desires for emotional comparison actually produced the differential affiliation levels would be desirable. An alternative possibility, for example, is that something about imminent threat makes an individual more apt to like someone facing the same threat, and as a result of greater interpersonal attraction (rather than desire for emotional comparison per se), visual affiliation increases (cf. Miller & Zimbardo, 1966).

***Summary.*** The available database on the effect of threat on visual affiliation for purposes of social comparison is so limited that it is difficult to draw firm conclusions. Recent evidence suggests that higher threat may increase visual affiliation specifically among those facing the same threat (Gump & Kulik, in press). These results are generally consistent with Schachter's emotional similarity hypothesis, but there remains a lack of direct evidence that these patterns reflect emotional comparison goals. Also generally lacking are studies that examine visual affiliation under acute threat when verbal affiliation is not prohibited.

---

[1]An unpublished study by Epley (1973; cited in Cottrell & Epley, 1977) likewise found that pairs of subjects under higher threat (of electric shock) looked at each other more than did pairs under lower threat. However because Epley did not explicitly manipulate (or even indicate) to subjects whether their partners faced the same or a different threat, it is unclear whether this increased affiliation was specific to partners who were believed to face the same situation. If Epley's subjects presumed their partners were facing the same situation, which seems to us quite likely, the finding that visual affiliation was greater under high than low threat is consistent with Gump and Kulik's finding that subjects who faced high threat looked more than did subjects who faced low threat at others they believed were facing the same situation (*M*s = 12.88 vs. 5.83 s, $p < .05$).

Given that the vast majority of threat situations faced outside of laboratory experiments probably do not restrict verbal affiliation, this is potentially an important external validity concern. It is conceivable that visual affiliation patterns are different when verbal affiliation is an option. The only study of which we are aware that examined both visual and verbal affiliation in the same experiment did produce results that are broadly consistent with the foregoing studies in that visual affiliation was again greater among high threat than low threat pairs (Kulik, Mahler, & Earnest, 1994). However, more attention to when and why visual affiliation parallels or diverges from verbal affiliation under threat is needed.

## VERBAL AFFILIATION IN THE FACE OF ACUTE THREAT

Morris et al. (1976) appear to have been the first to take a social comparison approach to the study of verbal affiliation patterns that occur in acute threat situations. Their study was not intended specifically to test Schachter's emotional similarity hypothesis, in that there was no explicit comparison of verbal affiliation under high versus low threat or with a similar versus dissimilar other. Instead, they examined the hypothesis that individuals facing a fear-inducing situation would spend more time affiliating for purposes of social comparison than would individuals facing either embarrassing or ambiguous situations. Groups of five individuals at a time arrived at the experimental room where they found props and materials intended to create fear (electric shock generators and "shock release" forms), embarrassment (contraceptive devices, nude photos), or ambiguity (two cardboard boxes filled with unidentified computer cards). Although not mentioned specifically by the authors, the results indicated that the greatest proportion of time in all three conditions was spent during the 20-minute waiting period in threat-irrelevant affiliation (e.g., talking about a recent movie). Beyond that, the results indicated also that time spent in "verbal information seeking (e.g., asking others if they know what is going on)," was greatest for the fear groups, least for the embarrassment groups, and intermediate for the ambiguity groups. This pattern of results is again roughly consistent with the affiliate-choice study by Sarnoff and Zimbardo (1961) that showed fear increased the desire to wait with others whereas embarrassment diminished the desire. However, because the Morris et al. study did not include a no or low-threat control group, the results do not demonstrate directly that fear increases verbal affiliation or that embarrassment decreases verbal affiliation, only that the two types of threat probably differ in their effects. It is interesting that although Morris et al. conceptualized the ambiguity condition as a third type of stressor, it seems quite plausible from their description that it was actually experienced as a low-threat condition. If so, the intermediate affiliation observed in the ambiguity condition would suggest that fear increases whereas embarrassment decreases verbal affiliation. Regardless, the aggregated manner in which verbal interaction was coded leaves completely unclear whether fear subjects were affiliating for purposes of emotional comparison, cognitive clarity, or other reasons.

A recent laboratory study by Kulik et al. (1994), mentioned briefly in our discussion of visual affiliation, was intended to test more explicitly the emotional similarity hypothesis in the context of verbal affiliation. To accomplish this, we recorded the verbal affiliations of subjects who faced either high or low threat (the prospect of strong versus negligible cold pressor pain) with someone who was either awaiting the same threat or who had already experienced the threat. Of interest was whether verbal affiliation would be greater under higher than lower threat principally with the similarly inexperienced affiliate. The study also was designed to explore the nature of the interactions that took place, that is, for example, the extent to which topics of conversation and questions focused on details of the experiment proper, experienced emotions, or "irrelevant" topics. The emotional similarity hypothesis in strongest form would appear to predict that higher threat should increase overall affiliation particularly with someone currently facing the same threat, or in weaker form, that affiliation for purposes of emotional comparison should be greatest with such a person under higher threat. On the other hand, if the desire for cognitive clarity is normally an important determinant of affiliation under threat when discussion is not artificially constrained, one might anticipate the most discussion specifically about the experiment when higher threat subjects wait with an experienced rather than inexperienced partner.

As was the case with the Morris et al. (1976) study, the results indicated that in absolute terms, more time was spent talking about threat-irrelevant topics than threat-relevant topics. Of more immediate interest, the results also generally did not support the emotional similarity hypothesis and in certain respects ran counter to it. First, although the threat manipulation differentially induced fear as intended, there was no evidence that high compared to low threat produced greater verbal affiliation either overall or specifically with a similarly threatened other; this was the case whether affiliation was defined in terms of total time talking or separated into time talking about threat-relevant versus threat-irrelevant topics. Second, threat-relevant affiliation did differ as a function of partner characteristics, but such that subjects and their partners engaged in more threat-relevant affiliation when the partners were threat-experienced rather than similarly inexperienced. More fine-grained analyses generally produced an overall picture with respect to threat-relevant affiliation that had subjects asking more factual (e.g., how long does it last?) and evaluative (how bad is it?) questions related to the threat situation and receiving more threat-relevant responses from experienced partners compared to inexperienced partners. Given that experienced partners would be expected to have greater information value than inexperienced partners, this pattern appears generally consistent with the hypothesis that cognitive clarity concerns differentiated actual verbal affiliations under threat. The desire for emotional comparison, theoretically best served by affiliation with others currently facing similar threat (Schachter, 1959), does not seem to be a viable explanation for these results.

From the foregoing laboratory studies we might expect that preoperative patients would (a) spend more time talking about threat-irrelevant than threat-relevant topics with their roommates, and (b) engage in more threat-relevant affiliation with a roommate who had already had the same surgery compared to a roommate who was awaiting the same surgery. In an initial attempt to test these predictions, Kulik, Moore, and Mahler (1993) conducted a study in which men scheduled for hernia, bladder–prostate, or open-heart (valve) surgery the next morning were asked to estimate the total number of minutes they had spent talking to their roommate and, additionally, the number of minutes that they had spent talking about each of five health-related topics (the medical staff, their own operation and health, their roommate's operation and health, their own past hospital experiences, their roommate's past hospital experiences) and each of five nonmedical topics (family and friends, military experiences, sports, current events and news, and "other"). A separate data collection examined interpatient agreement on these judgments and found quite acceptable reliabilities. Roommates were classified with respect to operative status (preoperative, postoperative, or nonsurgical) and the similarity of their health problem to that of the subjects. The question of immediate concern was whether patients faced with such a real world, physical threat would affiliate most with someone currently facing similar threat (and therefore presumably of similar emotional status).

Consistent with the Morris et al. (1976) and Kulik et al. (1994) laboratory experiments, the results indicated first that individuals under threat generally spent more time talking about nonthreat-relevant (nonmedical) topics than about threat-relevant (medical) topics. Partial support also was found for the emotional similarity hypothesis in that patients spent significantly more time talking to roommates who were, like themselves, preoperative rather than postoperative; however, there was no indication that this difference was specific to or more pronounced if the roommate had either a similar or a dissimilar health problem. It may be that the failure of the similarity of the roommate's health problem to exert significant effects on verbal affiliation stemmed from a lack of power, however. That is, it turned out that so few subjects had roommates with similar health problems that the test of the roommate similarity factor was probably weakened substantially.

Although the Kulik et al. (1993) study had the virtue of examining verbal affiliation in an acute, real world situation, there are several other limitations of note for present purposes. First, because all patients faced imminent threat, the study was not designed specifically to examine the extent to which threat per se played a part in determining affiliation. Kulik et al. (1993) also did not attempt to differentiate affiliations that might have involved emotional comparison, cognitive clarity, or other motivations. To address these issues, we have recently completed a study that compares the hospital roommate affiliations of 73 patients scheduled to undergo coronary-artery bypass graft (CABG) surgery to those of 82 patients scheduled to undergo transurethral prostatectomy (TURP) surgery.[2] Patients were assigned before surgery to a roommate who had either a similar or dissimilar surgical problem and who was either similar (preoperative) or dissimilar (postoperative) in surgical status. The night before their surgery, patients also completed privately a short (10-item) form of the state version of the State-Trait Anxiety Inventory (STAI; Spielberger, Gorsuch, & Luschene, 1970) to assess preoperative anxiety. TURP surgery, although no walk in the park, clearly does not pose the life-threatening risks of CABG surgery. And, as expected, TURP patients reported experiencing significantly less preoperative anxiety than CABG patients ($p < .01$). Although patients were obviously not randomly assigned to their surgery, we may thus consider the TURP patients to be faced with a relatively low threat situation compared to CABG patients.

Patients also completed a questionnaire the night before surgery that was designed to determine overall affiliation (minutes spent talking to the roommate) and, more specifically, the extent to which patients had engaged in affiliations involving emotional comparison, cognitive clarity, and emotional support. To assess emotional comparison activity, patients were asked to indicate on separate 4-point scales ranging from 1 (*not at all*) to 4 (*very much so*), the extent to which they had (a) mentioned to their roommate how they felt about their operation (e.g., how calm or nervous), (b) thought about how nervous their roommate

[2]The data relevant to the coronary-bypass sample are described and analyzed more fully in Kulik, Mahler, and Moore (1996).

seemed compared to themselves, and (c) had been told by their roommate how he felt about his operation (e.g., how calm or nervous). Relevant to cognitive clarity, patients also indicated the extent to which they had (a) discussed with their roommate how it will feel after surgery; (b) discussed ways to make recovery easier; (c) learned things by watching their roommate that would be helpful for their own recovery; (d) learned things by talking to their roommate that would be helpful for their own recovery; and (e) had come to have "a better idea of what to expect after surgery" because of their roommate. Finally, to assess emotional support affiliations, patients indicated the extent to which (a) their roommate had said things to them in an effort to make them feel better about their operation (e.g., "things will be all right"); (b) they had said things to their roommate in an effort to make him feel better about his operation; and (c) they liked to joke with their roommate about their operations.

For present purposes, the issue of primary interest is the extent to which patients engaged in affiliations that reflected emotional comparison, cognitive clarity, or emotional support as a function of threat level (i.e., the patient's surgery), the similarity of the roommate's surgical problem, and the similarity of the roommate's surgical status. In this context, the emotional similarity hypothesis would predict that affiliation (either overall or specifically involving emotional comparison) should be highest for CABG (high threat) patients paired with a roommate who is also awaiting CABG surgery. A somewhat different pattern would be expected for affiliation involving efforts to achieve cognitive clarity or information about the threat situation. Because a roommate who has already been through the same surgery is *perceived* as having the greatest information value with respect to the threat (Kulik & Mahler, 1989), we might expect that affiliations directed toward obtaining information about what to expect and how best to cope with the surgery (i.e., cognitive clarity) would be greatest for patients paired with roommates already recovering from similar surgery. If desire for cognitive clarity increases with threat, we might also expect this pattern to be more pronounced for the CABG patients compared to the TURP patients. Finally, Schachter's (1959) hypothesis that threatened individuals also might be motivated to affiliate with similarly threatened others for anxiety reduction suggests that evidence of emotionally reassuring affiliations should be greatest for patients paired with roommates who are awaiting the same surgery.

A Surgical Threat (TURP vs. CABG surgery) × Roommate Surgical Problem (similar vs. dissimilar) vs. Roommate Surgical Status (preoperative vs. postoperative) analysis of covariance that controlled for exposure time (number of hours spent in the room with the roommate) indicated no significant effects on total affiliation beyond a positive relationship with exposure time ($p < .001$). Thus there was no support for the strongest form of the emotional similarity hypothesis. With respect to affiliations specifically relevant to emotional comparison, however, there were some condition effects. First, high threat patients were more likely than low threat patients to mention their nervousness to their roommates (*Ms* = 2.15 vs. 1.69, $p < .02$) and to have been informed of the roommate's nervousness (*Ms* = 1.91 vs. 1.57, $p < .05$). Patients also were more likely to have mentioned how nervous they felt to a roommate who had a similar compared to dissimilar surgical problem, ($p < .02$). These main effects were not significantly qualified by the surgical status of the roommate, and there were no significant condition effects at all in the tendency of patients to report having compared how nervous they felt compared to their roommate.

The fact that the higher threat (CABG) patients engaged in significantly more affiliation concerning their own and their roommate's emotional status than did the lower threat (TURP) patients may constitute the most direct evidence to date that threat prompts verbal affiliation for purposes of emotional comparison. However, the rather indiscriminate influence of increased threat on discussions of emotional state is not consistent with even the weaker form of the emotional similarity hypothesis. That is, there was no indication that threat increased discussion of emotions specifically or primarily with a roommate who was awaiting the same surgery (and who therefore was presumably most relevant for emotional comparison). One possibility is that under such high threat, patients view anyone who is facing or has recently faced surgery as able to provide feedback that would be helpful for determining the appropriateness of their emotional response to the situation. That is, perhaps under threat people are not so well calibrated to the finer distinctions between affiliate characteristics implied by the emotional similarity hypothesis. An alternative possibility is that patient discussions of their emotional states did not reflect emotional comparison efforts per se but something else. Perhaps increased fear prompts individuals to mention their nervousness inadvertently, because it is so salient that it "slips out." Or perhaps high threat patients mention how nervous they feel hoping for sympathy or reassurance from any quarter. Clearly more work is needed to clarify these issues.

The separate finding that patients were more apt to discuss their emotions with someone who had a similar compared to dissimilar health problem is somewhat easier to reconcile with the emotional similarity hypothesis, if certain assumptions are made. First, it may be that beyond a certain level of threat, increasing levels of threat simply do not translate monotonically into greater desires for emotional comparison.

Even the low threat (TURP) patients were faced with a level of threat that substantially exceeds that of any laboratory threat. Second, and more interesting, the long-held presumption that emotional comparison requires that the potential affiliate be facing the same threat currently and thereby be in an emotionally similar state may be incorrect so long as verbal affiliation is not restricted. After all, a potential affiliate who has already experienced the same threat ordinarily can still tell the threatened individual how he or she felt prior to the threatening event. There is no obvious reason why such information would be any less useful to threatened individuals for determining the appropriateness of their emotional reactions than if obtained from someone currently facing the same threat.

As noted previously, fear and affiliation-choice studies historically have tended to require threatened subjects to choose affiliates under conditions where verbal affiliation was completely restricted or limited to threat-irrelevant topics. In so doing, the researchers removed any potential for engaging in emotional comparison through verbal affiliation and, as a result, may have inadvertently overemphasized the importance of absolute emotional similarity at the moment of affiliation. That is, if we wish to engage in emotional comparison but are prohibited for some reason from doing so through direct discussion, the nonverbal expressions of someone currently facing the same threat might well provide a better emotional gauge than the nonverbal expressions of someone who has already experienced the threat. However, so long as verbal affiliation is not restricted (which is almost always the case in the real world), it may be that the key is more simply whether or not the potential affiliate has first-hand experience with a similar threat. Such affiliates, whether they are currently experiencing or have already experienced the threat, may be viewed as capable of reducing uncertainties about one's emotional reactions and thereby motivate relevant verbal affiliation for that purpose.

The separate cognitive clarity items were averaged to form an overall index for simplicity and because separate item analyses yielded similar conclusions. The primary results indicate first a main effect of threat ($p < .01$), such that patients facing the greater (CABG) threat engaged in more cognitive clarity affiliation than did patients facing the smaller (TURP) threat. Patients overall also engaged in more cognitive clarity affiliations with roommates who had similar compared to dissimilar surgical problems ($p < .0001$). This makes sense in that all else being equal, a roommate with a similar compared to dissimilar surgical problem should have more threat-relevant information and therefore be better able to enhance the patient's cognitive clarity for the situation. These two main effects were qualified, however, by their interaction ($p$

< .02), which indicated that the tendency to engage in more cognitive clarity affiliation with a roommate who had a similar rather than dissimilar problem was greater under high threat (*M*s = 2.40 vs. 1.55) than under low threat (*M*s = 1.73 vs. 1.53). This effect, displayed in Fig. 8.1, held regardless of whether the roommate was preoperative or postoperative (three-way interaction $F < 1$).

This is not to say that the surgical status of the roommate did not matter, because the results also reveal a simple main effect ($p = .05$) that indicates patients generally engaged in more cognitive clarity affiliation with postoperative roommates than with preoperative roommates. This suggests that some cognitive clarity may be gained also by affiliation with a postoperative roommate even if that roommate has undergone a different surgery; certain important aspects of postoperative recovery are common across different surgeries (e.g., nausea and discomfort symptoms, the need to ambulate and to perform deep breathing exercises). The effect of the affiliate's surgical status on cognitive clarity is qualified in two respects, however. First, as indicated in Fig. 8.2, the tendency to engage in more cognitive clarity affiliation with a roommate who was postoperative rather than preoperative was found specifically for high threat patients (*M*s = 2.22 vs. 1.73, $p < .05$) rather than for low threat patients (*M*s = 1.64 vs. 1.62, *ns*). Second, the effect of the roommate's surgical status also depended substantially on the similarity of the roommate's problem ($p < .002$). Figure 8.3 shows that across threat levels, patients engaged in significantly ($p < .05$) more cognitive clarity affiliations with roommates who were already recovering from similar surgeries ($M = 2.41$) than with those awaiting similar surgery ($M = 1.72$), awaiting a different surgery ($M = 1.63$), or recovering from a different surgery ($M = 1.46$).

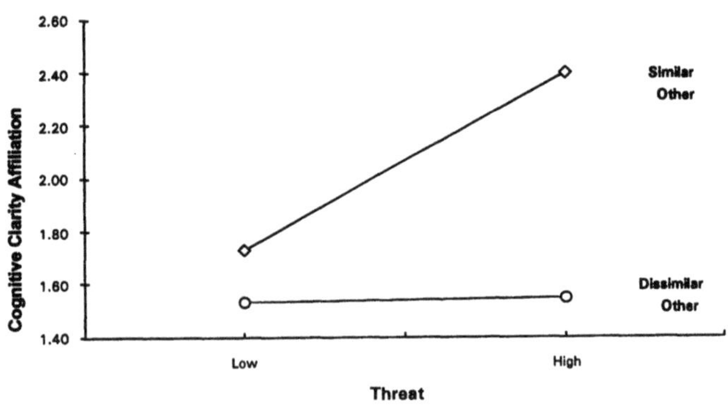


FIG. 8.1. Cognitive clarity affiliation as a function of threat level and similarity of roommate's health problem.

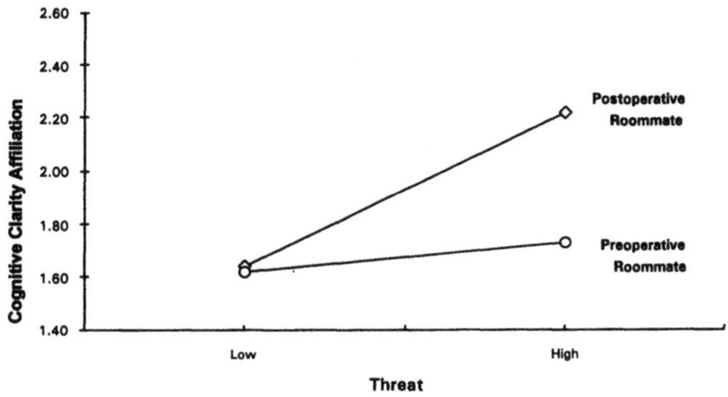


FIG. 8.2. Cognitive clarity affiliation as a function of threat level and roommate's surgical status.

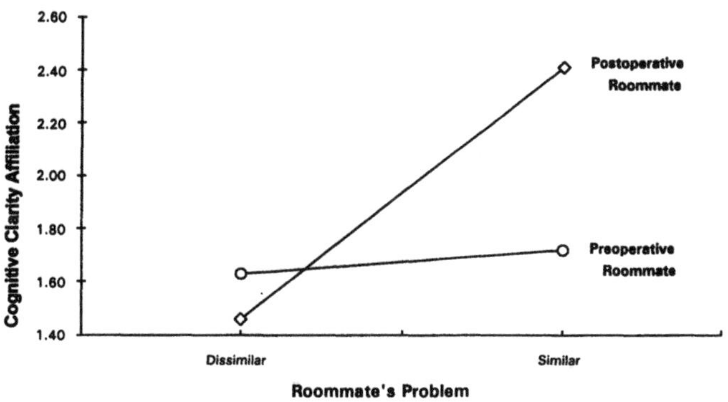


FIG. 8.3. Cognitive clarity affiliation as a function of similarity of roommate's health problem and roommate's surgical status.

Thus the overall picture we see with respect to cognitive clarity affiliations is very interesting. Regardless of threat level, patients engaged in more cognitive clarity affiliations with the person who is likely to have the greatest information about the particular threat they face (i.e., someone who is already recovering from a similar operation). Such an individual may be such an optimal resource for gaining a better understanding of what to expect and do that, given such ready access, even individuals facing relatively low threat avail themselves of the opportunity to learn more. The effect of absolute threat level on cognitive clarity affiliations instead showed up more subtly in the greater extent to which high threat compared to low threat patients engaged in cognitive clarity affiliations when the roommate's information value was suboptimal. Thus, under higher threat, patients engaged in more cognitive clarity affiliation if the affiliate had a relatively similar problem, whether or not the affiliate had already experienced the threat. Higher threat likewise produced more cognitive clarity affiliation if the affiliate was threat-experienced rather than inexperienced, whether or not the affiliate's surgical problem was the same.

With respect to emotionally supportive affiliations, patients did not differ significantly by condition in their tendency to extend verbal reassurances to their roommate (sample mean = 2.07). There were differences in the receipt of reassurances from the roommate, however. Thus, patients tended to receive more emotional reassurances from roommates who had similar compared to dissimilar surgical problems (*Ms* = 2.51 vs. 1.97, $p < .01$). This indirectly supports Schachter's notion that anticipation of anxiety reduction (via emotional reassurance) may motivate desire to await threat in the presence of similarly threatened others, but again fails to support the necessity that the affiliate be currently facing the threat. Indeed, an additional main effect of the roommate's surgical status indicated that roommates who were postoperative gave more reassurances than roommates who were preoperative (*Ms* = 2.47 vs. 2.02, $p < .03$). These effects were qualified by their interaction ($p < .04$), however. As Fig. 8.4 indicates, it was principally a roommate who was recovering from a similar surgery who was likely to provide emotional reassurances ($M = 2.96$) compared to a roommate who was awaiting the same surgery ($M = 2.07$) or to roommates who were either recovering or awaiting dissimilar surgery (*Ms* = 1.99 and 1.96).

It seems likely that individuals faced with imminent threat may be focused primarily on coping with their own problems. The emotional support results suggest that someone who has recently experienced and weathered an acute threat such as surgery may be relatively more

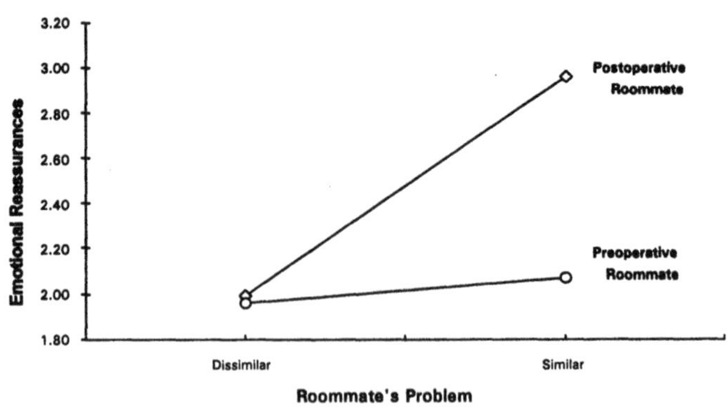


FIG. 8.4. Emotional reassurances received from roommate as a function of similarity of roommate's health problem and roommate's surgical status.

inclined to extend reassurances to those currently facing threat, particularly if it is a threat similar to the one they themselves confronted. Thus an interesting possibility that warrants future research attention is that, as a byproduct of a recent threat experience, there is an increased likelihood that individuals will in effect assume a role, that of emotional cheerleader, to those about to follow in their footsteps (cf. Helmreich & Collins, 1967). As far as we know, this idea has not been addressed directly, but there are several strands of evidence from the social support literature that are roughly consistent. For example, it appears that a major reason patients join support groups is the desire to help (similar) others (Taylor, Falke, Shoptaw, & Lichtman, 1986). There is also evidence that individuals who are better off sometimes seek affiliation with worse off others for altruistic reasons (Helgeson & Mickelson, 1995), which presumably could include extending emotional reassurances. In the context of surgical threat, it seems likely that a patient who is postoperative will view a patient who is preoperative for a similar surgery as worse off. Even if true, this would not explain why the postoperative patient might be more inclined to issue reassurances specifically to a patient who is preoperative for the same surgery. One general possibility of course is that for some reason it makes the postoperative patient feel good to offer such reassurances. Interestingly, it has been suggested that the positive feeling that one is helping others may in fact be one means by which support groups benefit members' emotional well-being (Yalom & Greaves, 1977). Exactly why reassuring similar others might make us feel good is an interesting question in its own right. It would seem that threat-experienced individuals, by virtue of knowing first-hand the relevant concerns, are in the optimal position to know what specific reassurances are likely to be most desirable or effective; as a result, they may be more inclined to offer them. If we know (or think we know) what to say to make someone feel better, we are more likely to say it. And to the extent we believe that our reassurances are effective, we should have a greater sense of being helpful, which in turn may lead us to feel better about ourselves. An equally interesting but alternative view would focus more on the part played by the individual who is faced with threat. Perhaps such an individual tries to elicit more reassurances specifically from the individual who has already experienced the same threat. Reassurances from those who already have experienced the threat we face may be particularly desirable because their expertise gives the reassurances greater credibility. Clearly, to address such issues, it will be necessary to have more online verbal affiliation data than are currently available.

***Summary.*** The degree to which the emotional similarity hypothesis predicts verbal affiliations that occur in the face of imminent physical threat so far appears modest. There was no evidence that higher compared to lower fear produced more verbal affiliation among individuals facing the same laboratory situation (Kulik et al., 1994). Under threat of imminent surgery, patients did talk more to roommates who were also awaiting surgery (and therefore presumably more similar emotionally) than to those who had already had surgery, but this effect was not specific to roommates facing the same type of surgical threat (Kulik et al., 1993). The best evidence that verbal affiliation follows predictions generated from the emotional similarity hypothesis was found in our comparison of the verbal affiliations of patients facing different levels of surgical threat. However, here too the support was partial. Although patients did discuss their emotions more when they faced higher compared to lower surgical threats and when their roommate had a similar rather than dissimilar surgical problem, discussions of emotions were not more pronounced specifically under high threat with a roommate facing the same surgery. Additional efforts to measure emotional comparison processes directly are clearly needed, and it is entirely possible that such efforts will yield stronger support. It is sobering, however, that the question that appears to us most directly reflective of emotional comparison (viz., the extent to which patients had considered how nervous they were compared to their roommate) yielded null results and, anecdotally, appeared to strike a number of patients as a bit odd. It may well be that people under threat do not deliberately or consciously compare their emotional states to others. If so, asking them whether their verbalizations about emotions were motivated by desires for emotional comparison may produce frustrations familiar to cognitive-dissonance researchers who frequently tried, and just as frequently failed, to find evidence that subjects consciously experienced feelings of dissonance or inconsistency (cf. Nisbett & Wilson, 1977).

In comparison, the results to date make a clearer case for the notion that fear-inducing threats increase verbal affiliations directed at achieving cognitive clarity for the situation. As noted in our discussion of affiliate-choice studies, this conclusion is quite compatible with current conceptualizations of stress and coping that emphasize the importance of cognitive appraisal processes (e.g., Cohen & Lazarus, 1983; Lazarus & Folkman, 1984) and with models of social comparison that propose threat increases affiliation for purposes of self-improvement (Taylor & Lobel, 1989; Buunk & Ybema, chapter 12, this volume; Wood & VanderZee, chapter 10, this volume; cf. Rofe, 1984). The verbal affiliation results more generally also appear in accord with our earlier argument that much of the classic work within the fear and affiliate-choice paradigm used methods that probably led to an overemphasis on the importance of emotional comparison and to a premature dismissal of the importance of cognitive clarity as a determinant of affiliation under threat (for similar views, see also Kirkpatrick & Shaver, 1988; Kulik & Mahler, 1990; Rofe, 1984; Shaver & Klinnert, 1982). At the same time, it would be a mistake to argue that cognitive clarity is the sole or preeminent determinant of verbal affiliation under threat. In the three studies for which relevant data are available (Kulik et al., 1993; Kulik et al., 1994; Morris et al., 1976), it is noteworthy that in absolute terms, most of the verbal affiliation that occurred was not threat-related. It would seem that neither cognitive clarity nor emotional comparison motivations are likely to account for the bulk of verbal affiliation that actually occurs under threat. Thus it might be more precise to suggest that one factor that distinguishes threat-relevant verbal affiliation may be a desire for cognitive clarity, and that this desire may increase with threat. That is clearly not the same as saying that desire for cognitive clarity (or self-improvement) is the (sole) determinant of verbal affiliation in the face of threat.

The importance of this point becomes more apparent when one considers the rather oversimplified, if not false sense of knowledge of affiliation under threat that has been generated by traditional affiliate-choice research. That is, judging by the fear and affiliate-choice work, we might have expected that people facing a novel physical threat in the presence of another would spend the preponderance of time affiliating for purposes of achieving emotional comparison. But when we look at what people actually do, the picture (as usual) is much more complicated, and as yet is not close to filled in. Probably a variety of factors that are likely important in mundane, nonthreat situations also influence verbal affiliation in threat situations, e.g., prior relationship, personality, affiliate attractiveness and demographic similarity. These possibilities remain largely to be explored, as does the influence of the affiliate's goals in the situation. The affiliate-choice paradigm, by focusing exclusively on the presumed affiliation motivations of the individual facing threat, has ignored this issue entirely. Presumably, however, a given level of motivation to affiliate with someone will produce different levels of actual affiliation depending on whether that person is receptive or not. As already mentioned, an interesting possibility is that threat-experienced individuals in effect occupy a particular role in relation to threat-inexperienced individuals. Perhaps threat-experienced individuals feel some sense of obligation or desire to impart their knowledge or reassurances to "help this person through" and, perhaps as a result, direct more discussion toward the threat (cf. Helmreich & Collins, 1967).

The amount of variance in affiliative behavior thus accounted for by the threatened individual's desires for cognitive clarity or emotional comparison may thus be more modest than commonly appreciated. This does not mean that such affiliations are unimportant to coping efforts. Emerging evidence, principally collected in the context of surgical threat, in fact suggests just the opposite conclusion. In the next section, we consider that research after first reviewing laboratory studies relevant to social comparison and emotional convergence.

## AFFILIATION, EMOTIONAL CONVERGENCE, AND COPING IN ACUTE THREAT SITUATIONS

One of the more interesting aspects of Schachter's (1959) extension of social comparison theory is the way others might influence our emotional reactions to a threat situation. As noted previously, Schachter proposed that a primary reason for affiliating when facing novel threat situations is to use the emotional responses of others as a gauge for evaluating the intensity, nature, or appropriateness of our emotional responses. In order to enable maximally informative and stable self-evaluations, the comparison others should be facing a similar threat situation and reacting emotionally in a fairly similar manner (cf. Festinger, 1954). One interesting implication of this idea is that if discrepancies in emotional responses to the same situation exist, there will be pressures toward reducing those discrepancies, that is, toward convergence in emotional responses among affiliates. Thus Schachter's view is that emotional convergence should occur as a function of emotional comparison primarily, if not exclusively, when facing a novel threat situation in the presence of another person who is facing the same threat. If we are not facing a novel threat situation, emotional comparisons would presumably be unnecessary. And if we are facing a novel threat but with an affiliate who faces an altogether different threat, emotional comparisons presumably would be largely irrelevant.

This social comparison position can be contrasted with the recent argument for "primitive emotional contagion," which proposes that people may quite generally and nonconsciously mimic the facial expressions, vocalizations, posture, and body movements of those around them and, as a result of afferent feedback, converge emotionally (Hatfield, Cacioppo, & Rapson, 1993). Thus emotional convergence or contagion may be a byproduct of social comparison under certain conditions, but it also may often be a byproduct of a more general mimicry mechanism. In the primitive emotional contagion view, there is no explicit implication either that threat or the similarity of the situation faced by the affiliate specifically influence the amount of emotional contagion that will occur.

Although not designed to test these alternative views of when and how emotional convergence occurs, there are a few early studies that provide results relevant to our present concerns. A study by Wrightsman (1960), for example, was intended to test Schachter's view that social comparison processes mediate emotional emergence. Wrightsman began by threatening multiple groups of subjects with the prospect of painful injections. Group members then waited either together or separately (alone). Anxiety ratings that were obtained both before and after the waiting period showed some evidence of greater uniformity of anxiety reactions among those individuals who waited together compared to those who waited alone. The evidence was modest, however, in that the obtained effects were limited to first-borns, and when certain procedural confounds were eliminated in a subsequent study by MacDonald (1970), the effects were not replicated. For present purposes, it also is important to note that because threat was not varied, the specific role of threat is indeterminate. Likewise, because all subjects faced the same threat, the impact of affiliate similarity was not assessed. As such, Wrightsman's (1960) results are also consistent with a primitive emotional contagion view that would emphasize a mimicry mechanism rather than an emotional comparison mechanism (cf. Reisenzein, 1983; Schachter & Singer, 1962).

Sullins (1991) conducted a study designed to determine whether emotional convergence is greater specifically with an affiliate facing a similar or a dissimilar situation. Before completing an opinion survey, subjects waited either alone, with someone believed to be "a second subject" (similar other), or with someone believed to be "taking a makeup exam" (dissimilar other). The degree of emotional convergence (defined as the ratio of postwait to prewait mood discrepancy scores) in these three conditions was compared, and it was found that emotional convergence occurred only in the similar partner condition. This finding is consistent with the similarity pattern that would be predicted by the emotional comparison hypothesis, but it is ambiguous with respect to the role of threat. On the face of it, the anticipation of completing an opinion survey would not seem to represent a novel threat situation. If so, the finding of emotional convergence without threat is consistent with the primitive emotional contagion view, although the fact that the convergence occurred only among individuals facing the same situation is not. On the other hand, one could argue that being a subject in any experiment represents a novel threat situation. Even if this is true, however, the fact that threat was not explicitly manipulated or varied still renders unclear the extent to which emotional convergence is influenced by threat. Further complicating interpretation, Sullins also found an inexplicable emotional divergence in the alone and dissimilar-other conditions. Such a divergence is not readily reconciled with either a social comparison or primitive emotional contagion view.

Recent work by Gump and Kulik (Experiment 1, in press), described briefly in our discussion of visual affiliation, was designed to consider more explicitly the emotional comparison and primitive emotional contagion views. To review, subject pairs were told over headphones that they would be performing an ischemia task, which was described either as quite painful (high threat) or as a mild pressure sensation (low threat). Independent of threat level, subjects also were led to believe either that the other subject would be performing the same task or a completely different task. Videotaped recordings of subjects' facial expressions were made while subjects listened to the audiotapes. As noted previously, manipulation checks supported both the threat and the perceived situational similarity manipulations. The pertinent results indicated, first of all, that high-threat subjects reported more anxiety after listening to the tapes than did low-threat subjects ($p < .001$), as one would expect. More interesting, and independent of the threat effect, subjects were more anxious the more anxious their affiliates were ($p < .01$). This emotional convergence was not qualified significantly either by threat level or situational similarity.

The fact that the observed emotional convergence was unqualified by threat level or situational similarity does not support the emotional comparison perspective. Rather, the results are more suggestive of a primitive emotional contagion effect that is perhaps mediated by non-verbal mimicry. Consistent with this possibility, additional evidence indicated that there was a substantial, positive relationship ($p < .001$) between the expressions exhibited by subject pairs while listening to the audiotapes (where expressions were indexed by the amount of time spent smiling minus amount of time spent frowning). Direct mediational tests, however, failed to show significant evidence that the observed emotional convergence was a direct function of such behavioral mimicry. Thus it is clear that much more work is needed to document the conditions under which emotional convergence occurs and to understand the underlying mechanisms.

One might ask of what practical relevance are issues of emotional convergence to the individual faced with an acute medical threat such as imminent major surgery? Perhaps more than has been generally realized. In a small initial study of coronary-bypass patients, one of our interests was in how patients' preoperative anxiety levels might be affected by assignment to a roommate who was either a cardiac or noncardiac patient and either preoperative or postoperative (Kulik & Mahler, 1987). The results indicated that patients assigned to a roommate who was postoperative compared to preoperative were significantly less anxious before their operations. This result was recently replicated in a larger sample of coronary-bypass patients (Kulik et al., 1996), and in another study involving patients facing hernia, open-heart (valve), or bladder-prostate surgeries (Kulik et al., 1993). The latter study also found that the anxiety levels of patients awaiting surgery with a roommate who was being treated medically (i.e., not facing surgery) were not different from those assigned a roommate who was postoperative, but were likewise significantly lower than those of patients assigned a roommate who was preoperative.

These results collectively suggest that patient affiliations before a major medical threat may have important consequences for emotion-focused coping, that is, for efforts to regulate or control emotional responses to the stressful situation (e.g., Cohen & Lazarus, 1979; Lazarus & Folkman, 1984; see also Wills, chapter 6, this volume; Tenner & Affleck, chapter 9, this volume). We have so far found no compelling evidence that patients' verbal affiliations toward the roommate or from the roommate are directly involved, however (Kulik et al., 1993; Kulik et al., 1996), although logistical and ethical obstacles to a comprehensive assessment of verbal affiliation leave this possibility open. Another interesting possibility is that the observed differences in patient anxiety levels reflect some type of emotional contagion effect. Preoperative patients are generally more anxious than postoperative and nonsurgical patients (e.g., Auerbach, 1973). Therefore the roommates of preoperative patients who are likewise preoperative generally should be more anxious than roommates who are postoperative or nonsurgical. If so, it may be that the roommate's anxiety level influenced our patients, although exactly how this might have happened remains to be determined. It is noteworthy in this regard that in none of these studies did the similarity of the roommate's problem significantly impact patient anxiety. Patients were more anxious preoperatively with a roommate who was preoperative rather than postoperative whether the roommate's health problem was similar or not. Thus if emotional contagion was involved, we found no evidence that it followed the specific pattern that would be expected from an emotional comparison mechanism. The pattern instead again is more consistent with the notion of primitive emotional contagion. Preoperative patients clearly believe that a roommate who is likely to be anxious by virtue of facing the same surgery may increase their own anxiety (Kulik & Mahler, 1989). What they may not realize is that a roommate who anxiously awaits a different surgery may also exacerbate their anxiety, perhaps because of a nonconscious tendency to mimic (either verbal or nonverbal) aspects of their roommate's behavior. Direct evidence for such mimicry is presently lacking but would be fascinating.

In addition to affecting emotion-focused coping, we have found evidence suggesting that preoperative patients' problem-focused coping efforts also may be influenced by their roommates. Problem-focused coping efforts are generally conceptualized as involving direct actions to change or reduce the demands of a stressful situation or to enhance one's resources for dealing with the situation (e.g., Cohen & Lazarus, 1979; Lazarus & Folkman, 1984). In the context of imminent surgery, problem-focused coping might include, for example, efforts to speed hospital release by obtaining information relevant to the recovery process and by walking and moving about after surgery to prevent various complications. We have already discussed evidence that suggests preoperative (prostate and coronary bypass) patients engage in information-seeking or cognitive clarity affiliation with their roommates in relation to the roommate's threat-relevant information value (Fig. 8.3). More dramatic and of practical importance, we have found in addition that coronary-bypass patients were significantly more ambulatory postoperatively and were released from the hospital significantly sooner if assigned before surgery to a roommate who was postoperative compared to preoperative (Kulik & Mahler, 1987; Kulik et al., 1996) and cardiac compared to noncardiac (Kulik et al., 1996).

The fact that the same roommate conditions in Kulik et al. (1996) that showed greater evidence of cognitive clarity affiliation were the same conditions that produced greater ambulation and quicker recovery after surgery raises the possibility that these preoperative affiliations directly mediated recovery. A fairly substantial literature suggests that practitioner-delivered efforts to provide a better conception of what to expect and do postoperatively may reduce length of stay and patient distress (Devine, 1992; Mumford, Schlesinger, & Glass, 1982; Suls & Wan, 1989, for relevant reviews). Thus fellow patients may serve as an unrecognized adjunct to professionally delivered, preoperative preparations. To test this idea, Kulik et al. (1996) examined the effects of preoperative roommate conditions on postoperative length of stay, controlling for cognitive clarity affiliations (as indexed by the five affiliation items previously described). The results indicated first that the more cognitive clarity affiliation before surgery the patient engaged in with the roommate, the more quickly the patient was released from the hospital after surgery ($p = .04$). In addition, when controlling for cognitive clarity affiliation levels, the significant effects of the similarity of the roommate's surgical problem and of the roommate's surgical status were reduced to nonsignificance. This overall pattern is consistent then with the notion that the relative benefits for coronary-bypass recovery of having a roommate before surgery who was a cardiac patient as compared to a noncardiac patient and who was postoperative compared to preoperative, respectively, were due at least in part to their relatively greater information value for the patient.

***Summary.*** The evidence for emotional convergence as a function of emotional comparison processes is at this point sketchy. The overall pattern of emotional convergence that would be predicted by an emotional comparison mechanism—specifically, greater emotional convergence under high than low threat when the other faces the same versus a different situation—has yet to be shown convincingly. There is a need to look also for more direct evidence that emotional comparison processes are involved when evidence of emotional convergence is found. That is, even if emotional convergence were found to be most pronounced under threat and specific to affiliation with a similarly threatened other, this would not in itself constitute evidence of emotional comparison or rule out mimicry mechanisms. It could be for example that people under threat spend more time attending to a person facing the same threat (perhaps in hopes of obtaining cognitive clarity, ideas for escape or coping). All else being equal, greater attention to another affords greater opportunity to mimic that person. There then would be an increased likelihood of greater emotional convergence through some sort of mimicry mechanism. The little relevant evidence that exists suggests that such an etiology, which seems qualitatively quite different from the emotional comparison processes depicted originally by Schachter, is at least plausible and worthy of additional study.

A better understanding of the mechanisms that give rise to emotional contagion under threat is of more than theoretical interest, given the evidence that the emotion-focused coping of preoperative surgery patients can be significantly influenced by affiliations with their roommates. At this point there is no evidence that verbal affiliation is directly involved, but it is too early to say that this possibility has been ruled. On the other hand, there is at least one piece of evidence suggesting that preoperative patients' problem-focused coping can be influenced directly by verbal affiliation with their roommates. That is, preoperative coronary-bypass patients who had roommates with greater threat-relevant information value engaged in more cognitive clarity affiliation and, apparently as a result of such affiliation, had shorter postoperative hospital stays (Kulik et al., 1996). From a practical standpoint, the magnitudes of differences in average length of stay that were found (1.1 to 2.4 days, depending on conditions) appear clinically significant, particularly when one considers that hospital costs range up to $1,000 or more per day and more than 300,000 coronary-bypass surgeries are performed yearly in the United States (American Heart

Association, 1993). A cost-effective policy for coronary-bypass surgery thus may entail systematic exposure of patients to fellow patients who are already recovering from the same operation. Logistically, of course, this may not always be possible. A postoperative coronary-bypass patient may not always be available, and bed constraints or staffing requirements may preclude such roommate assignments. An open question of practical importance then is whether something like simply bringing the postoperative cardiac patient by to talk to the preoperative cardiac patient would have beneficial effects. Whether similarly significant roommate effects would be found with women patients, for other major surgeries, in other hospitals, and under different payment structures are additional questions of practical importance that remain to be determined (see Kulik & Mahler, 1990, for an extended discussion of these issues).

For the present, we conclude that fellow patients, in the form of roommates prior to surgery, can exert a largely unrecognized but systematic influence on coronary-bypass patients' hospital experiences. As part of coping with the impending threat of this major surgery, preoperative patients apparently can use their roommates, to varying degrees and with good effect, as adjuncts to professionally delivered, preoperative preparations.

## GENERAL SUMMARY AND CONCLUSIONS

We have suggested classic work that relied on the fear and affiliate-choice paradigm has not made a convincing case that affiliation so indexed is motivated by the desire for emotional comparison (cf. Cottrell & Epley, 1977). We have further suggested that this early work has likely led to an overemphasis of the importance of emotional comparison and to an underemphasis of the importance of cognitive clarity desires as determinants of affiliation in the face of novel, physical threat situations (cf. Rofe, 1984; Shaver & Klinnert, 1982; Suls, 1977).

Similar conclusions apply to more recent efforts to examine both the actual affiliative behaviors exhibited in acute threat situations and the implications of those behaviors for health outcomes. Although much more work is needed, to date we are more impressed with the degree to which both visual and verbal affiliations in acute threat situations appear systematically directed toward affiliates who can better provide information needed for cognitive clarity or self-improvement than toward affiliates who theoretically can provide better referents for emotional comparison. We are also more impressed with how cognitive clarity rather than emotional comparison affiliations seem to be related to health outcomes. There is intriguing evidence for example that our emotional reactions to both laboratory and medical threats may converge with the emotional reactions of our affiliates, but the most directly relevant work so far suggests that a mimicry mechanism is more likely the mediator than an emotional comparison mechanism. On the other hand, there is remarkably direct evidence that cognitive clarity affiliations may influence such medical outcomes as recovery from surgery. Both the work on emotional contagion and surgical recovery require and we believe merit considerable future attention.

How important then are social comparison processes for affiliation and coping with acute threat situations? The answer depends on whether one considers efforts to obtain cognitive clarity from others as a social comparison activity. As we noted previously, Schachter (1959) originally emphasized social comparison for purposes of self-evaluation (i.e., emotional comparison) and preferred to view cognitive clarity efforts as relatively asocial and not relevant directly to social comparison. If we consider only evidence bearing on emotional comparison or self-evaluation processes, we then would have to conclude that the evidence does not indicate a major role of social comparison either as a determinant of affiliation in the face of acute threat or of coping success.

On the other hand, more recent extensions of social comparison theory have tended to posit additional goals of social comparison besides self-evaluation (see Helgeson & Mickelson, 1995). Most notably, it has been argued that threat also may increase the desire for self-improvement and thereby motivate social comparison activity in the form of information seeking from better-off or more knowledgeable others (e.g., Brickman & Bulman, 1977; Taylor & Lobel, 1989; Wood, 1989; Wood & Taylor, 1991). This idea is itself reminiscent of Festinger's (1954) original notion of a unidirectional drive upward that leads us generally to seek out others with abilities slightly better than our own for self-improvement. Presumably, social comparison processes are involved in determining which potential affiliates are likely to have more or less relevant information by which to improve our performance. As such, it would seem that the cognitive clarity affiliations that we observed, which may be viewed as a specific case of seeking information for self-improvement, did indeed involve social comparison activity. If so, then our conclusion regarding the importance of social comparison processes for affiliation and coping with acute threat situations changes considerably. Although cognitive clarity affiliations in absolute terms may constitute a small subset of the total affiliative behavior exhibited in acute threat situations, the fact that they account for a significant portion of the variance in something like surgical recovery suggests they nevertheless can be quite important.

## ACKNOWLEDGMENTS

This chapter was supported by grant HS06348 from the Agency for Health Care Policy and Research and by grant HL43654 from the National Heart, Lung, and Blood Institute of the National Institutes of Health.

We thank Bram Buunk, Rick Gibbons, Bill Gerin, and Tony Ahrens for helpful comments.

## REFERENCES

American Heart Association. (1993). *Heart and stroke facts.* Dallas, TX: Author.

Ajzen, I., & Fishbein, M. (1977). Attitude-behavior relations: A theoretical analysis and review of empirical research. *Psychological Bulletin, 84,* 888–918.

Argyle, M., & Dean, J. (1965). Eye-contact, distance, and affiliation. *Sociometry, 28,* 289-304.

Auerbach, S. M. (1973). Trait-state anxiety and adjustment to surgery. *Journal of Consulting and Clinical Psychology, 40,* 264–271.

Brickman, P., & Bulman, R. J. (1977). Pleasure and pain in social comparison. In J. M. Suls & R. L. Miller (Eds.), *Social comparison processes: Theoretical and empirical perspectives* (pp. 149-186). Washington, DC: Hemisphere.

Buck, R. W., & Parke, R. D. (1972). Behavioral and physiological response to the presence of a friendly or neutral person in two types of stressful situations. *Journal of Personality and Social Psychology, 24,* 143–153.

Buunk B. P. (1994). Social comparison processes under stress: Towards an integration of classic and recent perspectives. In W. Stroebe & M. Hewstone (Eds.), *European review of social psychology* (Vol. 5, pp. 211-241). New York: Wiley.

Buunk B. P. (1995). Comparison direction and comparison dimension among disabled individuals: Toward a refined conceptualization of social comparison under stress. *Personality and Social Psychology Bulletin, 21,* 316–330.

Cohen, F., & Lazarus, R. S. (1979). Coping with the stresses of illness. In G. C. Stone, F. Cohen, & N. E. Adler (Eds.), *Health psychology-A handbook* (pp. 77–112). San Francisco: Jossey-Bass.

Cohen, F., & Lazarus, R. S. (1983). Coping and adaptation in health and illness. In D. Mechanic (Ed.), *Handbook of health, health care, and the health professions* (pp. 608–635). New York: Free Press.

Cottrell, N. B., & Epley, S. W. (1977). Affiliation, social comparison and socially mediated stress reduction. In J. M. Suls & R. L. Miller (Eds.), *Social comparison processes: Theoretical and empirical perspectives* (pp. 43–68). Washington, DC: Hemisphere.

Darley, J. M. (1966). Fear and social comparison as determinants of conformity behavior. *Journal of Personality and Social Psychology, 4,* 73–78.

Darley, J. M., & Aronson, E. (1966). Self-evaluative vs. direct anxiety reduction as determinants of the fear-affiliation relationship. *Journal of Experimental Social Psychology, 2*(Suppl. 1), 66–79.

Devine, E. C. (1992). Effects of psychoeducational care for adult surgical patients: A meta-analysis of 191 studies. *Patient Education and Counseling, 19,* 129–142.

Epley, S. W. (1973). *The effect of the presence of a companion upon the speed of escape from electric shock.* Unpublished doctoral dissertation, University of Iowa, Iowa City.

Festinger, L. A. (1954). A theory of social comparison processes. *Human Relations, 7,* 117–140.

Firestone, I. J., Kaplan, K. J., & Russell, J. C. (1973). Anxiety, fear, and affiliation with similar-state versus dissimilar-state others: Misery sometimes loves nonmiserable company. *Journal of Personality and Social Psychology, 26,* 409–414.

Gerard, H. B., & Rabbie, J. M. (1961). Fear and social comparison. *Journal of Abnormal and Social Psychology, 62,* 586–592.

Gerard, H. B. (1963). Emotional uncertainty and social comparison. *Journal of Abnormal and Social Psychology, 66,* 568–573.

Gibbons, F. X., & Gerrard, M. (1991). Downward comparison and coping with threat. In J. M. Suls & T. A. Wills (Eds.), *Social comparison: Contemporary theory and research* (pp. 317–346). Hillsdale, NJ: Lawrence Erlbaum Associates.

Gump, B., & Kulik, J. A. (in press). Patterns of affiliation and emotional contagion: Revisiting social comparison theory. *Journal of Personality and Social Psychology.*

Hakmiller, K. L. (1966). Threat as a determinant of downward comparison. *Journal of Experimental Social Psychology, 2*(Suppl. 1), 32–39.

Hatfield, E., Cacioppo, J. T., & Rapson, R. L. (1993). Emotional contagion. *Current Directions in Psychological Science, 2,* 96–99.

Helgeson, V. S., & Mickelson, K. D. (1995). Motives for social comparison. *Personality and Social Psychology Bulletin, 21,* 1200–1209.

Helgeson, V. S., & Taylor, S. E. (1993). Social comparisons and adjustment among cardiac patients. *Journal of Applied Social Psychology, 23,* 1171–1195.

Helmrich, R. L., & Collins, B. E. (1967). Situational determinants of affiliative preference under stress. *Journal of Personality and Social Psychology, 6,* 79–85.

Kirkpatrick, L. A., & Shaver, P. (1988). Fear and affiliation reconsidered from a stress and coping perspective: The importance of cognitive clarity and fear reduction. *Journal of Social and Clinical Psychology, 7,* 214–233.

Kulik, J. A., & Mahler, H. I. M. (1987). Effects of preoperative roommate assignment on preoperative anxiety and postoperative recovery from coronary-bypass surgery. *Health Psychology, 6,* 525–543.

Kulik, J. A., & Mahler, H. I. M. (1989). Stress and affiliation in a hospital setting: Preoperative roommate preferences. *Personality and Social Psychology Bulletin, 15,* 183–193.

Kulik, J. A., & Mahler, H. I. M. (1990). Stress and affiliation research: On taking the laboratory to health field settings. *Annals of Behavioral Medicine, 12,* 106–111.

Kulik, J. A., Mahler, H. I. M., & Earnest, A. (1994). Social comparison and affiliation under threat: Going beyond the affiliate-choice paradigm. *Journal of Personality and Social Psychology, 66,* 301–309.

Kulik, J. A., Mahler, H. I. M., & Moore, P. (1996). Social comparison and affiliation under threat: Effects on recovery from major surgery. *Journal of Personality and Social Psychology, 71,* 967–979.

Kulik, J. A., Moore, P., & Mahler, H. I. M. (1993). Stress and affiliation: Hospital roommate effects on preoperative anxiety and social interaction. *Health Psychology, 12,* 119–125.

Lazarus, R. S., & Folkman, S. (1984). *Stress, appraisal, and coping*. New York: Springer.
Lewin, K. (1948). *Resolving social conflicts*. New York: Harper.
MacDonald, A. P. (1970). Anxiety affiliation and social isolation. *Developmental Psychology, 3*, 242–254.
Miller, N., & Zimbardo, P. G. (1966). Motives for fear induced affiliation: Emotional comparison or interpersonal similarity. *Journal of Personality, 34*, 481–503.
Molleman, E., Pruyn, J., & van Knippenberg, A. (1986). Social comparison process among cancer patients. *British Journal of Social Psychology, 25*, 1–13.
Morris, W. N., Worchel, S., Bios, J. L., Pearson, J. A., Rountree, C. A., Samaha, G. M., Wachtler, J., & Wright, S. L. (1976). Collective coping with stress: Group reactions to fear, anxiety, and ambiguity. *Journal of Personality and Social Psychology, 33*, 674–679.
Mumford, E., Schlesinger, H. J., & Glass, G. V. (1982). The effects of psychological intervention on surgery and heart attacks: An analysis of the literature. *American Journal of Public Health, 72*, 141–151.
Nisbett, R. E., & Wilson, T. D. (1977). Telling more than we can know: Verbal reports on mental processes. *Psychological Review, 84*, 231–259.
Reisenzein, R. (1983). The Schachter theory of emotion: Two decades later. *Psychological Bulletin, 94*, 239–264.
Rofe, Y. (1984). Stress and affiliation: A utility theory. *Psychological Review, 91*, 235–250.
Sarnoff, I., & Zimbardo, P. G. (1961). Anxiety, fear, and social isolation. *Journal of Abnormal and Social Psychology, 62*, 356–363.
Schachter, S. (1959). *The psychology of affiliation*. Stanford, CA: Stanford University Press.
Schachter, S., & Singer, J. E. (1962). Cognitive, social, and physiological determinants of emotional state. *Psychological Review, 69*, 379–399.
Shaver, P., & Klinnert, M. (1982). Schachter's theories of affiliation and emotions: Implications of developmental research. In L. Wheeler (Ed.), *Review of personality and social psychology* (Vol. 3, pp. 37–71). Beverly Hills, CA: Sage.
Spielberger, C. D., Gorsuch, R. L., & Lushene, R. E. (1970). *Manual for the State-Trait Anxiety Inventory*. Palo Alto, CA: Consulting Psychologists Press.
Sullins, E. S. (1991). Emotional contagion revisited: Effects of social comparison and expressive style on mood convergence. *Personality and Social Psychology Bulletin, 17*, 166–174.
Suls, J. M. (1977). Social comparison theory and research: An overview from 1954. In J. M. Suls & R. L. Miller (Eds.), *Social comparison processes: Theoretical and empirical perspectives* (pp. 1–20). Washington, DC: Hemisphere.
Suls, J., & Wan, C. K. (1989). Effects of sensory and procedural information on coping with stressful medical procedures and pain: A meta-analysis. *Journal of Consulting & Clinical Psychology, 57*, 372–379.
Taylor, S. E., Buunk, B., & Aspinwall, L. (1990). Social comparison, stress, and coping. *Personality and Social Psychology Bulletin, 16*, 74–89.
Taylor, S. E., Buunk, B., Collins, R. L., & Reed, G. M. (1992). Social comparison and affiliation under threat. In L. Montada (Ed.), *Life crisis and experiences of loss in adulthood* (pp. 213–227). Hillsdale, NJ: Lawrence Erlbaum Associates.
Taylor, S. E., Falke, R. L., Shoptaw, S. J., & Lichtman, R. R. (1986). Social support, support groups, and the cancer patient. *Journal of Consulting and Clinical Psychology, 54*, 608–615.
Taylor, S. E., & Lobel, M. (1989). Social comparison activity under threat: Downward evaluation and upward contacts. *Psychological Review, 96*, 569–575.
Thornton, D. A., & Arrowood, A. J. (1966). Self-evaluation, self-enhancement, and the locus of social comparison. *Journal of Experimental Social Psychology, 2* (Suppl. 1), 40–48.

Wicker, A. W. (1969). Attitudes versus action: The relationship of verbal and overt behavior responses to attitude objects. *Journal of Social Issues, 25,* 41–78.

Wills, T. A. (1981). Downward comparison principles in social psychology. *Psychological Bulletin, 90,* 245–271.

Wood, J. V. (1989). Theory and research concerning social comparisons of personal attributes. *Psychological Bulletin, 106,* 231–248.

Wood, J. V., & Taylor, K. L. (1991). Serving self-relevant goals through social comparison. In J. Suls & T. A. Wills (Eds.), *Social comparison: Contemporary theory and research* (pp. 23–50). Hillsdale, NJ: Lawrence Erlbaum Associates.

Wrightsman, L. S. (1960). Effects of waiting with others on changes in level of felt anxiety. *Journal of Abnormal and Social Psychology, 61,* 216–222.

Yalom, I. D., & Greaves, C. (1977). Group therapy with the terminally ill. *American Journal of Psychiatry, 134,* 396–400.

Zimbardo, P. G., & Formica, R. (1963). Emotional comparison and self-esteem as determinants of affiliation. *Journal of Personality, 31,* 141–162.

# CHAPTER 9

# Social Comparison as a Coping Process: A Critical Review and Application to Chronic Pain Disorders

Howard Tennen
Glenn Affleck
*University of Connecticut Health Center*

Chronic pain and disability give people many opportunities to draw conclusions about how their situation compares to that of others (social comparison), and to use their own state at an earlier time as a comparison target (temporal comparison). The many dimensions on which they can compare include the intensity of pain, its duration, one's ability to carry out daily activities, and adaptation to living with a chronic burden. In this chapter we examine the view that pain-related social comparison, particularly downward comparison, functions as an emotion-focused coping strategy. We argue that although individuals with chronic pain disorders may at times use downward comparison to regulate their emotions or to provide a more comforting view of themselves or the future, their expression of downward comparisons may also reflect a conclusion or outcome derived from available evidence, an accurate or inaccurate belief, or a pain-related thought that is not specifically intended to help them adapt to the pain or limitations it imposes. Many contributors to the social comparison literature now assume that when individuals facing threatening circumstances acknowledge worse possible situations or others to whom their circumstance compares favorably, they are engaging in emotion-focused coping (e.g., Gibbons & Gerrard, 1991; Langston, 1994; Taylor, Wayment, & Carrillo, 1995; Wills, 1987; Wills, chapter 6, this volume; Wood & VanderZee, chapter 10, this volume). Our principal goal in this chapter is to show that this view is limited and limiting, and that a broader conceptualization of social comparisons among people experiencing chronic pain and facing other chronically threatening situations is likely to enhance our understanding of both social comparison and the coping process.

We begin with an overview of how people cope with chronic pain. We then offer a brief history of how social comparison theory has been applied to health and illness and how its evolution has led theorists to view such comparisons, particularly downward comparisons, as emotion-focused coping strategies. Drawing on the broader coping literature, we then ask "what might we reasonably expect from a coping strategy?" If a behavioral or cognitive process is deemed a coping strategy, what should we expect it to look like, and how should we expect it to behave? Our answers to these questions set the stage for a review of the few studies of social comparison phenomena among individuals with chronic pain disorders. Our chapter ends with a proposal that investigators turn to within-person study designs to best capture coping processes, their antecedents, and their consequences. We provide an illustration of idiographic procedures for social comparison research from an ongoing study of the daily lives of individuals with fibromyalgia, a generalized pain syndrome.

## COPING WITH CHRONIC PAIN: AN OVERVIEW

Individuals living with chronic pain experience both misery and significant functional limitations. The following descriptions offered by participants in our studies of rheumatoid arthritis capture the experience well:

> I can't do things that I used to take for granted. I have little energy and strength. I come home from shopping feeling as if I had run a marathon. Besides not having energy, I'm in terrible pain.
>
> There are times when I'm downright miserable, like when I can't even pick up a pot off the stove. Every once in a while, I have to miss work for a week or two because I simply can't keep my knee in a position to drive a car.
>
> There are a lot of things I'm not able to do anymore. Even turning a faucet gives me a lot of pain. A lot of things that most people take for granted, like scraping snow off the car windows, are impossible for me.
>
> It's hard to describe how bad the pain is or how helpless you feel. You're constantly aware that you have to walk with your feet and that they're always in pain. Getting up in the morning is sheer torture. Sometimes it takes hours to get out of bed and dressed.

> Any bump or pull might cause my hands to swell. I might not be able to walk very well. I dread having to turn a doorknob. The pain can be excruciating. It's a burning pain. It's like torture.

These descriptions capture the central characteristics of chronic pain disorders: the misery of intense and sometimes unrelenting pain, the emotional drain and physical exhaustion associated with activities previously taken for granted, and the numerous adjustments and accommodations required to get through the day. And unlike individuals experiencing acute pain episodes related to a recent injury, those with chronic pain disorders must also adjust to an uncertain future. Each of these features of chronic pain disorders poses a threat to self-esteem (Gentry & Owens, 1986) and to one's sense of self-efficacy and optimism (Turk & Holzmam, 1986). The threat to esteem, the uncertainty, and the emotional distress associated with chronic pain disorders make them an ideal context in which to study coping processes. The threat to self-esteem inherent in the chronic pain experience is particularly important because Wills's (1981) downward comparison theory maintains that downward comparisons are characteristic of individuals who face threats to their self-esteem.

Pain researchers and clinicians rely heavily on coping theory to study chronic pain disorders and to develop cognitive and behavioral interventions. Most self-management programs include coping strategies as their centerpiece (e.g., Hansen & Gerber, 1990), and stress the importance of shifting from pain elimination or reduction as a primary goal to pain coping and accommodation (Gentry & Owens, 1986). In this pain coping literature, distinctions have been made among *cognitive coping strategies,* which are conscious, purposeful, attempts to manage pain or make it more tolerable; *pain cognitions,* which are adaptive or maladaptive pain-related thoughts not specifically intended to help one deal with a pain episode; and *pain related beliefs or attitudes* (Hanson & Gerber, 1990; Turk, Meichenbaum, & Genest, 1983). The distinctions among pain coping strategies, pain related thoughts, and pain beliefs or attitudes parallel distinctions we make here between coping and adaptive beliefs.

Cognitive strategies for coping with pain include those that attempt to alter the appraisal of the painful situation and those that attempt to divert attention from the pain. Diversion strategies include creating mental images incompatible with pain, interpreting pain sensations as something other than pain, ignoring pain sensations, and refocusing attention away from the pain through activities like work or social activity (Turk et al., 1983). A common and effective reappraisal strategy is transforming the pain experience into a teacher or reminder. This strategy has been successfully taught and employed during episodes of intense pain (Hanson & Gerber, 1990).

Where do pain-related social comparisons fit in the matrix of pain beliefs, pain-related thoughts, and pain coping strategies? Jensen, Turner, Romano, and Karoly (1991), in an extensive review of the literature on coping with chronic pain, distinguish beliefs, which they define as people's cognitions about their pain problem, from coping, which they define as active strategies to manage or vitiate a stressful encounter. They categorize comparative evaluations as coping strategies based on the assumption that when experiencing a stressful encounter, people compare themselves favorably to other people or situations "*in an effort* to make themselves feel comparatively fortunate, and thereby buffer themselves against the effects of the stressor" (Jensen et al., 1991, p. 276, italics added). Throughout this chapter we question the effortful nature of downward comparisons.

## SOCIAL COMPARISON: FROM SOURCE OF SELF-RELEVANT INFORMATION TO EMOTION-FOCUSED COPING STRATEGY

Over the past 15 years there has been a distinct shift in how social comparisons are conceptualized. This shift, which Wheeler (1991) called "neo-social-comparison theory," was fueled by innovations in social psychological theory (cf. Gibbons & Gerrard, 1991) as well as changes in the definition and measurement of coping processes. These changes, in turn, converged on a new conceptualization of downward comparison as an effort to modulate one's emotional reactions to a threatening encounter. We now review briefly how this change unfolded and suggest that its potential to provide insights into the nuances of coping remains largely unfulfilled (see also Buunk, Gibbons, & Reis-Bergan, chapter 1, this volume).

Festinger's (1954) focus on accurate self-evaluation and comparisons "upward" was extended first by Hakmiller (1966) to threatening circumstances and downward comparisons, and later by Goethals and Darley (1977), who argued explicitly that when people experience threats to their self-esteem, comparisons to disadvantaged others might serve an adaptive end (cf. Gruder, 1977). Gibbons and Gerrard (1991) described three further developments in the social comparison literature that led them to view such comparisons, and particularly downward comparisons, as coping strategies. First was Brickman and Bulman's (1977) convincing argument that although comparing oneself to superior others can be informative, it can also be threatening. They, like Goethals and Darley (1977) and Gruder (1977), argued that individuals facing a threatening encounter may be inclined to compare themselves to others who are worse off.

The other two influences mentioned by Gibbons and Gerrard were Wills' (1981) important article linking downward comparison and subjective well-being, and Taylor and her colleagues' (Taylor, Wood, & Lichtman, 1983; Wood, Taylor, & Lichtman, 1985) studies of comparative evaluations among individuals facing life-threatening circumstances. Wills' (1981) theory of downward comparison processes formed the foundation of what has become the prevailing view that social comparison is a coping strategy. Wills argued that downward comparisons are not only adaptive but common among people facing threatening events. He suggested that the goal of such comparisons was to help the threatened individual experience her or his own situation as less aversive. In a subsequent chapter, Wills (1987) explicitly defined such comparisons as coping strategies. At the same time, Taylor, Wood, and associates (Taylor et al., 1983; Taylor & Lobel, 1989; Wood et al., 1985) provided some of the earliest systematic evidence of downward comparisons beyond the laboratory. In their study of women with breast cancer, Taylor et al. (1983) found an unexpectedly high prevalence of passive downward comparison (i.e., taking advantage of opportunities to compare oneself with less fortunate others; see also Wood & VanderZee, chapter 10, this volume). When asked how well they were adapting compared to other women with breast cancer, eighty percent of the participants, even those who by all available evidence were not doing well, reported adjusting somewhat better or much better than others. And those who didn't know another woman with a more serious affliction chose to imagine others who were not adapting as well.

Wills' persuasive arguments and Taylor et al.'s provocative findings led Gibbons and Gerrard (1991) to describe downward comparison as an emotion-focused coping strategy. They explicitly linked the phenomenon of downward comparison with other emotion-focused coping strategies such as seeking social support and efforts to appraise a threatening situation in a less threatening light. As an emotion-focused coping strategy, the aim of downward comparison is to reduce emotional discomfort.[1]

At the same time, however, changes were taking place in coping

[1]As defined in the literature, the superordinate concept of emotion-focused coping is perhaps excessively broad. It includes attempts to reduce emotional distress, positive reappraisals, and a host of other efforts that are not aimed directly at the circumstance causing the problem. In this chapter we accept this broad definition, and leave it to others to determine if a more focused construct would better serve the field. Later in the chapter we describe some of the unintended consequences of this broad definition.

theory. One such change among investigators who worked from more traditional coping models was the inclusion of social comparison in the taxonomy of coping strategies (Menaghan, 1982; Pearlin & Schooler, 1978). Most important, however, were the distinctions being drawn among well learned adaptive behaviors that do not require effort and concentration, beliefs, and coping strategies. Largely owing to the influence of Richard Lazarus (Lazarus, 1991, 1993a, 1993b; Lazarus & Folkman, 1984), but anticipated by others (Coelho, Hamburg, & Adams, 1974), coping researchers began to appreciate that "not all adaptive processes are coping. Coping is a subset of adaptational activities that *involves effort* and does not include everything that we do in relating to the environment" (Lazarus & Folkman, 1984, p. 132, italics added). The effortful nature of coping is also captured in Haan's (1977, 1992) distinction between coping and defending. Haan (1992) concluded, "People should be able to describe their coping efforts because a hallmark of coping is conscious choice" (p. 268). Despite Lazarus and Folkman's (1984) care to focus on the effortful and strategic nature of coping, they too defined seemingly effortless positive comparisons and worse possible outcomes as examples of emotion-focused coping.

This more restricted and clearly articulated definition of coping excludes higher order beliefs, including existential beliefs, which can be held without corroborating evidence. These beliefs help people create meaning in threatening situations, which in turn can enhance emotional well-being (Bulman & Wortman, 1977) and health outcomes (Affleck, Tennen, & Rowe, 1991). Although adaptive, these beliefs are not coping strategies as they are now commonly defined. The current definition of coping also excludes situational appraisals such as the perception of control. Although perceived control often has positive adaptive value (see Burger, 1989, for exceptions), it too is not a coping strategy. Finally, automatized adaptive behavior, that is, well learned behavior that requires neither concentration nor effort, does not qualify as coping.

Many investigators share this view of coping as conscious and effortful. Aldwin (1994), for example, is adamant in her conviction that coping strategies reflect conscious decision making. Parker and Endler (1996), Schwarzer and Schwarzer (1996), and Zeidner and Saklofske (1996) share this conviction. But certainly not all investigators and theorists agree that coping strategies require conscious effort. Houston (1987), for example, finds this requirement "curious." Others (e.g., Janoff-Bulman, 1992; Janoff-Bulman & Timko, 1987) are less concerned about distinctions between defense mechanisms and coping strategies. And still others (e.g., Sackeim, 1983) use the term "strategies" to describe self-deceptive positive illusions.

Most recently, Coyne and Gottlieb (1996) have argued that a

definition of coping that excludes automatized behaviors and thoughts is too restrictive. They hold, as do Thomas Wills (chapter 6, this volume) and Hart Blanton (personal communication, December 1995) that over time, individuals with chronic medical conditions routinize effective coping strategies so that they are no longer conscious or effortful.[2] These authors also remind us that some ways of adapting to stressful circumstances, such as defensive pessimism (Cantor & Norem, 1989), may not always be recognized as strategies by those who engage in them (and we might add that they may be effective precisely because they are not so recognized). Coyne and Gottlieb conclude that to understand why particular coping strategies are employed, and whether such strategies are adaptive, we must also consider habit and (unconscious) routine. We agree. We also believe that situational appraisals (e.g., loss, threat, challenge, control) and beliefs (Moos & Schaefer, 1992) are critical to our understanding of coping. Yet we do not equate these appraisals and beliefs with coping efforts, because current conceptualizations posit a causal relation between beliefs and coping, and appraisals and coping (Bandura, 1986; Lazarus & Folkman, 1984). In differentiating coping from other adaptive responses, we are not denying the existence of fundamental assumptions held out of awareness, nor are we disagreeing with Coyne and Gottlieb's portrayal of how conscious efforts might become automatized behavior. It is because we embrace these concepts that we wish to differentiate them from, and understand their relation to, coping strategies.

To anticipate our position and place downward comparison within this definition of coping, consider the situation of a woman with a recently diagnosed pain disorder. If this woman actively scans her environment for evidence of less fortunate others, she is coping. If she takes the time to remind herself that her pain is less intense than it is for others, she is coping. But if she simply reports the conclusion that she is fortunate compared to others when provided the opportunity during an interview, she is not necessarily coping. That her conclusion may

[2]Although Coyne and Gottlieb (1996) highlight effective coping efforts that evolve into routinized "coping" behavior, they do not explain how automatic responses remain constrained so as not to evolve into overgeneralized coping (i.e., coping behavior maintained after the termination of the stressor), stereotypic coping (i.e., coping behavior used routinely and indiscriminately in response to diverse stressors). The automatic quality of the responses described by these authors seem to make them vulnerable to both overgeneralization and stereotypy. Individuals with intermittent chronic pain often develop compensatory strategies that evolve into automatic responses. These responses can create new problems (e.g., walking with a limp) when they are no longer regulated by conscious processes. A more complete discussion of overgeneralized and stereotypic coping appears in Lepore and Evans (1996) and Cohen, Evans, Stokols, and Krantz (1986).

have been reached through selective evaluations or is biased by objective standards is irrelevant to its status as a coping strategy. Its adaptive function is equally irrelevant to whether it is a copying strategy. If coping requires conscious effort, evidence of such effort is required. Throughout the remainder of this chapter we evaluate the social comparison literature related to chronic pain disorders keeping in mind a distinction we first made in 1988 between comparison conclusions and comparison coping (Affleck, Tennen, Pfeiffer, & Fifield, 1988). Related distinctions are made in other chapters of this volume (e.g., Ahrens & Alloy, chapter 13; Buunk & Ybema, chapter 12; Wood & VanderZee, chapter 10). We differentiate downward comparison as a coping strategy (*comparison coping*), downward comparison as an inference (*comparison conclusion*), and downward comparison as a motivated appraisal that enhances a sense of esteem and psychological control (*secondary control comparison*). We take the position that although downward comparisons typically benefit those who offer them, the literature provides scant evidence that these comparisons function as coping strategies.[3]

## WHAT MAY WE REASONABLY EXPECT OF A COPING STRATEGY?

Having described the consensus (though not universal) definition of coping, we can articulate expectations for the "behavior" of coping strategies. Put simply, if social comparison is a coping strategy, it should behave like one. We offer three conceptually reasonable expectations for how comparisons should behave as a coping strategy: (a) they should be effortful; (b) through their influence on commitment patterns they should affect more than emotional well-being; and (c) in response to situational demands they should change in predictable ways.

### Coping as Effortful

Lazarus's (1993b) definition of coping as "cognitive and behavioral efforts to manage psychological stress" (p. 237) fits well with what we usually consider a *strategy,* that is, a plan or technique for achieving some end. Carver et al. (1989) followed the spirit of this definition and

[3]It is tempting to surmise that a comparison conclusion is itself evidence that comparison coping took place. Lessons learned from evolutionary biology (cf. Gould, 1985) about the dangers of positing adaptive explanations (in this case adaptive efforts) for observed outcomes should constrain our enthusiasm for linking comparison coping with comparison conclusions.

of their theory of engagement (investing effort) and disengagement when they selected items for the COPE, an inventory to assess coping. Similarly, Hobfoll, Dunahoo, and Ben-Porath (1994) generated items for the P-SAC by culling the well-developed strategy literature related to military maneuvers, chess, and bridge. And Stone and Neale's (1984) Daily Coping Inventory is "intention oriented in that it . . . asks if anything was thought or done with the intention of accomplishing the function . . ." (Stone, Neale, & Shiffman, 1993). These investigators appreciate the effortful nature of coping.

Are social comparisons effortful? Theoretical analyses of social comparisons hint at an effortful process (Levine & Resnick, 1993), and we are certain that comparisons can be effortful. We are equally certain, however, that they are not necessarily effortful as typically measured. An individual with rheumatoid arthritis facing an extended period of intense pain may try to think of less fortunate others as a way of making the pain more bearable. He or she may try to recall an earlier time when the pain was worse or when he or she felt less well equipped to endure it. These efforts at social and temporal comparison can justifiably be called cognitive coping strategies. They capture the intentional, strategic quality of coping and in this way are like other pain coping strategies such as diverting attention or reinterpreting pain sensations (Rosenstiel & Keefe, 1983). Other comparison processes are not as clearly intentional. A comparison to a manufactured or "mythical" other (Taylor, Wood, & Lichtman, 1983), for example, relies on an illusion or successful self-deception (Lazarus & Folkman, 1984; Suls, 1983; Taylor, 1989). Because the adaptational benefits of such comparisons turn on their plausibility, we suspect that few people would say that they tried to invent from whole cloth less fortunate others in order to compare themselves favorably. Individuals may, however, try to convince themselves that there must be others whose pain is worse than their own. But we are aware of only one field study (Jensen & Karoly, 1992) in which downward comparisons have been assessed so as to capture their effortful nature. Although studies have examined the need for comparison, its direction and frequency, the conclusion of how well one fares compared to others, and the emotional antecedents and consequences of comparison, they have not pursued effortful comparisons intended to alleviate distress (i.e., comparison coping).

This conceptual and operational confusion between comparison as a potentially adaptive conclusion and comparison as a coping process is not unique to the social comparison literature. The Coping Strategies Questionnaire (Rosenstiel & Keefe, 1983), designed to evaluate pain coping strategies, includes items that measure "catastrophizing," that is, negative statements such as "I worry all the time about whether it will end." Similarly, rumination has been described as an emotion-focused coping strategy (Nolen-Hoeksema, Parker, & Larson, 1994). Consider as well the concept of *positive focus*. Dunkel-Schetter, Feinstein, Taylor, and Falke (1992) factor analyzed the Ways of Coping Inventory (Folkman & Lazarus, 1988) among cancer patients and derived five strategies. One of these strategies was positive focus, "characterized by *efforts* to find meaning in the experience by focusing on personal growth" (Taylor & Aspinwall, 1992, italics added). We can imagine someone with cancer trying to find meaning in the illness experience or trying to grow as a person from the experience. But items measuring positive focus do not measure such efforts. Rather, they measure conclusions (e.g., "I came out of the experience better than I went in"). And to the extent that such conclusions are veridical, we should be neither surprised nor impressed if they are associated with positive psychological or health outcomes. The confusion between comparison as a coping strategy and comparison as a conclusion thus reflects the same confusion in the broader coping literature that has only rarely (e.g., Aldwin & Revenson, 1987) been addressed.

We have demonstrated in our work on adaptation to rheumatoid arthritis (Affleck, Urrows, Tennen, & Higgins, 1992; see also Affleck & Tennen, 1993) that theoretical and measurement distinctions among appraisals, beliefs, and coping are not trivial. For example, we found that the prospectively measured daily use of a positive reappraisal strategy is bimodal: although most individuals rarely employed this tactic, a few relied on it almost every day as a way of contending with their daily pain. However, responses to a reliable indicator assessing positive reappraisal of the chronic pain experience (a conclusion) did not differentiate those who used this strategy frequently from those who used it rarely. This underscores empirically the distinction between conclusions (or beliefs) and coping strategies.

**Adaptational Consequences of Comparison Coping**

In addition to being effortful, we would expect downward comparisons to have adaptational consequences beyond emotional well-being. Yet in keeping with what may be too narrow a conception of emotion-focused coping, most studies have limited their focus to the relation between downward comparisons and well-being. Although it is clear that people make efforts to regulate their mood (Catanzaro & Mearns, 1990; Mayer, Salovey, Gomberg-Kaufman, & Blainey, 1991; Thayer, Newman, & McClain, 1994), it is far less clear that they employ downward comparisons to achieve such self-regulation. One reason why emotion-focused strategies are sometimes inversely correlated with one another is that strategies serving functions other than emotional regulation are lumped with actual mood regulation strategies (Carver et al., 1989). In fact, Lazarus now seems to reserve the term *emotion-focused* coping for mood regulation strategies. Other strategies aimed at changing the meaning of a threatening situation he calls "cognitive coping" (Lazarus, 1991, 1993b). This shift is far more than a lexical nuance. It represents an acknowledgment that strategies implemented to change the significance of a threatening event are not simply mood regulation strategies. Rather, they lead to "internal restructuring . . . to the point of changing a commitment pattern that can't be actualized" (Lazarus, 1991, p. 112; see also Smith & Lazarus, 1993). If downward comparisons are efforts to change the significance of a threatening event, they should do more than regulate emotions.

The definition and functions of emotion-focused coping are complicated further when we attempt to distinguish problem-focused from emotion-focused coping among individuals with chronic pain disorders. When someone diverts attention from his or her pain to alleviate distress, the reallocation of attention may well reduce the pain itself. The same is true for ignoring pain sensations. Someone who ignores the pain so as to get on with his or her day may actually experience less pain. And consider the following remark from a participant in our study of rheumatoid arthritis pain:

> There are certain things you just can't do. And once you accept that, you can reduce the pain.

This comment suggests that for individuals experiencing chronic pain, emotion-focused beliefs or strategies are intertwined with problem-focused behaviors.

## Coping As an Unfolding Process

Aside from being effortful and predicting more than mood regulation, cognitive coping strategies typically change over time. Temporal change is inherent in Lazarus and Folkman's (1984) description of coping as "constantly changing efforts." Yet field studies of comparison processes have paid scant attention to the issue of change. With few exceptions (e.g., Gibbons et al., 1991) change in comparisons over time has been assumed because individuals who have been facing a stressor for a longer time report making fewer downward comparisons than those facing the stressor for a shorter time. Aside from our concerns about the reliability of retrospectively reported coping strategies—a concern we address later in this chapter—we suspect that any genuine decline in the deployment of downward comparisons as a coping strategy may reflect an unmeasured change in the comparison target from others to oneself (i.e., a shift from social to temporal comparison, cf. Affleck & Tennen, 1991). That is, early on people have no real opportunity to make temporal comparisons (Albert, 1977; Suls & Mullen, 1983), because they haven't had sufficient experience with the stressor. Over time, the most reliable and informative comparisons can be made with one's own previous experience rather than the experience of others. Later in this chapter we provide preliminary evidence that adaptive comparison activity may shift from others to the self over time. The spontaneous comments of our research participants with rheumatoid arthritis suggest how this process might unfold and how it can reflect a belief as easily as a coping effort:

> The first year was very difficult, not really knowing when it would stop or if it would, and how I would end up. . . . I've learned how to pick things up and open things up so I can limit the pain I experience.

> I've learned that I can do this instead of that. I can do what has to be done by making certain adjustments. It takes time to get to that point.

> Over the years, I've learned with trial and error that I could control it; that the pain didn't have to control me.

> Over time I've figured out that I can do things to bring on the pain and things that could limit it. I also figured out that my flares won't last forever, although while they're happening it seems like forever. It took quite a while to figure that out.

These comparisons to prior and more difficult experiences, which offer no indication that they reflect coping efforts, needed time to emerge, and they suggest that for those whose pain has grown worse over time, temporal comparisons on other dimensions are readily available. When such comparisons did emerge, they reflected not only that things could have been worse, but that they actually had been worse. Such comparisons appear to have far greater "assurance potential" than comparisons to less fortunate others and can be made without the excess baggage of moral ambivalence noted by Brickman and Bulman (1977) and Wills (1981) for downward social comparisons. And they do not carry the liability inherent in the long-term reliance on downward comparison (Aspinwall & Taylor, 1993; Crocker & Major, 1989), nor the risks of upward comparisons. We suspect that once they emerge, downward temporal comparisons are far more durable and helpful than are downward social comparisons and more prevalent than upward comparisons.

## DOWNWARD COMPARISONS AS SECONDARY CONTROL BELIEFS

We expect social comparison as a coping strategy to be effortful, to influence more than emotional well-being, and to change in predictable ways. But even if these conceptual expectations are only occasionally met by social comparisons, comparison conclusions might still function as self-protective beliefs or defensive appraisals. These too should change in ways anticipated by theory. We have found, for example, that event appraisals (such as experiencing benefit or meaning in the event) are associated with psychological and physiological responses to a wide range of stressful health events including a first heart attack (Affleck, Tennen, Croog, & Levine, 1987; Affleck, Tennen, & Rowe, 1991), the birth of a medically fragile infant (Affleck, Tennen, Urrows, & Higgins, 1991), impending coronary artery bypass surgery (Fitzgerald, Tennen, Affleck, & Pransky, 1993), and impaired fertility (Tennen, Affleck, & Mendola, 1991), and that the association is independent of coping efforts (Litt, Tennen, Affleck, & Klock, 1992).

Rothbaum, Weisz, and Snyder (1982) speculated that such appraisals are "secondary control" beliefs, which through a process of accommodation, provide an alternative to feelings of helplessness in the face of an uncontrollable event. Rothbaum et al.'s formulation echoes Wills (1981, 1987) and Taylor et al.'s (1995) position that social comparisons should emerge when a threat cannot be overcome through instrumental action, and for events that are uncontrollable. If secondary control represents a "fallback" position after attempts to control an aversive situation have failed, it follows that secondary control, including downward comparisons, should increase as primary control appraisals diminish. There have been similar suggestions in the coping literature that emotion-focused and cognitive coping efforts are more likely to occur when an individual believes that nothing more can be done to change a threatening situation (Lazarus & Folkman, 1984). Although careful to avoid a stage model in which a lost sense of personal control invariably leads to secondary control appraisals, Rothbaum et al.'s model predicts that secondary control reappraisals should increase as perceived control or optimistic expectancies decrease.

Of the secondary control beliefs described by Rothbaum et al., interpretive control has received the greatest theoretical and empirical attention. In *interpretive control,* a person reevaluates a threatening event in a more positive light or ascribes a less threatening meaning to it. One manifestation of interpretive control is construing benefits. The conceptual similarities between construing benefits and making downward comparisons is captured by Buunk (1994) who convincingly classifies both as manifestations of "selective evaluation." The similarities are equally well depicted by Schulz and Decker (1985) who found that individuals disabled by spinal cord injury rated their situation in relatively favorable terms compared to those who were not disabled. These disabled persons supported their self-enhancing comparisons by citing intellectual accomplishments, positive social relationships, and sensitivity to others—benefits of their injury. Applying the logic of Rothbaum et al.'s two-process model, Lazarus and Folkman's stress and coping model, and Wills' downward comparison theory, we would predict that construing benefits and perceiving worse possible outcomes or less fortunate others should increase as perceived control or optimistic expectancies decrease.

We are aware of only one study that has addressed this prediction longitudinally. McLaney, Tennen, Affleck, and Fitzgerald (1995) found that among men and women with impaired fertility, finding benefits was inversely related to changes in outcome expectancy, such that a more pessimistic expectancy over time was associated with an increase in perceived benefits. This type of dynamic relation between outcome expectancies and secondary control beliefs is precisely the one predicted by downward comparison theory for the relation between perceived control or perceived mutability and downward comparisons. To our knowledge, there is no longitudinal evidence for such a relation. Empirical tests are needed to clarify the place of social comparison among theoretically related secondary control constructs.

Just as downward comparison theory makes predictions regarding the temporal relation between downward comparisons and changes in personal control, it makes a clear prediction about the adaptational consequences of downward comparisons in situations in which control is limited or absent (Major, Testa, & Bylsma, 1991; Taylor et al., 1995; Wood & VanderZee, chapter 10, this volume). Specifically, "when one perceives that one's situation may change and that one has little control over that change, the prospect of getting worse may be especially salient, thus enhancing the negative affective consequences of downward social comparisons" (Taylor et al., 1995, p. 15). This straightforward prediction has received preliminary support in a study by Buunk, Collins, Taylor, Van Yperen, and Dakof (1990), who found that cancer patients who believed that they had little control over their symptoms reported feeling worse after they made downward comparisons. Conceivably, the comparison evoked in these patients the possibility that they might become less fortunate in the future.

The population of individuals who are HIV-positive provides an ideal context for evaluating this prediction. Clearly, these people's situation may change. And there is likely to be considerable variation in how much control afflicted individuals believe they can exert over this change. For those who anticipate little control, downward comparison theory predicts that comparisons should have negative affective consequences. Rothbaum et al.'s two-process theory, on the other hand, predicts that for those who anticipate less control, secondary control beliefs should have a salutary effect. Among a group of HIV-positive men Thompson, Nanni, and Levine (1994) examined primary control and a manifestation of secondary control described by Rothbaum et al. (1982) in which the threatened individual accepts outcomes that cannot be personally influenced. The findings were consistent with a "fallback" interpretation of secondary control: for those who experienced less personal control, greater acceptance was associated with less distress. These findings are, of course, opposite to those predicted for downward comparisons, which following Buunk et al. (1990), should be associated with greater rather than less distress for those who experience less control.

These conflicting predictions and findings present a conceptual problem for three reasons. First, there is no evidence that, like other secondary control appraisals, downward comparisons increase as perceived control or optimistic expectancies decrease. Second, if Buunk et al.'s (1990) findings are replicated, they suggest that what is true for other secondary control beliefs is not true for downward comparisons. Finally, current theory seems to predict that downward comparisons are most likely to occur and least adaptive for individuals who experience little control, making them harmful for those in greatest need of emotional buffering.

In summary, downward comparisons do not seem to adhere to any of our expectations for coping strategies nor do they behave like secondary control appraisals. Our tentative conclusion is that if something doesn't look like a coping strategy or secondary control belief, and doesn't act like a coping strategy or secondary control belief, it may typically function as something other than a coping strategy or secondary control belief. We urge investigators to study a wide array of adaptational outcomes and to clarify when and how downward comparison functions as a conscious, effortful strategy or as an adaptive belief. This aspect of coping has been given inadequate attention even by those who differentiate coping from other adaptive processes. We now turn to studies that have examined downward comparison among individuals with chronic pain to discern how well comparisons have been evaluated as coping strategies.

## SOCIAL COMPARISON IN CHRONIC PAIN DISORDERS: STRATEGY OR CONCLUSION?

There is now an ample literature relating social comparison processes to health, illness, and disability. A search of the literature using PsychLit from 1987 to mid-1996 produced more than 40 references that examined comparisons among various patient groups across the life span. Nine of these studies examined individuals with chronic pain disorders, and eight of the pain-related studies involved rheumatoid arthritis.

Rheumatoid arthritis (RA) is a relatively common, chronic, and incurable disease. Its physical signs and symptoms include severe joint pain and stiffness, fatigue and, short of surgery, irreversible joint damage and immobility. Many affected individuals face increasing disability as the disease progresses. Still, a confident prognosis for most patients is difficult to make, and many patients experience fluctuating symptoms of disease activity, that is, flares and remissions. The ambiguity of this illness and its many threats to self-esteem and well-being make it a useful context in which to study social comparisons and other selective evaluations.

Affleck, Tennen, Pfeiffer, Fifield, and Rowe (1987) found that in response to a structured interview, RA patients tended to rate their illness as less severe than that of the average patient and their adjustment as being better than average. Patients who rated their illness as comparatively less severe actually had a less active disease than other patients in the sample and those rating their adjustment as better than average were judged by their care providers as adjusting better to their illness. These findings suggest that these social comparison conclusions may have some degree of accuracy and may even signal differences in psychosocial adjustment to rheumatoid arthritis.

In a second report (Affleck, Tennen, Pfeiffer, & Fifield, 1988), we made a more direct examination of the accuracy of patients' responses to a social comparison questionnaire and the specific association between their social comparison conclusions and their psychosocial adjustment as rated by health care providers. Although we highlighted the distinction between social comparison as a coping strategy and as a conclusion, we did not directly measure comparison coping. Accuracy was examined by computing intraclass correlations with criterion measures of disease activity, functional status, and psychosocial adjustment. Significant, but only modest statistical agreement was found for the disease activity and disability comparisons but not for the coping–adjustment comparison. Patients who expressed more favorable views of their comparative disease activity were rated as adjusting better to their illness, independent of their age, education, income, illness duration, actual disease activity, and the accuracy of their disease activity comparison.

Investigators at the University of North Carolina have been examining RA patients' use of social comparisons and their preferences for information that could be used to make these comparisons. Blalock, DeVellis, DeVellis, and Sauter (1988) and Blalock, DeVellis, and DeVellis (1989) examined RA patients' reported use of social comparisons under two conditions: when they were encountering difficulties in tasks involving manual dexterity and when they were setting standards for desired functioning in this area. Participants said that they more often compared themselves to other individuals with RA when they were encountering performance difficulties, but they compared themselves to disease-free individuals when they were setting performance standards. Furthermore, those who were most likely to describe this contextual difference in social comparison were more satisfied with their ability to perform the manual tasks. Satisfaction, in turn, was related positively to emotional well-being. In another study, Blalock, Afifi, DeVellis, Holt, and DeVellis (1990) extracted social comparison statements from interviews with RA patients. They found that most patients made unprompted comparisons, and that patients who emphasized their similarity to individuals not affected by RA exhibited better psychological adjustment. Although these investigators explicitly described these comparisons as coping strategies, it is not clear whether these were intentional or effortful comparisons.

In another study from the North Carolina group, DeVellis et al. (1990) examined RA patients' preferences for information that could be used to make a downward or an upward social comparison. In addition to summarizing their information preferences on a questionnaire, participants were also given the choice of selecting a folder in which they could read about a patient who was "doing better" or "doing worse" than they were. Consistent with downward comparison theory (Wills, 1981), most participants preferred information on patients whose illness was more severe than their own. This pattern was reversed, however, for informational preferences concerning other patients' coping and adjustment to the illness. Three times as many patients wanted to learn about others with RA whose spirits were "high more often than low" as they did about others whose spirits were "low more often than high," and nine times as many desired information about others who led active lives with this illness as desired information about others who led inactive lives. Although these findings are consistent with Taylor and Lobel's (1989) demonstration that the use of downward social comparisons for self-enhancement can and does coexist with the desire to interact with similar others who are contending admirably with the problem, these comparison preferences do not reveal whether comparisons function as coping strategies.

DeVellis et al. (1991) exposed women with RA to unavoidable social comparison information through a slide–tape presentation. When separate ratings were made for their own adjustment to RA and that of the target, participants who viewed someone who was adapting well rated her as dealing satisfactorily with the illness and, compared to the self-adaptation rating, better than they were themselves. Those exposed to someone managing less well rated her as adapting more poorly compared to their self-adaptation rating. However, when asked later to compare themselves directly with the same comparison target, only 5% of those who had been exposed to the target adapting well acknowledged they might be adapting less well than the target. We agree with DeVellis et al.'s conclusion that individuals are able to extract self-enhancing information from social comparisons, even when the comparison target and dimension are constrained and the target is superior on the selected dimension. We also believe that people can extract hopeful conclusions from comparing themselves accurately with better functioning individuals. Yet we see no evidence in this study that comparisons are coping strategies.

Giorgiano, Blalock, DeVellis, DeVellis, Keefe, and Jordan (1994) examined both social and temporal comparisons among men and women who had been first diagnosed with RA within 1 year prior to participation in their study. Comparisons were again conceptualized as coping strategies and were measured separately for leisure activities, household activities, and pain. In each of these areas, participants were asked to identify a person they might think about when they were having difficulty in that area. They were also asked who came to mind if they were thinking about how easily they would like to be able to perform each activity. Temporal comparison measures paralleled those for social comparison, with oneself at some earlier time as the comparison target. These newly diagnosed patients made more downward social and temporal comparisons for pain than for leisure and household activities, demonstrating that comparisons are not necessarily comparable across all aspects of a chronic illness. If the comparison target was rated as having moderate difficulty performing a task, the participant was thought to be making a stronger downward comparison than if the target was rated as having modest difficulty. One can imagine, however, that whether this is true depends on the relation between one's own and the target's performance difficulty. This issue aside, there is again no evidence that comparisons functioned as coping strategies.

In the only investigation of social comparison and chronic pain that did not study individuals with RA, Jensen and Karoly (1992) interviewed former inpatients at a multidisciplinary pain program, the majority of whom suffered from chronic low back pain or headache. This is also the only study to assess comparisons as cognitive coping strategies. That is, use of selective focus as an effortful strategy was queried with the item: "When in pain, I remind myself about things that I have going for me that other people don't have, such as intelligence, good looks, and good friends." Creation of worse possible worlds was assessed with the item: "When in pain, I remind myself that things could be worse." To assess the setting of manufactured normative standards, participants were asked how frequently they reminded themselves that they were adjusting to their pain better than the average pain patient. And the indicator of downward comparisons asked participants how often they remind themselves that there are people who are worse off. Combining these indicators into a composite measure of comparative self-evaluation, Jensen and Karoly found that after controlling for demographic and pain-related variables, the tendency to use downward comparisons was associated with fewer depressive symptoms, particularly for those with the shortest pain duration. Contrary to current theory, however, participants who believed they had greater control over their pain were those who most strongly endorsed comparative coping. To explain this anomaly, the authors suggested that when patients experience sufficient personal control over their illness, favorable comparisons may no longer represent coping efforts, but rather reflect accurate appraisals. Although we believe that this distinction is critical for the advancement of social comparison theory and for the emergent coping paradigm, Jensen and Karoly's care to measure comparative coping makes us doubt their interpretation. We are also convinced that any cross-sectional association between social comparison and well-being cannot inform us about the use or effectiveness of such comparisons to cope with pain and other chronic illnesses. To answer these questions, individuals need to be studied intensively over time. We next address the promise and challenges of such an approach to coping processes.

## AN IDIOGRAPHIC-NOMOTHETIC APPROACH TO COPING PROCESSES

Jensen et al. (1991) concluded their comprehensive review of the pain coping literature with three concerns that we believe apply equally well to the broader stress and coping literature and particularly to investigations of downward comparison as a coping strategy. First, they remind us that although our theoretical models describe causal relations among stress, coping and well-being, the correlational findings of field studies cannot even establish the temporal precedence of presumed causal factors. Laboratory studies, which allow causal inference, are typically far removed from the everyday lives of research participants. Jensen et al. also remind us that whereas theories, such as Wills' (1981, 1987) theory of downward comparison, posit moderators of stress–coping–adaptation relations, with few exceptions (e.g., self-esteem as a moderator of the relation between threat and social comparison) research has not aggressively pursued tests of moderational models. Finally, Jensen et al. call for more single subject designs, because they are "uniquely suited to understanding an individual's coping process over time" (p. 280). We now describe an *idiographic–nomothetic* approach to the study of daily stress, coping, and comparison processes that has the potential to address each of Jensen et al.'s concerns: it strengthens our causal inferences while remaining true to "real-world" experience, it evaluates relevant moderators, and it examines individuals intensively over time. Our description focuses on key features of the approach and those most relevant to the study of social comparisons. A more complete and statistically oriented description is provided elsewhere (Tennen & Affleck, 1996).

Behavioral research is dominated by the nomethetic approach, in which the investigator asks whether there are lawful relations among variables across individuals. The idiographic approach, which appears infrequently, takes the individual as the unit of analysis and focuses on the relations of variables across situations and over time in that individual's life (Allport, 1937). Its examination of individuals over time makes the idiographic approach uniquely suited to capture the "constantly changing cognitive and behavioral efforts" that define coping processes (Lazarus & Folkman, 1984), as well as the trait-like qualities of coping that have been less well demonstrated. We endorse and have applied (Affleck, Tennen, Urrows, & Higgins, 1994; Tennen & Affleck, 1996) an approach to coping that combines the strengths of both the idiographic and nomothetic strategies. This approach was first advanced by Epstein (1983) and has been applied more recently by Larsen (e.g., Larsen & Kasimatis, 1991).

### The Potential Contribution of Idiographic Assessment to Coping and Comparison Processes

Intensive idiographic assessment brings three unique capacities to the study of coping and social comparisons. This approach (a) captures stressors and coping efforts closer to their actual occurrence; (b) tracks change in rapidly fluctuating processes like social comparisons and mood; and (c) minimizes recall error inherent in field studies of social comparisons, coping, and well-being (Tennen & Affleck, 1996). These features of idiographic assessment ensure reliability and are essential to the study of stress and coping. In most investigations, including our own previous work on coping and social comparison (Affleck, Tennen, & Rowe, 1991; Stanton, Tennen, Affleck, & Mendola, 1992) participants complete a questionnaire such as the Ways of Coping Scale (Folkman & Lazarus, 1988), the COPE (Carver, Scheier, & Weintraub, 1989), the CISS (Endler & Parker, 1990) or in studies of coping with pain, the Coping Strategies Questionnaire (Rosenstiel & Keefe, 1983) or the Vanderbilt Pain Management Inventory (Brown & Nicassio, 1987). These questionnaires ask research participants to summarize their coping activities retrospectively. None inquire about social comparisons. Intensive assessment of individuals over time allows us to examine day-by-day changes in what presumably is a process. Indeed, if we believe that emotional well-being and physical adaptation change in response to coping efforts, including effortful social comparisons, then we need to measure coping and its emotional and physical consequences near to the time they occur. And day-by-day prospective assessment should minimize random and systematic recall bias and thus provide superior data than that obtained via recall for the same time period.

We know of two studies that compared directly daily coping reports with retrospectively reported coping over the same period of time. In one of these studies, part of our investigation of daily coping with rheumatoid arthritis (Affleck, Tennen, Urrows, & Higgins, 1991), we compared participants' recollection of the number of days they had used each of seven pain coping strategies (not including social comparison) with the tally of strategies taken from their daily reports over the same thirty days. The prospective (daily) data yielded a far richer description of pain coping than was apparent from the retrospective appraisals. Participants reported using more forms of coping from day to day than they recalled having used. And strategies that were used less than 5 days that month were most likely to be missed in the retrospective appraisal, although these less frequently employed strategies may signal efforts to cope with unusual demands.

Our concern here is not only with inaccuracy, but also its source. One potential source of inaccuracy is some measured (or worse, unmeasured) personality characteristic. There is good reason to believe that individuals use different cognitive heuristics to assist their recall (Neisser, 1991; Ross, 1989), and that the same personal characteristics that lead someone to under-report instances of social comparison, for example, may also influence his or her symptom reports (cf. Larsen, 1992). The outcome of the coping process may also influence coping recall (Ptacek, Smith, Espe, & Raffety, 1994). Because people systematically bias their recall so that it is consistent with and thus maintains their self-image (Ross & Fletcher, 1985; Snyder, Higgins, & Stucky, 1983), it is quite possible, as Ptacek et al. (1994) suggest, that a positive outcome motivates people to take credit for the outcome through the selective recall of a problem-focused strategy. Similarly, a negative outcome may lead to disavowing the use of problem-focused strategies. Such a process could be contributing to the rather consistent association between reports of problem-focused coping and indicators of positive well-being. Just how such a process might influence reports of downward comparisons or its relation to psychological well-being isn't clear, because existing coping measures do not assess comparative evaluations. But it's not hard to imagine someone who successfully navigates a threatening encounter recalling favorable comparisons to others and also reporting enhanced well-being.

A second recent study comparing daily and retrospective coping reports suggests that it will not be easy to assuage concerns about the biased recall of coping strategies, even over brief periods. Ptacek et al. (1994) followed college students every day for a week as the students recorded their coping strategies in preparing for an exam. Five days after the test they were asked to recall how they had coped during the same one week daily assessment period, using a retrospective coping scale containing the same coping categories as the daily measure. Each of the three coping dimensions measured in this study showed only moderate concordance between daily and retrospective reports. Aggregated daily reports of problem solving efforts shared merely 34% common variance with their retrospectively reported counterparts. Avoidance and Support Seeking shared only 22% and 24% variance with their respective scales. Worse yet, these investigators were unsuccessful in their well conceived attempt to evaluate which aspects of the coping process were captured by retrospective reports. Participants were no more successful at recalling the strategies they used most frequently nor those used for the longest period of time. Their retrospective reports did not reflect how they coped when the stress was most intense or what they did early or late in the coping process. So it seems that people's retrospective descriptions of their coping efforts (i.e., the descriptions obtained in nearly all studies of coping and social comparison) reflect an unreliable aggregated recollection that captures neither what they did most frequently nor what they did during the most threatening moments of the stressful encounter.

Although the reliability of intensive idiographic data is a significant advantage, there are other reasons to favor an idiographic–nomothetic approach to coping and social comparison: (a) a within-person design eliminates potential sources of between-person confounding by stable dispositions; (b) these designs preserve temporal sequences, which in turn (c) strengthens our causal inferences (Tennen & Affleck, 1996). It is common in the coping literature, including studies of social comparison under threat, to draw within-person inferences from between-person associations. For example, that individuals who report more downward comparisons also report less distress tells us nothing about the effect of such comparisons on distress nor does it speak to affective states that prompt comparisons. Yet investigators typically translate a between-person finding in the form "individuals who engage in more downward comparisons are less distressed" as if it were a within-person finding in the form "*when* individuals compare themselves favorably to others they are less distressed" or "individuals engage in downward comparisons *when* they are distressed, and the comparison process alleviates the distress." Only intensive within-person (idiographic) designs can reliably address temporal associations because they preserve temporal sequences.

Two recent studies have applied intensive within-person assessments of social comparisons and have begun to address Wills' (1981) suggestion that investigators evaluate social comparisons as they occur in naturalistic settings. To examine how individuals cope on a daily basis with negative events and particularly the ways in which they capitalize or savor (Bryant, 1989) positive events, Langston (1994) followed a group of sorority members for 15 days. At the end of each day they described one negative and one positive event and described how they responded to the event. Social comparison responses were combined with other "emotion-focused" responses, so their prevalence cannot be evaluated. Yet as a group, these emotion-focused responses occurred more frequently in response to positive events than to negative events, providing indirect support for our contention that comparisons are not uniquely or even primarily associated with threatening situations. Just as we might seek social contact to help us savor a joyous experience as well as to support us when we feel threatened, harmed or have experienced loss, so may we compare ourselves to others when we feel fortunate as well when our esteem has been threatened. The point we wish to reiterate is that the act of making a downward comparison may or may not indicate its use as a coping strategy. The prevalence of such comparisons as part of the experience of savoring highlights this point.

Wheeler and Miyake (1992) examined social comparisons as they occurred in natural contexts. Unlike interview-based assessments, questionnaires, interval-contingent recording, and signal-contingent recording (Wheeler & Reis, 1991), this "event-contingent method" allows individuals to describe their comparison experiences in real time, thus avoiding the potential problems associated with recalled comparisons. Although their approach relies on participants' recollections of how they were feeling just prior to making a comparison, it represents a significant advance in the measurement of social comparisons in daily life by measuring comparisons as they occurred and by measuring comparison behaviors rather than the comparison conclusions frequently obtained in field studies.

College freshmen participated in this study every day for 2 weeks. They completed a measure of trait self-esteem and then kept a structured record of their everyday social comparisons. The most interesting finding was that these students made upward comparisons when their mood was more negative and they made downward comparisons when their mood was more positive. This pattern contradicts the motivational explanation for comparisons offered in downward comparison theory. According to the theory, people are inclined to compare themselves to less fortunate others when they are distressed. The pattern fits quite well, however, with the idea that our mood influences our interpretation of ambiguous situations (Bower, 1991; Forgas, Bower, & Moylan, 1990). This explanation of the findings, though quite consistent with the evidence, is simply inconsistent with an explanation that invokes coping to explain them.

But one does not have to posit alternative theories to argue that downward comparisons are not inherently coping strategies. If these comparisons are a form of coping, we would expect them to emerge only rarely in everyday life and to occur less frequently than lateral or upward comparisons (cf. Foddy & Crundall, 1993; Taylor et al., 1995). Yet in Wheeler and Miyake's (1992) study of everyday life, participants reported on average more than 23 comparisons over a 13-day period, and were more likely to make downward then lateral or upward comparisons. When combined with Langston's (1994) data suggesting that downward comparisons may be a regular feature of savoring, these two idiographic studies give reason to doubt that evidence of downward comparison is by itself evidence of a coping effort. We now describe an idiographic study of chronic pain patients in which we examined comparison coping and its relation to daily pain and daily mood.

### Within-Person Study of Daily Comparison Processes in Fibromyalgia

Fibromyalgia is a syndrome of widespread pain combined with unusual tenderness in multiple sites (Wolfe et al., 1990). It is accompanied by much psychological distress, sleep disturbance, and use of health care services (Boissevain & McCain, 1991). Although its pathogenesis is controversial, fibromyalgia is currently believed to be a pain-amplification disorder arising from diverse, perhaps multiple underlying causes (Smythe, 1989; Wilke & Mackenzie, 1985). We are conducting a prospective 30-day study of fibromyalgia patients, entailing time-intensive self-monitoring of daily symptoms, experiences, behaviors, emotions, and cognitions. In this section, we summarize preliminary findings from 25 study participants, describe their effortful daily use of social and temporal pain comparisons, and characterize the within-person relations of these comparison processes with pain intensity, mood states, pain "catastrophizing" (Keefe, Brown, Wallston, & Caldwell, 1989), perceived control over daily pain, and the perceived efficacy of daily pain coping efforts. The participants, all women, were on average 41 years old, and estimated their widespread pain to have started an average of 10 years earlier.

The self-monitoring methodology used in this study combines a nightly structured questionnaire with a computer-assisted "real-time" assessment of pain intensity and mood three times each day. The electronic diary was a PSION palmtop computer programmed to deliver auditory signals to complete an on-screen interview at randomly selected times during the midmorning, midafternoon, and midevening. The interview responses were time-stamped and stored in the palmtop computer for subsequent uploading to a desktop system. Shiffman and colleagues (Penner, Shiffman, Paty, & Fritzche, 1994; Shiffman et al., 1994) inspired our use of this self-monitoring method and have established their many advantages over traditional paper-and-pencil methods, including superior compliance encouragement and monitoring and mitigation of some systematic biases in experience sampling. The 25 participants fulfilled their responsibilities admirably: 747 of 750 nightly questionnaires (99.6%) and 2,241 or 2,250 electronic diary interviews (99.6%) were completed.

Two items on the nightly questionnaire measured the effortful use of downward social and temporal comparisons concerning that day's pain. Participants used a point scale ranging from 0 (*not at all*) to 6 (*very much*) to describe how much they had "reminded [themselves] that [their] pain today was not as bad as it is for others" (social comparison) and "that [their] pain today was not as bad as it had been at one time" (temporal comparison). The average daily mean for the social comparison question was 1.1 ($SD = 1.4$) and for the temporal comparison question was 1.8 ($SD = 1.8$). The mean percentage of days the average respondent reported making any social comparison was 36.5% ($SD = 37.3$); any temporal comparison, 48% ($SD = 34.7$). Figure 9.1 displays the frequency distribution of the number of days for which any comparison effort was reported. Clearly, these individuals differed considerably in how often they compared their pain to that of others who are worse off or to that of a time when they were worse off. For example, while nearly one quarter of the respondents never compared their pain to others' pain, an equal proportion did so on at least 2 of every 3 days.

Individuals with higher mean daily social comparison scores also had higher mean temporal comparison scores ($r = .73$, $p < .001$). This high concordance, however, cannot capture how social and temporal comparisons are patterned from day to day. The time plots of social and temporal comparison use by three subjects in Fig. 9.2 illustrate just how diversely these processes can be configured together over time. Subject 1 made temporal comparisons on several days, social comparisons on several days, but never both on the same day. Subject 2 also reserved some days for social comparison and other days for temporal comparison, but on other days she made both types of comparisons. Yet another pattern is evidenced for Subject 3, who occasionally made temporal comparisons without making social comparisons, but who never made social comparisons without also making temporal comparisons. These dissimilar configurations are a compelling invitation to explore their antecedents and consequences in other daily process measures.

To estimate the within-person relations of daily comparison efforts

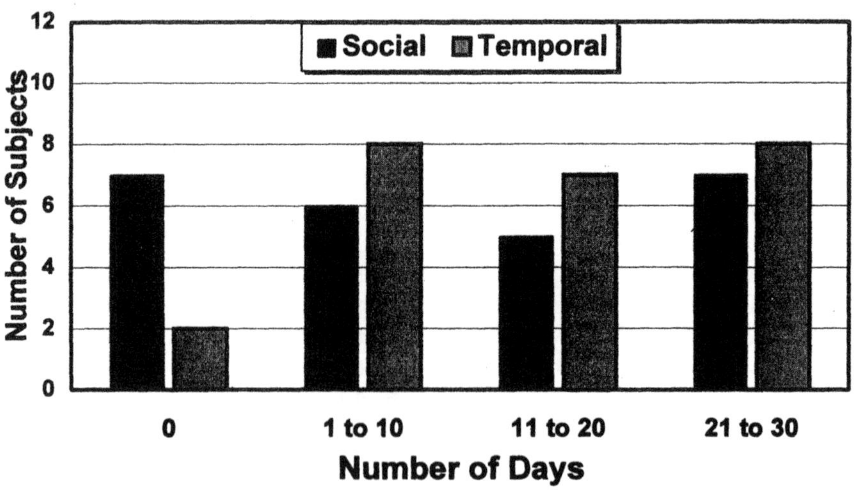


FIG. 9.1. Frequency distribution of daily use of social and temporal comparisons.

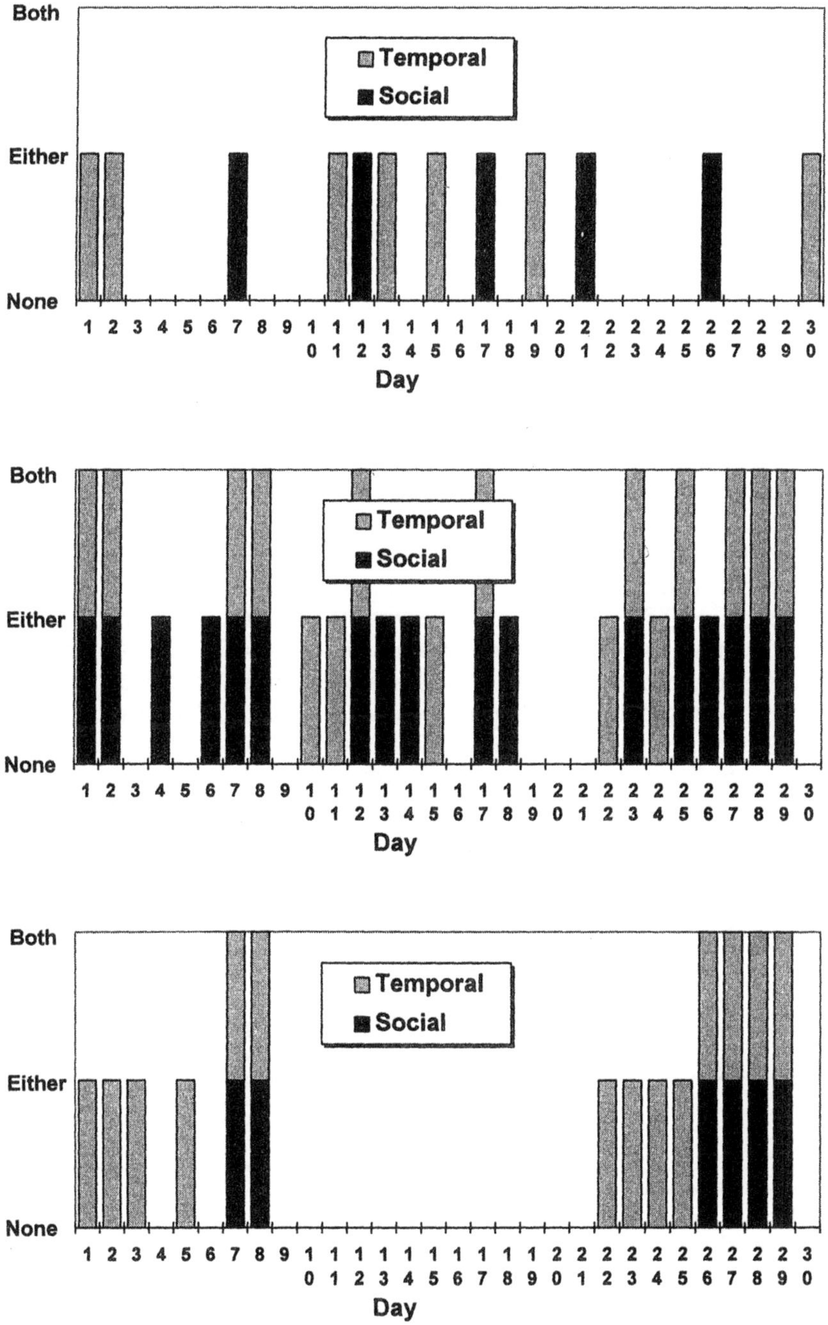


FIG. 9.2. Three illustrative patterns of daily use of social and temporal comparisons.

with other daily processes, the data were pooled across persons and days and subjected to a least squares dummy-variable multiple regression analysis (Jaccard & Wan, 1993). This strategy incorporates $N - 1$ dummy variables to capture subject identity in the regression equation, thereby adjusting within-person effects for across-person differences in the pooled data set. In testing the correlates of temporal comparisons (or social comparisons), eight subjects who never or always made such comparisons were excluded from the data matrix because they accounted for no within-person variance.

One set of within-person analyses related daily comparison reminding to average daily pain intensity, measured by the average daily ratings of 14 areas of the body, as well as the change in pain intensity from morning to evening. As Table 9.1 indicates, social comparison use and temporal comparison use were each more frequent on less painful days.

Other findings presented in Table 9.1 concern the pain-adjusted relations of social and temporal comparison with other variables measured once a day. The "fallback hypothesis" that downward comparisons would increase as perceptions of control over that day's pain decreased was not supported by these preliminary findings. Decreasing levels of daily pain catastrophizing (Keefe et al., 1989) measured by five items from the Coping Strategies Questionnaire (Lawson, Reesor, Keefe, & Turner, 1990) were accompanied by increasing social and temporal efforts. Finally, downward temporal comparisons were more likely on days when individuals rated their coping efforts that day to be more successful in improving their mood. Table 9.2 shows that greater use of temporal comparisons was more often associated with pain-adjusted improvement in daily mood in several of the eight mood

TABLE 9.1
Pooled Partial Within-Person Correlations Between Daily Downward Social and Temporal Comparisons and Other Daily Processes

| | *Downward Comparisons* | |
|---|---|---|
| | *Social* | *Temporal* |
| Daily pain intensity | −.12** | −.26*** |
| Within-day change in pain intensity[a] | −.05 | −.18*** |
| Daily catastrophizing[b] | −.19*** | −.22*** |
| Daily personal control of pain[b] | .01 | .02 |
| Perceived coping efficacy in reducing pain[b] | −.03 | .06 |
| Perceived coping efficacy in improving mood[b] | .06 | .23*** |

[a]Measured by evening report, covarying morning report.
[b]Controlling for daily pain intensity.
$^{**}p < .01$. $^{***}p < .001$.

TABLE 9.2
Pooled Partial Within-Person Correlations Relating Within-Day Change in Mood to Daily Downward Social and Temporal Comparisons, Adjusting for Morning and Evening Pain Intensity

| *Mood* | | *Downward Comparison* | |
|---|---|---|---|
| *Dimension* | *Descriptors* | *Social* | *Temporal* |
| Pleasant | Happy, cheerful | .06 | .17*** |
| Unpleasant | Sad, blue | −.04 | −.15*** |
| Aroused | Active, lively | .08* | .14*** |
| Unaroused | Passive, quiet | −.04 | −.07 |
| Pleasant-aroused | Peppy, stimulated | .08* | .15*** |
| Pleasant-unaroused | Calm, relaxed | .01 | .09* |
| Unpleasant-aroused | Anxious, nervous | −.01 | −.09* |
| Unpleasant-unaroused | Tired, drowsy | .01 | .00 |

*$p < .05$. ***$p < .001$.

circumplex categories (Larsen & Diener, 1992) captured by the indicated adjectives.

In summary, this preliminary within-person analysis of intentional daily comparisons concerning fibromyalgia pain adds credibility to our speculation that after years of living with chronic pain, downward temporal comparisons, occurring when the individual compares her current symptoms with a time when symptoms were worse, become more important as a potential cognitive coping strategy than do downward social comparisons. During the course of a day when the participants in this study reported using more downward temporal comparisons, they evidenced an abatement in pain and, independently, a brightening of their mood; they were more cheerful and more lively. These findings gain further significance by the ability of temporal comparisons to contribute to feelings of coping self-efficacy and to undercut catastrophizing responses to pain.

## CONCLUSION

The assumption that social comparison is an emotion-focused coping strategy has considerable intuitive appeal. Yet empirical support for the coping function of social or temporal comparisons remains ambiguous. We distinguished among comparison coping, comparison conclusions, and secondary control comparisons, and we have argued that current assessment techniques and research designs do not allow us to differentiate these aspects of comparisons. Cross-sectional studies of comparison conclusions, preferences, and responses to forced comparisons have added considerably to our knowledge of cognitive adaptation to chronic pain, but they have also obscured the coping function of comparison processes by equating adaptive responses with coping efforts. Within-person studies that measure intentional efforts at social and temporal comparisons hold considerable promise in evaluating the place of comparison processes in how people adapt to adversity.

## ACKNOWLEDGMENTS

The unpublished findings reported in this chapter come from a study funded by National Institute of Arthritis, Musculoskeletal, and Skin Diseases Grant #AR-20621 to the University of Connecticut Multipurpose Arthritis Center. We are grateful for Susan Urrows's and Micha Abeles's collaboration, for the aid of Jeffrey Siegel of National Technology Services for programming the electronic diary described in this article, for the assistance of Pamela Higgins and Debra Begin with data collection and management, and for the insightful comments of Thomas Ashby Wills, Hart Blanton, and Bram P. Buunk on an earlier version of this chapter.

## REFERENCES

Affleck, G., & Tennen, H. (1991). Social comparison and coping with major medical disorders. In J. Suls & T. A. Wills (Eds.), *Social comparison: Contemporary theory and research* (pp. 369–393). Hillsdale, NJ: Lawrence Erlbaum Associates.

Affleck, G., & Tennen, H. (1993). Cognitive adaptation to adversity: Insights from parents of medically fragile infants. In A. P. Turnbull, J. M. Patterson, S. K. Behr, D. L. Murphy, J. G. Marquis, & M. J. Blue-Banning (Eds.), *Cognitive coping, families, and disability: Participatory research in action* (pp. 135–150). New York: Brooks Publishers.

Affleck, G., Tennen, H., Croog, S., & Levine, S. (1987). Causal attribution, perceived benefits, and morbidity following a heart attack. *Journal of Consulting and Clinical Psychology, 55,* 29–35.

Affleck, G., Tennen, H., Pfeiffer, C., & Fifield, J. (1988). Social comparisons in rheumatoid arthritis: Accuracy and adaptational significance. *Journal of Social and Clinical Psychology, 6,* 219–234.

Affleck, G., Tennen, H., Pfeiffer, C., Fifield, J., & Rowe, J. (1987). Downward comparison and coping with serious medical problems. *American Journal of Orthopsychiatry, 57,* 570–578.

Affleck, G., Tennen, H., & Rowe, J. (1991). *Infants in crisis: How parents cope with newborn intensive care and its aftermath.* New York: Springer-Verlag.

Affleck, G., Urrows, S., Tennen, H., & Higgins, P. (1992). Daily coping with pain from rheumatoid arthritis: Patterns and correlates. *Pain, 51,* 221–229.

Affleck, G., Tennen, H,. Urrows, S., & Higgins, P. (November, 1991). *Coping with rheumatoid arthritis pain from day to day: Patterns and correlates.* Presented at the annual meeting of the Arthritis Health Professionals Association, Boston, MA.

Affleck, G., Tennen, H., Urrows, S., & Higgins, P. (1994). Person and contextual features of daily stress reactivity: Individual differences in relations of undesirable daily events with mood disturbance and chronic pain intensity. *Journal of Personality and Social*

*Psychology, 66,* 329–340.

Albert, S. (1977). Temporal comparison theory. *Psychological Review, 84,* 485–503.

Aldwin, C. M. (1994). *Stress, coping, and development: An integrative perspective.* New York: Guilford.

Aldwin, C. M., & Revenson, T. A. (1987). Does coping help? A reexamination of the relation between coping and mental health. *Journal of Personality and Social Psychology, 53,* 337–348.

Allport, G. W. (1937). *Personality: A psychological interpretation.* New York: Holt, Rinehart & Winston.

Aspinwall, L. G., & Taylor, S. E. (1993). Effects of social comparison direction, threat, and self-esteem on affect, self-evaluation, and expected success. *Journal of Personality and Social Psychology, 64,* 708–722.

Bandura, A. (1986). *Social foundations of thought and action: A social-cognitive theory.* Englewood Cliffs, NJ: Prentice Hall.

Blalock, S. J., Afifi, R. A., DeVellis, B. M., Holt, K., & DeVellis, R. (1990). Adjustment to rheumatoid arthritis: The role of social comparison processes. *Health Education and Research, 5,* 361–370.

Blalock, S. J., DeVellis, B. M., & DeVillis, R. F. (1989). Social comparison among individuals with rheumatoid arthritis. *Journal of Applied Social Psychology, 19,* 665–680.

Blalock, S. J., DeVellis, B. M., DeVellis, R. F., & Sauter, S. V. H. (1988). Self-evaluation processes and adjustment to rheumatoid arthritis. *Arthritis and Rheumatism, 31,* 1245–1251.

Boissevain, M., & McCain, G. (1991). Toward an integrated understanding of fibromyalgia syndrome II: Psychological and phenomenological aspects. *Pain, 45,* 239–248.

Bower, G. H. (1991). Mood congruity of social judgments. In J. P. Forgas (Ed.), *Emotion and social judgments* (pp. 31–53). Elmsford, NY: Pergamon Press.

Brickman, P., & Bulman, R. J. (1977). Pleasure and pain in social comparison. In J. M. Suls & R. L. Miller (Eds.), *Social comparison processes: Theoretical and empirical perspectives* (pp. 149–186). Washington, DC: Hemisphere.

Brickman, P., & Bulman, R. J. (1977). Pleasure and pain in social comparison. In J. M. Suls & R. L. Miller (Eds.), *Social comparison processes: Theoretical and empirical perspectives* (pp. 149–186). Washington, DC: Hemisphere.

Brown, G., & Nicassio, P. (1987). The development of a questionnaire for the assessment of active and passive coping strategies in chronic pain patients. *Pain, 31,* 53–65.

Bryant, F. B. (1989). A four-factor model of perceived control: Avoiding, coping, obtaining, and savoring. *Journal of Personality, 57,* 773–797.

Bulman, R. J., & Wortman, C. B. (1977). Attributions of blame and coping in the "real world": Severe accident victims react to their lot. *Journal of Personality and Social Psychology, 35,* 351–363.

Burger, J. M. (1989). Negative reactions to increases in perceived personal control. *Journal of Personality and Social Psychology, 56,* 246–256.

Buunk, B. P. (1994). Social comparison processes under stress: Towards an integration of classic and recent perspectives. In W. Stroebe & M. Hewstone (Eds.), *European review of social psychology* (Vol. 5, pp. 211–241). New York: Wiley.

Buunk, B. P., Collins, R. L., Taylor, S. E., Van Yperen, N., & Dakof, G. (1990). The affective consequences of social comparison: Either direction has its ups and downs. *Journal of Personality and Social Psychology, 59,* 1238–1249.

Cantor, N., & Norem, J. K. (1989). Defensive pessimism and stress and coping. *Social Cognition, 7,* 92–112.

Carver, C. S., Scheier, M. F., & Weintraub, J. K. (1989). Assessing coping strategies: A theoretically based approach. *Journal of Personality and Social Psychology, 56,* 267–283.

Catanzaro, S. J., & Mearns, J. (1990). Measuring general expectancies for negative mood regulation: Initial scale development and implications. *Journal of Personality Assessment, 54,* 546-563.

Coelho, C. V., Hamburg, D. A., & Adams, J. E. (Eds.). (1974). *Coping and adaptation.* New York: Basic Books.

Cohen, S., Evans, G. W., Stokols, D., & Krantz, D. S. (1986). *Behavior, health, and environmental stress.* New York: Plenum.

Coyne, J. C., & Gottlieb, B. H. (1996). The mismeasure of coping by checklist. *Journal of Personality, 64,* 959-991.

Crocker, J., & Major, B. (1989). Social stigma and self-esteem: The self-protective properties of stigma. *Psychological Review, 96,* 608-630.

DeVellis, R. F., Blalock, S. J., Holt, K., Renner, B. R., Blanchard, L. W., & Klotz, M. L. (1991). Arthritis patients' reactions to unavoidable social comparisons. *Personality and Social Psychology Bulletin, 17,* 392-399.

DeVellis, R. F., Holt, K., Renner, B. R., Blalock, S. J., Blanchard, L. W., Cook, H., Klotz, M., Mikow, V., & Harring, K. (1990). The relationship of social comparison to rheumatoid arthritis symptoms and affect. *Basic and Applied Social Psychology, 11,* 1-18.

Dunkel-Schetter, C., Feinstein, L., Taylor, S. E., & Falke, R. (1992). Patterns of coping with cancer and their correlates. *Health Psychology, 11,* 79-87.

Endler, N. S., & Parker, J. D. A. (1990). *CISS: Coping Inventory for Stressful Situations Manual.* Toronto: Multi-Health Systems.

Epstein, S. (1983). A research paradigm for the study of personality and emotions. In M. Page (Ed.), *Personality—Current theory and research: Nebraska Symposium on Motivation* (pp. 91-154). Lincoln: University of Nebraska Press.

Festinger, L. A. (1954). A theory of social comparison processes. *Human Relations, 7,* 117-140.

Fitzgerald, T., Tennen, H., Affleck, G., & Pransky, G. (1993). The relative importance of dispositional optimism and control appraisals in quality of life after coronary artery bypass surgery. *Journal of Behavioral Medicine, 16,* 25-43.

Foddy, M., & Crundall, I. (1993). A field study of social comparison processes in ability evaluation. *British Journal of Social Psychology, 32,* 287-305.

Folkman, S., & Lazarus, R. S. (1988). Manual for the Ways of Coping Questionnaire. Palo Alto, CA: Consulting Psychologists Press.

Forgas, J. P., Bower, G. H., & Moylan, S. J. (1990). Praise or blame? Affective influences on attributions for achievement. *Journal of Personality and Social Psychology, 59,* 809-819.

Gentry, W. D., & Owens, D. (1986). Pain groups. In A. D. Holzman & D. C. Turk (Eds.), *Pain management: A handbook of psychological treatment approaches* (pp. 100-112). New York: Pergamon Press.

Gibbons, F. X., & Gerrard, M. (1991). Downward comparison and coping with threat. In J. Suls & T. A. Wills (Eds.), *Social comparison: Contemporary theory and research* (pp. 317-346). Hillsdale, NJ: Lawrence Erlbaum Associates.

Gibbons, F. X., Gerrard, M., Lando, H. A., & McGovern, P. G. (1991). Social comparison and smoking cessation: The role of the "typical smoker." *Journal of Experimental Social Psychology, 27,* 239-258.

Giorgino, K. B., Blalock, S. J., DeVellis, R. F., DeVellis, B. M., Keefe, F. J., & Jordan, J. M. (1994). Appraisal of and coping with arthritis-related problems in household activities, leisure activities, and pain management. *Arthritis Care and Research, 7,* 20-28.

Goethals, G., & Darley, J. (1977). Social comparison theory: An attributional approach. In J. M. Suls & R. L. Miller (Eds.), *Social comparison processes: Theoretical and empirical perspectives* (pp. 259-278). Washington, DC: Hemisphere.

Gould, S. G. (1985). *The flamingo's smile: Reflections in natural history.* New York: Norton.

Gruder, C. L. (1977). Choice of comparison persons in evaluating oneself. In J. M. Suls & R. L. Miller (Eds.), *Social comparison processes: Theoretical and empirical perspectives* (pp.

21–41). Washington, DC: Hemisphere.

Haan, N. (Ed.). (1977). *Coping and defending: Processes of self-environment organization.* New York: Academic Press.

Haan, N. (1992). The assessment of coping, defense, and stress. In L. Goldberger & S. Breznitz (Eds.), *Handbook of stress: Theoretical and clinical aspects* (2nd ed., pp. 258–273). New York: Free Press.

Hakmiller, K. L. (1966). Threat as a determinant of downward comparison. *Journal of Experimental Social Psychology, 2* (Suppl. 1), 32–39.

Hanson, R. W., & Gerber, K. E. (1990). *Coping with chronic pain: A guide to patient self-management.* New York: Guilford.

Hobfoll, S. E., Dunahoo, C. L., & Ben-Porath, Y. (1994). Gender and coping: The dual-axis model of coping. *American Journal of Community Psychology, 22,* 49–82.

Houston, B. K. (1987). Stress and coping. In C. R. Snyder & C. Ford (Eds.), *Coping with negative life events: Clinical and social-psychological perspectives* (pp. 373–399). New York: Plenum.

Jaccard, J., & Wan, C. (1993). Statistical analysis of temporal data with many observations: Issues for behavioral medicine data. *Annals of Behavioral Medicine, 15,* 41–50.

Janoff-Bulman, R. (1992). *Shattered assumptions: Towards a new psychology of trauma.* New York: Free Press.

Janoff-Bulman, R., & Timko, C. (1987). Coping with traumatic life events: The role of denial in light of people's assumptive worlds. In C. R. Synder & C. Ford (Eds.), *Coping with negative life events: Clinical and social-psychological perspectives* (pp. 135–159). New York: Plenum.

Jensen, M. P., & Karoly, P. (1992). Comparative self-evaluation and depressive affect among chronic pain patients: An examination of selective evaluation theory. *Cognitive Therapy and Research, 16,* 297–308.

Jensen, M. P., Turner, J. A., Romano, J. M., & Karoly, P. (1991). Coping with chronic pain: A critical review of the literature. *Pain, 47,* 249–283.

Keefe, F., Brown, G., Wallston, K., & Caldwell, D. (1989). Coping with rheumatoid arthritis pain: Catastrophizing as a maladaptive strategy. *Pain, 37,* 51–56.

Langston, C. A. (1994). Capitalizing on and coping with daily life events: Expressive responses to positive events. *Journal of Personality and Social Psychology, 67,* 1112–1125.

Larsen, R. (1992). Neuroticism and bias in the encoding and recall of physical symptoms: Evidence from a combined prospective-retrospective study. *Journal of Personality and Social Psychology, 62,* 480–488.

Larsen, R., & Diener, E. (1992). Promises and problems with the circumplex model of emotion. In M. S. Clarke (Ed.), *Emotion* (pp. 25–59). Newbury Park, CA: Sage.

Larsen, R. J., & Kasimatis, M. (1991). Day-to-day physical symptoms: Individual differences in the occurrence, duration, and emotional concomitants of minor daily illnesses. *Journal of Personality, 59,* 387–424.

Lawson, K., Reesor, K., Keefe, F., & Turner, J. (1990). Dimensions of pain-related cognitive coping: cross-validation of the factor structure of the Coping Strategy Questionnaire. *Pain, 43,* 195–204.

Lazarus, R. S. (1991). *Emotion and adaptation.* New York: Oxford University Press.

Lazarus, R. S. (1993a). From psychological stress to the emotions: A history of changing outlooks. *Annual Review of Psychology, 44,* 1–21.

Lazarus, R. S. (1993b). Coping theory and research: Past, present and future. *Psychosomatic Medicine, 55,* 324–247.

Lazarus, R. S., & Folkman, S. (1984). *Stress, appraisal, and coping.* New York: Springer.

Lepore, S. J., & Evans, G. W. (1996). Coping with multiple stressors in the environment. In M. Zeidner & N. S. Endler (Eds.), *Handbook of coping: Theory, research, applications* (pp. 350–377). New York: Wiley.

Levine, J. M., & Resnick, L. B. (1993). Social foundations of cognition. *Annual Review of Psychology, 44,* 585-612.

Litt, M., Tennen, H., Affleck, G., & Klock, S. (1992). Coping and cognitive factors in adaptation to in vitro fertilization failure. *Journal of Behavioral Medicine, 15,* 171-187.

Major, B., Testa, M., & Bylsma, W. H. (1991). Responses to upward and downward social comparisons: The impact of esteem-relevance and perceived control. In J. Suls & T. A. Wills (Eds.), *Social comparison: Contemporary theory and research* (pp. 237-260). Hillsdale, NJ: Lawrence Erlbaum Associates.

Mayer, J. D., Salovey, P., Gomberg-Kaufman, S., & Blainey, K. (1991). A broader conception of mood experience. *Journal of Personality and Social Psychology, 60,* 100-111.

McLaney, M. A., Tennen, H., Affleck, G., & Fitzgerald, T. (1995). Reactions to impaired fertility: The vicissitudes of primary and secondary control appraisals. *Women's Health: Research on Gender, Behavior, and Policy, 1,* 143-159.

Menaghan, E. (1982). Measuring coping effectiveness: A panel analysis of marital problems and coping efforts. *Journal of Health and Social Behavior, 23,* 220-234.

Moos, R. H., & Schaeffer, J. A. (1992). Coping resources and processes: Current concepts and measures. In L. Goldberger & S. Breznitz (Eds.), *Handbook of stress: Theoretical and clinical aspects* (2nd ed., pp. 234-257). New York: Free Press.

Neisser, U. (1991). A case of misplaced nostalgia. *American Psychologist, 46,* 34-36.

Nolen-Hoeksema, S., Parker, L. E., & Larson, J. (1994). Ruminitive coping with depressed mood following loss. *Journal of Personality and Social Psychology, 67,* 92-104.

Parker, J. D. A., & Endler, N. S. (1996). Coping and defense: A historical overview. In M. Zeidner & N. S. Endler (Eds.), *Handbook of coping: Theory, research, applications* (pp. 3-23). New York: Wiley.

Pearlin, L. I., & Schooler, C. (1978). The structure of coping. *Journal of Health and Social Behavior, 19,* 2-21.

Penner, L., Shiffman, S., Paty, J., & Fritzche, B. (1994). Individual differences in intraperson variability in mood. *Journal of Personality and Social Psychology, 66,* 712-721.

Ptacek, J. T., Smith, R. E., Espe, K., & Raffety, B. (1994). Limited correspondence between daily coping reports and retrospective coping recall. *Psychological Assessment, 6,* 41-49.

Rosenstiel, A. K., & Keefe, F. J. (1983). The use of coping strategies in low-back pain patients. Relationship to patient characteristics and current adjustment. *Pain, 17,* 33-40.

Ross, M. (1989). Relation of implicit theories to the construction of personal histories. *Psychological Review, 96,* 341-357.

Ross, M., & Fletcher, G. J. O. (1985). Attribution and social perception. In Lindzey & Aronson (Eds.), *The handbook of social psychology* (3rd ed., pp. 73-122). Reading, MA: Addison-Wesley.

Rothbaum, F., Weisz, J., & Snyder, S. (1982). Changing the world and changing the self: A two-process model of perceived control. *Journal of Personality and Social Psychology, 42,* 5-37.

Sackeim, H. A. (1983). Self-deception, self-esteem, and depression: The adaptive value of lying to oneself. In J. Masling (Ed.), *Empirical studies of psychanalytical theories* (Vol. 1, pp. 101-157). Hillsdale, NJ: Lawrence Erlbaum Associates.

Schulz, R., & Decker, S. (1985). Long-term adjustment to physical disability: The role of social support, perceived control, and self-blame. *Journal of Personality and Social Psychology, 48,* 1162-1172.

Schwarzer, R., & Schwarzer, C. (1996). A critical survey of coping instruments. In M. Zeidner & N. S. Endler (Eds.), *Handbook of coping: Theory, research, applications* (pp. 107-132). New York: Wiley.

Shiffman, S., Fischer, L., Paty, J., Gnys, M., Hickcox, M., & Kassel, J. (1994). Drinking and smoking: A field study of their association. *Annals of Behavioral Medicine, 16,* 203-209.

Smith, C. A., & Lazarus, R. S. (1993). Appraisal components, core relational themes, and the emotions. *Cognition and Emotion, 7,* 233–269.

Smythe, H. (1989). "Fibrositis" as a disorder of pain modulation. *Clinics of Rheumatic Disease, 5,* 823–832.

Snyder, C. R., Higgins, R. L., & Stucky, R. J. (1983). *Excuses: Masquerades in search of grace.* New York: Wiley.

Stanton, A., Tennen, H., Affleck, G., & Mendola, R. (1992). Coping and adjustment to infertility. *Journal of Social and Clinical Psychology, 11,* 1–13.

Stone, A. A., & Neale, J. M. (1984). A new measure of daily coping: Development and preliminary results. *Journal of Personality and Social Psychology, 46,* 892–906.

Stone, A. A., Neale, J. M., & Shiffman, S. (1993). Daily assessments of stress and coping and their association with mood. *Annals of Behavioral Medicine, 15,* 8–16.

Suls, J. (1983). *Psychological perspectives on the self* (Vol. 1). Hillsdale, NJ: Lawrence Erlbaum Associates.

Suls, J., & Mullen, B. (1983). From the cradle to the grave: Comparison and self-evaluation across the life span. In J. Suls (Ed.), *Psychological perspectives on the self* (Vol. 1, pp. 97–125). Hillsdale, NJ: Lawrence Erlbaum Associates.

Taylor, S. E. (1989). *Positive illusions: Creative self-deception and the healthy mind.* New York: Basic Books.

Taylor, S. E., & Lobel, M. (1989). Social comparison activity under threat: Downward evaluation and upward contacts. *Psychological Review, 96,* 569–575.

Taylor, S. E., Wood, J. V., & Lichtman, R. R. (1983). It could be worse: Selective evaluation as a response to victimization. *Journal of Social Issues, 39,* 19–40.

Taylor, S. E., & Aspinwall, L. G. (1992). Coping with chronic illness. In L. Goldberger and S. Breznitz (Eds.), *Handbook of stress: Theoretical and clinical aspects* (2nd ed., pp. 511–531). New York: Free Press.

Taylor, S. E., Wayment, H. A., & Carrillo, M. (1995). Social comparison and self-regulation. In R. M. Sorrentino & E. T. Higgins (Eds.), *Handbook of motivation and cognition* (pp. 3–27). New York: Guilford.

Tennen, H., & Affleck, G. (1996). Daily processes in coping with chronic pain: Methods and analytic strategies. In M. Zeidner & N. S. Endler (Eds.), *Handbook of coping* (pp. 151–177). New York: Wiley.

Tennen, H., Affleck, G., & Mendola, R. (1991). Causal explanations for infertility: Their relation to control appraisals and psychological adjustment. In A. Stanton & C. Dunkel-Schetter (Eds.), *Infertility: Perspectives from stress and coping research* (pp. 109–132). New York: Plenum.

Thayer, R. E., Newman, R., & McClain, T. M. (1994). Self-regulation of mood: Strategies for changing a bad mood, raising energy, and reducing tension. *Journal of Personality and Social Psychology, 67,* 910–925.

Thompson, S. C., Nanni, C., & Levine, A. (1994). Primary versus secondary and central versus consequence-related control in HIV-positive men. *Journal of Personality and Social Psychology, 67,* 540–547.

Turk, D. C., & Holzman, A. D. (1986). Commonalities among psychological approaches to in the treatment of chronic pain: Specifying the meta-constructs. In A. D. Holzman & D. C. Turk (Eds.), *Pain management: A handbook of psychological treatment approaches* (pp. 257–267). New York: Pergamon.

Turk, D. C., Meichenbaum, D., & Genest, M. (1983). *Pain and behavioral medicine: A cotnitive-behavioral perspective.* New York: Guilford.

Turk, D. C., Meichenbaum, D., & Genest, M. (1983). *Pain and behavioral medicine: A cognitive-behavioral perspective.* New York: Guilford.

Wheeler, L. (1991). A brief history of social comparison theory. In J. Suls & T. A. Wills (Eds.), *Social comparison: Contemporary theory and research* (pp. 3–22). Hillsdale, NJ:

Lawrence Erlbaum Associates.
Wheeler, L., & Miyake, K. (1992). Social comparison in everyday life. *Journal of Personality and Social Psychology, 62,* 760–773.
Wheeler, L., & Reis, H. T. (1991). Self-recording of everyday events: Origins, types, and uses. *Journal of Personality, 59,* 339–354.
Wilke, W., & MacKenzie, A. (1985). Proposed pathogenesis of fibrositis. *Cleveland Clinics Quarterly, 52,* 147–154.
Wills, T. A. (1981). Downward comparison principles in social psychology. *Psychological Bulletin, 90,* 245–271.
Wills, T. A. (1987). Downward comparison as a coping mechanism. In C. R. Snyder & C. Ford (Eds.), *Coping with negative life events: Clinical and social-psychological perspectives* (pp. 243–268). New York: Plenum.
Wolfe, F., Smythe, H., Yunus, M., Bennett, R., Bombardier, C., Goldenberg, D., Tugwell, P., Campbell, S., Abeles, M., Clark, P., Fam, A., Farber, S., Fiechtner, J., Franklin, C., Gatter, R., HAmaty, D., Lessard, J., Lictbroun, A., Masi, A., McCain, G., Reynolds, J., Romano, T., Russell, J., & Sheon, R. (1990). The American College of Rheumatology 1990 criteria for the classification of fibromyalgia. *Arthritis and Rheumatism, 33,* 160–172.
Wood, J. V., Taylor, S. E., & Lichtman, R. R. (1985). Social comparison in adjustment to breast cancer. *Journal of Personality and Social Psychology, 49,* 1169–1183.
Zeidner, M., & Saklofske, D. (1996). Adaptive and maladaptive coping. In M. Zeidner & N. S. Endler (Eds.), *Handbook of coping: Theory, research, applications* (pp. 505–531). New York: Wiley.

# CHAPTER 10

# Social Comparisons Among Cancer Patients: Under What Conditions Are Comparisons Upward and Downward?

Joanne V. Wood
*University of Waterloo*

Karen VanderZee
*University of Groningen*

About one quarter of the people in the United States will be diagnosed with cancer at some point in their lives (Haney, 1984). Although advances in medical treatment have greatly improved survival rates for many types of cancer, many patients contend with the threat of a possible recurrence. Treatments for cancer, which may include surgery, chemotherapy, radiation, and hormonal treatments, are often time-consuming, disfiguring, painful, or quite toxic. Besides fears for one's life and physical well-being, cancer may introduce many other stressors, such as disruptions in one's job performance and strains in one's families and friendships (Wortman & Dunkel-Schetter, 1979). How do people who have been diagnosed with cancer cope with all these stressors? Certainly, the answer to this question depends on the type of cancer a person has and its stage at diagnosis, which determines treatment and prognosis. However, we believe that virtually all people coping with cancer or the threat of its recurrence will be interested to some degree in social comparison. They may compare themselves with others to evaluate their disease, to learn about treatment, to evaluate how well they are coping, to feel better about their own situation, to learn from others who are coping well, and for many other reasons.

Do people who have been diagnosed with cancer make predominantly upward comparisons—with people who are better off than themselves—or downward comparisons—with people who are worse off? The first study that addressed this question found, in interviews, that many breast cancer patients made remarks such as the following:

> I had just a comparatively small amount of surgery on the breast, and I was so miserable, because it was so painful. How awful it must be for women who have had a mastectomy. . . . I just can't imagine it, it would seem to be so difficult. (Wood, Taylor, & Lichtman, 1985, p. 1178)

Respondents overwhelmingly compared themselves with others who were less fortunate than themselves or inferior in some way, which strongly supported Wills' (1981) theory of downward comparisons. Wills proposed that when people experience misfortune or threat, they frequently compare themselves with someone who is inferior to or less advantaged then themselves, in an attempt to feel better. Considerable additional evidence of downward comparisons among threatened populations has emerged since then (see Gibbons & Gerrard, 1991; Wood, 1989, for reviews).

In a review of social comparisons of cancer patients, however, Taylor and Lobel (1989) proposed a theoretical perspective that challenged Wills' (1981) downward comparison theory. They argued that certain types of comparisons—specifically, comparisons involving information seeking and affiliation—are typically upward, rather than downward. In this chapter, we describe Taylor and Lobel's (1989) perspective and then propose a reconciliation between Wills' (1981) and Taylor and Lobel's (1989) models: We argue that cancer patients seek both upward and downward comparison information, but under different circumstances. We then review the literature on cancer patients' social comparisons to see how well the evidence supports this argument.

## CONFLICTING THEORETICAL PERSPECTIVES

### Taylor and Lobel's Model

Observing that there exist several ways of operationalizing social comparison and that these operationalizations may not all mean the same thing (cf. Wood, 1989), Taylor and Lobel (1989) proposed that two main categories of these operationalizations diverge under threat. Specifically, they included under "explicit self-evaluations" "comparative ratings," in which respondents rate themselves relative to others, and "free-response" comparisons—in which respondents make remarks of a comparative nature that are not in response to any specific interview question (Wood et al., 1985). Under "contacts," they included measures that tap into people's preferences for information about others as well as their preferences for people with whom to affiliate. Taylor and Lobel's

(1989) thesis is that "in certain groups under threat, there is a strong preference to evaluate the self against less fortunate others (*downward* evaluations) but a desire for information about and contact with more fortunate others (. . . *upward* contacts)" (p. 569).

Taylor and Lobel's explanation for this discrepancy between the two types of measures is that the uncertainty and unpleasant emotions aroused in threatening circumstances lead people to have two primary coping motivations (Lazarus & Folkman, 1984): to solve the problems that the threat poses (e.g., learn about treatments) and to regulate one's emotional states. Taylor and Lobel proposed that upward contacts serve both needs: People who are doing better than oneself provide information that may assist one's problem-solving efforts, and their examples provide hope and inspiration. Downward evaluations, Taylor and Lobel argued, serve primarily to regulate emotions, because people feel better when they can focus on how advantaged they are relative to others (see also Buunk, Gibbons, & Reis-Bergan, chapter 1, this volume).

Because the evidence Taylor and Lobel cited in support of their analysis concerned cancer patients and because their paper has been influential in the study of social comparisons and coping more generally, it merits close examination in this chapter. Among the many strengths of Taylor and Lobel's (1989) provocative analysis is that, with respect to measures of "contacts," it challenged what had become entrenched in contemporary social comparison theorizing, namely that threat leads to downward comparisons. In addition, by showing that different measures seem to contradict each other within the same group of people, Taylor and Lobel made a very convincing case that different operationalizations of comparison are not interchangeable. Taylor and Lobel (1989) also made the critical observation that victims have desires not only to enhance their self-perceptions but also to improve themselves, another motive that may be served by social comparison (Festinger, 1954; Wood, 1989); people under threat desire to learn how to manage their problems and to cope better with them. Moreover, Taylor and Lobel made it clear that these various motives, and hence preferences for different types of social comparison, can coexist within the same individuals.

Considerable evidence is consistent with the pattern that Taylor and Lobel identified: Many studies indicate that on comparative rating measures, people ordinarily rate themselves as superior to others (see Taylor & Brown, 1988, for a review; see also Klein & Weinstein, chapter 2, this volume), and many studies indicate that on comparison selection measures, by far the greatest tendency is to seek information about others who are superior—that is, to make upward comparisons (see

Wood, 1989, for a review). Similarly, previous studies of affiliation have indicated that people ordinarily choose to affiliate with others who are superior (Miller & Suls, 1977; Nosanchuk & Erickson, 1985).

However, the evidence just cited concerns nonthreatening conditions, rather than threatening conditions. Under threatening conditions, evaluations are often downward, as both Taylor and Lobel and Wills (1981) predict. However, studies of information-seeking and affiliation under threat often contradict Taylor and Lobel's predictions. This is especially true of measures of information-seeking: Most earlier studies that have employed such measures have indicated that threat leads to downward comparisons—or, at least, to comparisons that are less upward than under nonthreatening conditions (see Collins, 1996; Wheeler & Miyake, 1992, for corrections to earlier reviews by Wills, 1981; Wood, 1989). The evidence concerning affiliation measures is less consistent (see Buunk, 1994, Rofé, 1984, for reviews). Some evidence indicates that people under threat avoid affiliating with others who are worse off, as Taylor and Lobel (1989) concluded. But there is also some evidence that people under threat seek affiliates who are worse off, as well as some evidence that people under threat avoid affiliating altogether (Gerrard, Gibbons, & Sharp, 1985; Gibbons, Gerrard, Lando, & McGovern, 1991).

In summary, although Taylor and Lobel (1989) are in agreement with Wills (1981) with respect to downward evaluations, Taylor and Lobel's prediction that people under threat seek upward information and affiliations is at odds with Wills's prediction that they seek downward information and affiliation. Taylor and Lobel's prediction concerning these so-called contacts is also inconsistent with some prior evidence, especially involving information seeking. These contradictions constitute the main focus of our chapter. Before attempting to reconcile these discrepancies, however, we briefly summarize studies on cancer patients' "explicit-self evaluations," at least those involving comparative rating measures.

**Comparative Ratings Made by Cancer Patients**

As both Taylor and Lobel (1989) and Wills (1981) predicted, cancer patients rate themselves as superior to other cancer patients on coping dimensions (Jenkins & Pergament, 1988; Wood et al., 1985) and on physical dimensions (VanderZee, Buunk, DeRuiter, Tempelaar, Van-Sonderen, & Sanderman, in press). In addition, the more favorably cancer patients rate themselves, the better adjusted they are (Jenkins & Pergament, 1988; VanderZee et al., in press). These findings are consistent with the idea that downward evaluations are self-enhancing. These findings are also consistent, however, with the possibility that favorable adjustment leads to downward evaluations, and with the possibility that general tendencies to present oneself favorably lead to both downward evaluations on the comparative rating and better adjustment on the adjustment measures. In addition, when the comparative rating itself concerns coping or adjustment (Jenkins & Pergament, 1988), any association with adjustment may suggest that patients' comparative ratings are veridical—that people who rate themselves as better adjusted than others are better adjusted—rather than that the patient was engaging in downward comparisons as a coping strategy. Ambiguities such as these concerning comparative ratings led Wood (1996) to argue that comparative ratings often may not reflect social comparisons at all.

### Reconciling the Wills (1981) and Taylor and Lobel (1989) Perspectives on Contacts

How can we reconcile Taylor and Lobel's (1989) upward information- and affiliation-seeking prediction with Wills's (1981) downward information- and affiliation-seeking prediction and with prior evidence that people under threat sometimes do not prefer upward affiliations and that they nearly always prefer less upward—or even downward—information about others? Clues are provided by recent theoretical and empirical work conducted by two teams of investigators: Major and her colleagues (Major, Testa, & Blysma, 1991; Testa & Major, 1988), and Taylor, Buunk, Collins, and their colleagues (Buunk, Collins, Taylor, Van Yperen, & Dakof, 1990, Study 1).

According to both groups of researchers, both downward and upward comparisons can have both negative and positive effects. As Buunk et al. (1990) put it,

> Learning that another is better off than yourself provides at least two pieces of information: (a) that you are not as well as everyone and (b) that it is possible for you to be better than you are at present. . . . Those able . . . to focus on the positive aspect of this information may feel better about themselves as a result of an upward comparison. Those who focus on the negative aspect may feel worse. Conversely, learning that another is worse off than yourself also provides at least two pieces of information: (a) that you are not as badly off as everyone and (b) that it is possible for you to get worse. Focusing on the fact that one is better off than others may lead one to feel better about oneself as a result of a downward comparison, but focusing on the possibility of getting worse may produce negative feelings about oneself. (p. 1239)

What determines which reactions a person will have? Many factors have been proposed (Major et al., 1991; Taylor, Wayment, & Carillo, in press). The factors that are most important in understanding the literature on cancer patients' social comparisons seem to boil down to one: the individual's subjective perception of whether he or she may improve or decline on the dimension of comparison. In the case of an upward comparison, if one believes that one will improve and perhaps attain the target's level, the comparison will be pleasing and inspiring; if one believes that one is unlikely to improve, the comparison may be demoralizing and may arouse envy. In the case of a downward comparison, the more one believes that it is possible to worsen on the dimension, the more threatening the comparison will be; if one has no fear that one's status on the dimension will worsen, the comparison is likely to be self-enhancing.[1]

The individual's subjective perception of whether he or she may improve or worsen on the dimension may be determined by many factors. An especially important factor that Major and her colleagues proposed concerns people's perceptions of the controllability of the dimension under evaluation (Major et al., 1991; Testa & Major, 1988; cf. Buunk et al., 1990; Taylor et al., in press); their beliefs about whether they will improve or worsen on the dimension certainly depend on whether they believe that they, their physicians, or God can control their standing on that dimension.

A second determinant of people's perception of whether they will improve or worsen on the dimension involves the degree to which the comparison involves a process of contrast versus what Collins (1996) has called *assimilation* or what Ybema (1994) and Buunk and Ybema (chapter 12, this volume) call *identification.* Traditional predictions about the effects of comparisons—namely, that downward comparisons make one feel good and upward comparisons make one feel bad—imply that one is contrasting oneself with the comparison target (see also Diener & Fujita, chapter 11, this volume). In assimilation or identification, however, we feel better the better off the comparison target is, and worse the worse off the comparison target is. This is because we assume similarity to the comparison target (Collins, 1996), and as a result the target's position on the comparison dimension influences our expectations of our own future standing on that dimension (Ybema, 1994). Hence, if we identify with an upward target, we believe that it is possible or likely

[1]Beyond the case of cancer patients, there are likely to be at least two important exceptions to these general rules. First, if one is competing with an upward target, an upward comparison may be aversive even when one believes that one will improve on the dimension; what is important is that right now one's rival is superior to oneself (cf. Wood, 1989). Second, if one has a close relationship with a downward target, one is not likely to feel self-enhanced as a result of the other's misfortune. Even if we have no fear that we will decline on the dimension, we may feel very fearful or sad for a friend.

that we will improve, whereas if we identify with a downward target, we believe that it is possible or even likely that we will worsen. Our tendency to identify or contrast ourselves with a comparison target may be influenced by many factors (Buunk & Ybema, chapter 12, this volume; Collins, 1996).[2]

People's perception of whether they may improve or worsen on the dimension may be determined by many additional factors, such as their dispositional level of optimism and self-esteem (see Buunk et al., 1990; Collins, 1996; Taylor et al., in press). The important point for the present analysis, however, is that the perception of whether a person may improve or decline on the dimension is the key factor in determining her or his reaction to comparisons.

### Reconciling Taylor and Lobel With Wills and With Past Research

From this perspective, Wills' (1981) and Taylor and Lobel's (1989) predictions concerning threatened people's comparison information seeking and affiliations conflict because they focused on different types of downward and upward comparisons. Wills (1981) seemed to have had in mind the type of downward comparison in which a person has little fear of worsening on the dimension of comparison. For example, if a happily married cancer patient compares herself favorably to another patient who is divorced, she is likely to feel fortunate rather than threatened. The type of downward comparison that Taylor and Lobel (1989) seem to have had in mind is the type in which people fear that they may worsen on the dimension of comparison. As we describe later, the evidence cited by Taylor and Lobel usually involved the dimension

---

[2]Buunk and Ybema (chapter 12, this volume) have proposed that vivid information about or direct contact with others in a similar situation also tends to instill identification. If this is true, it would support Taylor and Lobel's (1989) upward contact prediction; because it would be preferable to identify with an upward target than a downward target, one should prefer upward contacts. Looking again beyond the context of cancer, however, it seems to us that direct contact would instill identification only under noncompetitive circumstances. Competition invites contrast; one feels better as the other person's situation worsens. In addition, an individual may be more likely to identify with vivid information than with impoverished information, as Buunk and Ybema suggest, because contact and vivid information present the individual with more features with which to find similarities with the target. However, contact and vivid information also present more features with which to seize on differences, which would promote contrast. We suspect that under many circumstances, a large determinant of whether people identify or contrast themselves with a comparison target does not rest in the features of the comparison context. Rather, the individual's motivation to identify or contrast himself or herself with the target may play a large role.

of general physical condition. For example, they cited Collins, Dakof, and Taylor's (1988) study, in which 70% of the patients indicated that they found waiting in their physician's waiting room with other cancer patients "to be noxious, and one of the most common reasons given for this reaction was that the presence of others who were so obviously deteriorating physically upset them or made them depressed" (Taylor & Lobel, 1989, p. 571).

We suspect that most cancer patients have at best mixed feelings about downward comparisons on the dimension of general physical condition. On one hand, they may feel lucky that they are not as bad off as the less fortunate target; on the other hand, they may feel somewhat threatened because such comparisons may remind them that it is possible that their own condition could deteriorate (cf. Gibbons & Gerrard, 1991; Hemphill & Lehman, 1991). Although many cancer patients believe that they have some personal control over cancer, or that their physicians, treatments, or God will control their cancer—Taylor, Lichtman, and Wood (1984) found that 56% and 68% of patients, respectively, in their study had such beliefs—we suspect that even people with high beliefs in control have some fear, however small, that their cancer may recur. Thus they should prefer to avoid comparisons with others whose cancers have recurred or whose conditions are deteriorating.

The type of downward comparison that Taylor and Lobel (1989) focused on differs not only from the type that Wills (1981) predicted would be preferred by people under threat; it also contrasts with the downward comparisons available in most studies involving threat. For example, in one study, research participants were led to believe that they had either failed or succeeded on a test and were then given the opportunity to see the answer sheets of other participants (Pyszczynski, Greenberg, & LaPrelle, 1985, Study 1). Participants who had failed requested to see more answer sheets when they expected these to reveal that most other people had also failed than when they expected these to reveal that most others had performed well. In this case, the choice of the relatively downward comparison presented no threat to the participants; there was no danger that the participant could have become worse, because the testing was over. Instead, the "failure" answer sheets could have reminded the participants that they were not alone, and they had the potential to show participants that others were even inferior to themselves.

Not only were the downward comparisons in Taylor and Lobel's review different from the downward comparisons typically available in threat studies, but the available upward comparisons differed as well. Taylor and Lobel (1989) argued that cancer patients seek contact with superior others so as to learn from them and to draw inspiration from them. So, for example, when people with cancer compare themselves with others who are long-term cancer survivors, they may hope to learn how to avoid a cancer recurrence themselves. Similarly, upward comparisons with people who are coping well with their cancer may provide instruction in successful coping as well as hope that one's own spirits will improve. According to the reasoning presented above, however, and as noted in Taylor's later work (Taylor, Buunk, Collins, & Reed, 1992), such upward contacts are instructive and inspiring only if they occur on a dimension on which the cancer patient can hope to improve. This type of instructive and inspiring upward comparison, however, is very different from the type of upward comparison that is typically available in threat studies. For example, in the Pyszczynski et al. (1985) study just described, there was no opportunity for the participant's own inferiority to be remedied. Hence, the upward comparison available to participants could not have offered instruction or hope; it could only have reminded them of their inferiority.

We are suggesting, then, that the pattern that Taylor and Lobel (1989) identified on information-seeking and affiliation measures—namely, avoidance of downward contacts and seeking of upward contacts—was in large part based on downward and upward comparisons that differed from those typically available in studies of social comparisons under threat. When Taylor and Lobel argued that downward information seeking and downward affiliations were threatening, they neglected a type of downward contact that can be self-enhancing, namely when the individual has little fear of declining on the dimension. Likewise, Wills' (1981) emphasis on downward comparisons as the route to self-enhancement under threatening conditions neglected a type of upward comparison that can be inspiring and encouraging, namely when the individual hopes to improve on the dimension.

Our perspective—that the key determinant of whether comparisons are inspiring, demoralizing, threatening, or self-enhancing is the degree to which the individual expects to improve or decline on the dimension—offers not only predictions about the effects of comparison, but also, to a limited extent, predictions about when people should seek upward and downward comparisons. When people expect to improve on the dimension of comparison they should select upward comparisons because they should be inspiring and informative. Such upward comparisons should be attractive regardless of whether the individual is under threat, because people who are not threatened have self-improvement goals (Wood, 1989), and because people who are threatened, as Taylor and Lobel (1989) made clear, also have problem-solving needs. When people are under some type of threat, they should avoid downward comparisons along dimensions on which they fear that they may worsen, because such downward comparisons should compound their threat. They should, however, seek downward comparisons along dimensions on which they have little fear of worsening, because such downward comparisons should be self-enhancing. When people are not under threat, they should have much less interest in downward comparisons, although they may still make some (Wood & Taylor, 1991).

We said that this perspective offers predictions about comparison selections "to a limited extent" because it fails to specify the direction of comparison in one particular case. Specifically, we have argued that when people have hope of improving on a dimension, they seek rather than avoid upward comparisons and that when they have little fear of worsening on the dimension, they seek rather than avoid downward comparisons. When the dimension is one on which people both hope to improve and have little fear of worsening, which do they prefer: upward or downward comparisons? We suspect that the answer depends on which motive predominates: self-improvement or self-enhancement. When self-improvement predominates, people will prefer upward comparisons; when self-enhancement predominates, people will prefer downward comparisons. Although upward comparisons may be self-enhancing (Collins, 1996), downward comparisons may be generally a safer and more effective route to self-enhancement.[3] Hence, downward comparisons should be preferred over upward comparisons when self-enhancement needs override self-improvement needs. The question this raises, of course, is when do self-enhancement needs override improvement needs? We address this question later. First we review the empirical studies of cancer patients' social comparisons.

## COMPARISON INFORMATION-SEEKING AND AFFILIATION-SEEKING BY CANCER PATIENTS: THE EVIDENCE

Research on cancer patients' social comparisons includes studies that have attempted to examine cancer patients' selections of social compar-

[3]Upward comparisons may be useful for self-enhancement, when the individual assumes similarity with the upward target (Collins, 1996; Wood, 1989). Our hunch, however, is that upward comparisons are a much riskier route to self-enhancement than are downward comparisons and, hence, should be preferred only by people with high self-esteem. Recent evidence suggests that high self-esteem people are more likely to take risks to benefit their self-esteem than are low self-esteem people (e.g., Wood, Giordano-Beech, Taylor, Michela, & Gaus, 1994). Consistent with our hunch, Collins (1996) cited evidence that high self-esteem people are especially likely to experience the self-enhancing benefits of upward comparisons. They are probably the most likely to assume similarity with upward targets.

ison information and affiliations, and studies of cancer patients' reactions to affiliations and social information. We include the studies reviewed by Taylor and Lobel (1989), as well as studies that have appeared since then. We evaluate these studies for the degree to which cancer patients make downward comparisons and upward comparisons, and whether the evidence supports our proposed reconciliation of the Wills (1981) and Taylor and Lobel (1989) models.

We caution, however, that our ability to evaluate our perspective is severely limited, for several reasons. First, very few studies that speak to cancer patients' social comparisons have been conducted, and some of these were not even designed to examine social comparisons. We include such studies, however, if they were included in the Taylor and Lobel (1989) review. Second, no study of cancer patients has employed measures of comparison selections that are typically used in the laboratory (Wood, 1996). That is, investigators have not provided potential sources of information and then asked respondents to choose whether or not or which ones they wanted to see. Similarly, no study of cancer patients' reactions to comparisons have used measures of comparison reactions that are typically used in the laboratory (Wood, 1996), in that investigators have not presented comparison information to respondents and then measured their reactions. The measures that researchers have used are sometimes difficult to interpret, as we discuss where appropriate.

Our ability to evaluate our perspective is limited also by the fact that respondents in these studies were not asked whether they expected to improve or worsen on the dimension of comparison. Nor were they typically asked about possible moderators of respondents' expectations and fears about improving or worsening, such as respondents' perceptions of control over each dimension, the degree to which they identified or contrasted themselves with the target, and their general optimism. We can only speculate, then, about respondents' expectations and fears about improving and worsening. As we argued earlier, the dimension of general physical condition is one on which many cancer patients probably have some fear of declining.

### Social Comparison Selections by Cancer Patients

***Measures that May Reflect Either Explicit Self-Evaluations or Social Information-Seeking.*** Two studies employed measures that may be interpreted either as reflecting explicit self-evaluations or as measuring social comparison information or affiliation seeking. First, VanderZee et al. (in press) asked 475 patients suffering from various forms of cancer questions such as, "How often do you realize that you are in many respects better off as compared to other cancer patients?" and, "How often do you compare yourself with other cancer patients who are worse off?" A control group of 255 healthy people were asked similar questions, but the questions were modified so that the comparison targets were not cancer patients (e.g., "How often do you realize that you are in many respects better off as compared to other persons?"). These questions were combined in a measure of "cognitive downward comparisons."

What does this measure reflect? The first question quoted above resembles comparative ratings, but it also may ask how often respondents remind themselves of less fortunate comparison others. The second question may, but does not necessarily, tap into respondents' social comparison contacts (information or affiliations). The finding obtained with this measure was that the cancer patients reported engaging in these "cognitive downward comparison" activities more than did the control group. To the extent that this measure is a measure of explicit self-evaluations, it supports both Wills' (1981) and Taylor and Lobel's (1989) predictions of downward evaluations. To the extent that it taps into respondents' selections of comparison contacts, it offers support for the downward contact prediction.

The second study that may be interpreted as measuring either explicit self-evaluations or contacts is Wood et al.'s (1985) breast cancer study, which Taylor and Lobel (1989) grouped with measures of explicit self-evaluations. In that study, some free-responses did resemble comparative ratings, such as when interviewees remarked, "I am coping much better than most other people with cancer" (see Wood, 1996, for a more complete discussion). However, the majority of free-responses in the Wood et al. (1985) study involved specific other people with whom the respondents had direct contact, and hence we argue that they reflect social comparison contacts. We describe the findings first, and then return to this issue.

Wood et al. (1985) coded as "free-response comparisons" any comparative remarks that respondents made that were *not* in response to the interview questions that specifically inquired about social comparisons. Because the interview questions about social comparisons occurred near the very end of the interviews, and because they concerned only the dimension of coping, they could not have prompted virtually any of the comparisons that Wood et al. labeled "free responses." We acknowledge, however, that these responses are only "free" or "spontaneous" relative to responses to structured interview questions; clearly, these responses could have been affected by other interview questions or by the interview context. Moreover, it is not clear that the comparisons expressed in interviews are representative of those expressed in everyday life (Wood, 1996).

Wood et al. (1985) coded the free-response comparisons into many categories, including comparisons involving coping, physical condition, and life situation (e.g., marital status). They also coded each comparison according to whether they involved an upward, downward, or similar comparison target. In all categories, respondents overwhelmingly compared themselves with others who were less fortunate than themselves or inferior in some way. Here are two examples:

> I have never been like some of those people who have cancer and they feel well, this is it, they can't do anything, they can't go anywhere. . . . I just kept right on going. (p. 1173)

> I have heard stories where men walked out on their wives, couldn't accept it. My friend, her husband couldn't discuss it. He didn't want to hear anything about it. (p. 1174)

Of the 69 respondents who made free-response comparisons, only one made more upward than downward comparisons, 5 made an equal number of downward and upward comparisons, and 63 made more downward than upward comparisons. These results, then, support the downward comparison prediction.

But do these results suggest that these respondents specifically selected information about downward targets and chose to affiliate with downward targets? In a different context, Taylor and Lobel (1989) offered alternative possibilities that may apply here. First, cancer patients may invent downward comparison targets in their imagination. Although we agree, this does not seem to account for the majority of free-response comparisons, which involved people with whom the respondent had had personal contact. The second possibility is that cancer patients do not seek downward contacts but the latter are thrust on them by other sources, such as the media, physicians' waiting rooms, and stories that other people tell them about other cancer patients. However, it seems likely that upward comparisons would be forced on cancer patients as well. For example, the media "usually feature positive, upbeat cancer stories" (Taylor & Lobel, 1989, p. 572).

We argue that the preponderance of downward comparisons in Wood et al.'s respondents' free responses suggests that these cancer patients did selectively attend to downward contacts. They may not have sought to affiliate with less fortunate others, because affiliation entails other costs that may interfere with comparison seeking (Buunk, 1994; Wood, 1996), but we believe that these respondents selected information about others who were doing worse. By the phrase, "selected information about others who were doing worse," we mean not only that respondents looked for such information in their social environments. Even more likely, we believe, is that respondents had contact with both upward and downward targets, but they focused on the downward information available to them, and they frequently reminded themselves of this information, because it made them feel better. For example, women who had less disfiguring surgeries compared themselves favorably with others who had more disfiguring surgeries, yet women with more disfiguring surgeries did not express the corresponding upward comparison with others who had less disfiguring surgery. These women with more disfiguring surgeries certainly knew that other women had less disfiguring surgeries, yet they selectively focused on the downward comparisons available to them rather than the upward comparisons. Similarly, many older women compared themselves favorably with younger women, yet younger women did not express unfavorable comparisons with older women, when surely they had had contact with older women with breast cancer (in physicians' waiting rooms, if not elsewhere). Again, these younger women seemed to focus selectively on their contacts with others who were doing worse than them in some way, instead of their contacts with others who were more fortunate.

We argue, then, that the majority of respondents' free-response comparisons reflected comparison contacts and that they reflected a preference for contact with downward information in particular. We also believe that this preference for downward social information was in large part the basis for these respondents' free-response "downward evaluations."

Readers should be aware, however, of the possibility that social desirability biases may have inflated the downward comparisons in the Wood et al. study. Upward comparisons may be seen as complaints, so respondents may be reluctant to express them, whereas downward comparisons may be socially desirable because they may convey that the respondent is looking on the bright side. However, because "looking on the bright side" seems to be very common among victims (e.g., Taylor, Wood, & Lichtman, 1983; Thompson, 1985), Wood (1996) argued that the free-response method may at most exaggerate an already strong tendency to make downward comparisons.[4]

Two studies that arguably tap into selections of social comparison information and affiliations, then, suggest that cancer patients select downward comparisons.

---

[4]It should also be recognized that social desirability constraints may operate against downward comparisons as well as upward comparisons. People may not want to appear to be arrogant or to take pleasure in another's misfortune (Brickman & Bulman, 1977; Wills, 1981).

***Selections of Comparison Information and Affiliations.*** Next we turn to studies that involve measures that reflect selections of information and affiliations more clearly than explicit self-evaluations. However, these measures also pose problems of interpretation because researchers have relied largely on respondents' self-reports as to the persons with whom they have had contact or with whom they prefer to have contact. Such self-report measures of social comparisons are vulnerable to several problems (Wood, 1996). First, they may be inaccurate. Respondents are often selective about the events they report, their memory for events may be distorted by their moods and by recency effects, and they may have difficulty aggregating their information into a global impression (cf. Reis & Wheeler's (1991) discussion of such problems with global measures of social interactions). Second, self-reported social comparisons are vulnerable to social desirability biases. Wood (1996) reviewed studies suggesting that people often do not want to admit that they engage in social comparison. People also may not want to report that they have made certain types of comparisons, such as downward comparisons (Wills, 1981). Third, people may often be unaware that they are making social comparisons (Brickman & Bulman, 1977). Concerns for social desirability and a lack of awareness of one's comparative processes may explain why, in the Wood et al. (1985) study, when respondents were asked whether they compared themselves with others, many said no, yet they had spontaneously voiced numerous comparisons before they were asked about comparisons (Wood et al., 1985). These limitations regarding self-report measures should be kept in mind while evaluating the studies described next.

Molleman, Pruyn, and van Knippenberg (1986) asked 418 outpatients suffering from various forms of cancer with whom they preferred to interact. The response options ranged from fellow patients who were "much better off" to "much worse off" on the dimension of general physical condition. Molleman et al. reported "a marked preference- . . . for interaction with fellow-patients who are similarly or slightly better off" (p. 6). However, of the respondents who answered this question, about 68% preferred to interact with patients who were similar and only about 8% preferred to interact with someone slightly better. These findings, then, contradict the downward contact prediction, and although they suggest that people prefer upward contacts to downward contacts, they do not offer strong support for the upward contact prediction.

Taylor, Aspinwall, Guiliano, Dakof, and Reardon (1993, Study 1) examined the stories that people with various forms of cancer heard about other cancer patients. Of the respondents, 59% said they "never" seek out such stories and 20% said they did so only rarely. The finding that only 20% of the sample reported that they sought out stories at least "sometimes" offers little support for the idea that cancer patients seek out either upward or downward comparisons—at least those provided by stories from third parties. However, patients may be much more interested in comparisons they can make directly with other patients. In addition, as argued earlier, self-reports may be susceptible to social desirability distortions. Although it is not clear that admitting that one seeks out stories about other cancer patients carries the same negative implications as admitting that one seeks out social comparisons, it is possible that the self-report nature of these findings should not be trusted completely. In addition, as Taylor et al. (1993) argued, it is possible that these patients were so far past their diagnoses (an average of about 3 years previously) that their social comparison needs had diminished (cf. Wood et al., 1985). These factors may account for the apparently low interest in comparisons.

***Summary of Selection Studies.*** Of the four studies that speak to cancer patients' social comparison selections, none supported the upward contact prediction, two offered some support for the downward contact prediction, and two studies contradicted both the upward and downward contact predictions. However, it is clear that further research is needed. It is difficult to draw firm conclusions from so few studies, especially when some of the measures involved are difficult to interpret, and when one of the studies was not designed to examine social comparisons per se (Taylor et al., 1993).

Are these findings, such as they are, compatible with our proposed reconciliation? Because of the absence of findings pointing to upward comparisons, we focus on downward comparisons. We predict that cancer patients will seek downward comparisons on dimensions on which they are confident that they will not decline. It is unclear whether VanderZee et al.'s (in press) evidence of downward comparisons supports the reconciliation perspective, because the dimensions on which respondents made comparisons were not specified. The Wood et al. (1985) study does support our perspective, because respondents made downward comparisons on a variety of dimensions that are probably viewed as relatively controllable, such as coping and marital status (Buunk, 1994; Hemphill & Lehman, 1991).

We have suggested that cancer patients are likely to avoid downward comparisons on the dimension of physical health because they may have some fear of declining on that dimension and hence, downward comparisons on that dimension may serve as frightening reminders of one's own vulnerability. One of the studies that indicated that patients do not prefer downward comparisons did involve that dimension (Molleman et al., 1986). In addition, the study that offered the strongest support for the downward comparison prediction, the Wood et al. (1985) study, found that respondents did not seem to prefer downward comparisons on the dimension of general physical health. Several respondents, for example, spoke of how they tried to arrange their appointments with their physicians to be early in the day so that they did not have to sit in the waiting room with other cancer patients whose conditions were deteriorating. Wood et al. kept these "threatening" physical comparisons distinct from downward comparisons that seemed to have the potential to be self-enhancing, and found that over one-quarter of the respondents described these threatening physical comparisons. Although Wood et al.'s respondents typically seemed able to draw comfort or self-enhancement from downward comparisons, they appeared to find aversive downward comparisons on the dimension of physical condition.

However, our reconciliation perspective predicts that not all downward comparisons on the physical dimension need be threatening; if the comparisons involve physical dimensions on which the person has no fear that he or she will decline, they may be self-enhancing. An example of a potentially self-enhancing downward comparison on the physical dimension is that many respondents in the Wood et al. study compared their own surgeries (e.g., lumpectomies) favorably with those of acquaintances who had had more extensive surgeries.

### Reactions to Social Comparisons by Cancer Patients

Turning now to studies of the reactions of cancer patients to social comparisons, we first review studies of the informational consequences of comparisons and then the affective consequences. As was true for the selection studies, investigators have examined respondents' self-reports of the social comparisons that they have made and their reactions to them. Such self-reports again may be suspect, however, because people may not want to admit that they were influenced by social comparisons and because they may even be unaware that they have socially compared.

***Informational Consequences of Comparisons.*** The Taylor and Lobel (1989) model and our reconciliation perspective both predict that contacts with fellow cancer patients who are superior to or better off than oneself will be perceived as most informative. As Taylor and Lobel (1989) pointed out, research on the contacts of cancer patients with fellow patients (e.g., van den Borne, Pruyn, & van den Heuvel, 1987;

see van den Borne, Pruyn, & Van Dam-de May, 1986, for a review) suggests that such contact is associated with increased knowledge and information about cancer and its treatment. However, because most of these studies are correlational, the causal direction between contacts with fellow patients and increased information is unclear. It is possible, for example, that people who are especially active in seeking out information about their cancer also seek out more contact with fellow patients. Even if we can assume that contact with other patients was informative—as seems quite likely—it is not clear, as Taylor and Lobel (1989) pointed out, whether the benefits of contact with fellow patients were derived from patients who were better off, worse off, or similar to the respondents.

More pertinent is a study of social support by Taylor and Dakof (1988). Their sample included people with various types of cancer. Respondents were asked to describe the most helpful and the least helpful actions that they experienced in their interactions with other cancer patients. A commonly reported helpful action from others was the provision of useful information about cancer and its treatment. It seems quite possible that the cancer patients who provided information were better off than the respondents in some way—that is, upward—if only because they had information that the respondent lacked. It also seems quite likely that a great deal of social comparison occurs in such interactions. Because this study was not designed to study social comparisons, however, it is impossible to tell whether the helpful information was imparted primarily through social comparisons (in this case, the sharing of experiences) or through direct instruction and advice.

In the study that speaks most directly to the prediction that upward contacts are most informative, the Molleman et al. (1986) affiliation study described earlier also asked respondents to indicate the extent to which they experienced interaction with various categories of fellow patients as informative. Respondents rated cancer patients who were similar on the dimension of general physical health as most informative and more informative than those who were slightly better or much better off than themselves. This result contradicts the prediction that upward contacts would be most informative. Consistent with Taylor and Lobel's (1989) analysis, however, was the finding that patients who were much worse off were considered to be the least informative.

In summary, the evidence concerning the informational consequences of comparisons is very sparse, making it difficult to draw conclusions until further research is done. What little evidence there is points a bit toward upward comparisons, but the most direct evidence contradicts the prediction that upward comparisons are most informative. Instead,

Molleman et al.'s (1986) finding that similar others are experienced as most informative supports Festinger's (1954) original emphasis on similar others.

*Affective Reactions to Social Comparisons.* According to our reconciliation perspective, both upward and downward comparisons can have both negative and positive effects on people's mood and morale, depending on whether they believe they can improve or decline on that dimension (cf. Major et al., 1991; Taylor et al., in press).

Taylor and Lobel (1989) focused on four studies as the primary evidence in support of their upward contact prediction. In the Collins et al. (1988) study described earlier, over 70% of the cancer patients indicated that they found waiting in their physician's waiting room upsetting because there they would see others who were physically deteriorating. In the Molleman et al. (1986) affiliation study also mentioned earlier, respondents were asked not only with which targets they preferred to interact, but how they experienced the interactions they had with other cancer patients. Respondents reported that they experienced their interactions with patients who were much worse off on the dimension of physical health most negatively and that they experienced their interactions with patients who were much better off most positively.

A third study cited by Taylor and Lobel (1989) is the study that examined cancer patients' reactions to stories about other cancer patients (Taylor et al., 1993, Study 1). Earlier we described the findings from this study concerning patients' reports about the stories they sought out. The researchers also examined respondents' reactions to stories that they did not seek out but that were told to them. Of the respondents, 85% reported having been told such stories. The stories that cancer patients either sought out or were told to them by others were cross-tabulated according to whether the outcomes of the stories were positive or negative and whether the respondent perceived them to be helpful or not helpful. Positive stories were experienced as more helpful than negative stories.[5]

The fourth study cited by Taylor and Lobel (1989) was the one in which Taylor and Dakof (1988) asked cancer patients to describe helpful and unhelpful actions that they experienced in their interactions with

[5]However, 68% of the respondents reported that they were unaffected by the stories that were told to them, which may cast doubt on the importance of this evidence concerning reactions to comparisons. It is possible that respondents may not have wanted to report that stories about other cancer patients had impact on them, or that they were unaware of the impact of such stories.

other cancer patients. Earlier we described results from that study concerning informational consequences of comparison, but now we focus on the affective consequences. Commonly described helpful actions included acting as a good role model, coping well with cancer, or simply surviving (see Taylor & Dakof, 1988; Taylor & Lobel, 1989). The most common unhelpful interactions that cancer patients reported involved contacts with others who were coping poorly or continuing to engage in actions that threatened their health. These findings point to a clear preference for upward contacts over downward contacts. However, it is interesting to note that the most frequently reported helpful action was the fellow cancer patient's "ability to offer the special kind of understanding that one gets from sharing a similar experience" (Taylor & Dakof, 1988, p. 110). This finding may suggest that cancer patients feel best after contact with similar others, or at least that, regardless of the direction of comparison, it is the similarity of fellow patients that is experienced as most helpful.

In addition to these four primary studies, Taylor and Lobel (1989) also cited research on cancer patients' contacts with fellow patients (e.g., van den Borne et al., 1987; see van den Borne et al., 1986, for a review). This research suggests that contact with fellow patients is associated not only with a higher level of knowledge and information about cancer and its treatment, as described earlier, but also with a reduction in negative feelings. As Taylor and Lobel (1989) stated, this evidence is consistent with the idea that upward affiliations are a source of inspiration and hope. Again, however, most of these studies are correlational. Hence, it is not clear whether contacts with fellow patients reduce negative feelings, whether people in better moods seek out more contacts, or whether a third variable leads to both improved mood and increased contacts.[6] In their review of this literature, van den Borne et al. (1986) concluded that of the three studies that involved random assignment of patients to a self-help or control group, none found negative effects of participation in self-help groups and two found positive affective consequences, including less body image disturbance and a reduction in negative feelings. Although these three articles indicate that contacts with fellow patients can be beneficial, it is not clear that the benefits flowed from the social comparisons that took place in the group; they

[6]Indeed, it is not even clear that mood changed at all. Many of these studies are based on retrospective self-reports of mood change, which are vulnerable to people's implicit theories about whether mood should change in response to contact with others. Conway and Ross (1984), for example, showed that students who had joined a study skills group remembered their study habits as having been poorer before they entered the study skills class than they had judged them to be at that earlier time.

may have been due to the social support provided by such groups. (We should note that these studies were not designed to study social comparison.) Even if we could safely attribute some of the positive effects of contacts with fellow sufferers to social comparisons, we would not know whether the comparisons that had the positive effects were upward or downward (cf. Taylor & Lobel, 1989). These findings, therefore, cannot speak to predictions concerning upward and downward comparisons.

The final study we review is one that was published after Taylor and Lobel's (1989) paper. It tests most directly the idea that both upward and downward contacts can have positive and negative effects. Specifically, Buunk et al. (1990, Study 1) studied 55 people who had experienced various types of cancer. During an interview, respondents were told:

> Some people have told us that when they see cancer patients who are not doing as well as they are, it makes them feel lucky and grateful that they are not in worse shape themselves. Other people have told us that when they see cancer patients who are not doing as well as they are, it makes them feel worse. For these people, seeing cancer patients who are worse off only increases their fears and anxieties. (p. 1240)

Respondents were then asked to rate how frequently they had felt (a) lucky or grateful and (b) fearful or anxious when exposed to worse-off others (on a 4-point scale ranging from 1 [*never*] to 4 [*often*]). Respondents were then asked about their reactions to upward comparisons:

> Some people have told us that when they see cancer patients who are doing better than they are, it makes them feel frustrated or depressed. Other people have told us they feel inspired or comforted when they see other cancer patients who seem to be doing better than they are. (p. 1241)

As for the downward comparison questions, respondents were asked to rate the frequency of each of these reactions on the same 4-point scale.

These questions strike us as difficult to answer. The expected problems of self-reported social comparisons, including selectivity in reporting, biases in recall, social desirability concerns, and lack of awareness of comparisons, would likely be present here, and may be even compounded because respondents are required to estimate not only how many times they engaged in social comparison, but how they reacted to them. This concern is alleviated somewhat, however, by the fact that the authors asked respondents to provide examples of times they experienced these comparisons. For most of the categories of comparison experience, a high percentage of the sample did provide a clear example.

A second difficulty in interpreting these questions is that they may reflect selections of comparisons or reactions to comparisons. For example, if respondents say that they rarely had negative reactions to upward comparisons, is that because they did not encounter such upward comparisons, that they actively avoided upward comparisons, or that they made many upward comparisons but that they had no negative reactions, or that they made such comparisons but avoided feeling bad about them?

In any case, the results of these questions indicated that 82% of the respondents reported that they made downward comparisons and felt good, 59% made downward comparisons and felt bad, 78% made upward comparisons and felt good, and 40% made upward comparisons and felt bad. In terms of the frequency ratings, downward comparisons that resulted in positive affect were rated as occurring most commonly, although upward positive affect comparisons were almost equally common.

In summary, all five studies concerning affective reactions to upward and downward comparison indicated that downward contacts can be threatening, or at least experienced negatively. This supports Taylor and Lobel's (1989) argument that cancer patients avoid downward comparisons. In the study that assessed most directly the upward and the downward contact predictions (Buunk et al., 1990, Study 1), support for both predictions was found (with perhaps a slight edge for the downward contact prediction, according to the authors). Three of the five studies indicated that respondents reacted more positively to upward contacts than to downward contacts (Molleman et al., 1986; Taylor & Dakof, 1988; Taylor et al., 1993, Study 1). However, it is not always clear from these three studies whether respondents enjoyed their upward contacts or found their downward contacts aversive or both.

Another problem in interpreting these results is that studies of people's reactions to social comparisons may or may not point to the kind of information they seek. For example, people may react more positively to upward than to downward comparisons, but they may prefer to have no comparisons at all. To the extent that the Taylor et al. (1993, Study 1) story study tapped into social comparisons, this is what it suggested; respondents liked upbeat stories about others who were coping well and who were physically well-off more than they liked stories about others who had not done well, yet they said they did not seek out stories about other cancer patients. (Of course, as mentioned earlier, not wanting to hear stories about cancer patients may not imply that one is uninterested in social comparisons obtained through other means—means that may allow a greater exchange of information with the actual comparison target.) In addition, Molleman et al.'s (1986) affiliation study indicated that respondents enjoyed their upward contacts more than their downward ones, but it also indicated that respondents did not seek primarily upward affiliations—they sought similar ones. Studies of reactions to comparisons, then, do not necessarily point to which comparisons people seek.

***Evaluation of the Reconciliation Perspective in Studies of Affective Reactions to Downward and Upward Comparisons.*** Do these studies of cancer patients' reactions to social comparisons support the reconciliation perspective? They would if the avoidance of downward contacts occurred when the respondents feared that they could decline and reach the downward target's level, and if upward comparison-seeking occurred when respondents had hope of improving on the dimension of comparison.

In most of these studies the comparison dimension was typically general physical condition. That was the sole dimension in the Collins et al. (1988) and Molleman et al. (1986) studies, and it was the primary dimension in the Taylor et al. (1993, Study 1) story study, because two thirds of the stories told to respondents "were about others who had died or done poorly" (p. 707). General physical condition was also the most common dimension in the Buunk et al. (1990) study. Buunk et al. (1990) coded the examples respondents had provided for each category of comparison experience (i.e., upward-positive affect, downward-negative affect, and so forth), and comparisons on the dimension of prognosis were found to be the most frequent in each category (ranging from 52% to 67%).

However, the downward contacts in the Taylor and Dakof (1988) "helpful-unhelpful" study apparently did not involve the dimension of physical condition; they involved the dimensions of coping and engaging in actions that threaten one's health. Why would such downward comparisons be aversive—would patients fear declining on these dimensions? Downward comparisons with others who are engaging in actions that threaten their health are unlikely to be threatening because behavior is seen as relatively controllable. Are downward comparisons with someone who is coping poorly threatening? Possibly; such comparisons may remind one of one's own fears and distress, and hence of how scary cancer is, whereas comparisons with a person who is coping very well may imply that cancer is manageable and not so frightening. On the other hand, coping may be viewed as fairly controllable (Buunk, 1994), so downward comparisons to poor copers may not be threatening, and may even be self-enhancing (Wood et al., 1985). It is not clear, then, whether these downward comparisons would have been threatening. Recall, however, that the dependent variable in the Taylor and

Dakof study concerned whether the contacts were "helpful" or "unhelpful." Regardless of whether respondents experienced their contacts with poor copers or with people who did not take care of themselves as threatening, they were likely to experience them as unhelpful. These findings, then, may not be pertinent to our predictions about when downward contacts are avoided.

In any case, the vast bulk of the findings that point to the aversiveness of downward comparisons involved the dimension of general physical condition, which we have argued would be threatening to many cancer patients. However, a result from the Buunk et al. (1990) study may seem inconsistent with this argument. Specifically, the dimension of prognosis was found to be the most frequent in each category of comparison experience, which implies that downward comparisons involving general physical condition not only lead people with cancer to feel "fearful or anxious," they also may lead them to feel "lucky or grateful." As we argued earlier, however, it seems very possible that cancer patients may experience both reactions to observing another patient whose condition has deteriorated; they may feel lucky that they are not in that condition themselves and simultaneously fearful that they could reach that condition. Indeed, Buunk et al. noted that, "Many [respondents] referred to the same target in response to questions assessing both positive and negative reactions" (p. 1242). Our hunch is that on balance, even though cancer patients may feel somewhat lucky when they do encounter such downward comparisons, their preference would be to avoid them. The evidence from the other studies, which indicate that cancer patients typically have negative reactions to downward comparisons on the dimension of general physical condition, supports this reasoning. Additional support for the reconciliation perspective is Buunk et al.'s (1990) finding that respondents were less likely to feel threatened by downward comparisons the higher their perceptions of control.

Did respondents prefer upward comparisons under conditions predicted by our reconciliation perspective, namely when they feared that they could decline or when they believed that they could improve on the dimension? Upward comparisons should be preferred over downward on the dimension of general physical condition. In support of the reconciliation perspective, the upward contacts suggested by these studies often involved others who have simply survived long term (Taylor & Dakof, 1988; Taylor et al., 1993; and perhaps Buunk et al., 1990; Molleman et al., 1986). Long-term survivors should offer hope and perhaps helpful information to most cancer patients. The upward contacts also often involved the dimension of coping (Taylor & Dakof, 1988; Taylor et al., 1993), which is likely to be perceived as relatively controllable (Buunk, 1994), and hence is one on which people could hope to improve.

## CONCLUSION AND RECOMMENDATIONS FOR FUTURE RESEARCH

In this chapter, we focused not on Taylor and Lobel's (1989) observation of the striking discrepancy between measures of "evaluations" and what they called *contacts*—measures of information seeking and affiliation seeking. Rather, we focused on the discrepancy between Taylor and Lobel's (1989) prediction of upward information seeking and affiliation seeking and Wills' (1981) prediction of downward information seeking and affiliation seeking. We offered a possible reconciliation of these two models, drawn from recent research, and examined its viability in studies of cancer patients. The evidence points to three main conclusions. First, Taylor and Lobel (1989) were right in challenging the view that people under threat always prefer downward comparisons: Cancer patients do appear to find some downward comparisons to be threatening rather than self-enhancing, and they often avoid them. On this point, the evidence is very convincing.

Our second conclusion, however, is that there is little evidence that cancer patients seek upward comparisons. Studies of cancer patients' reactions to comparisons clearly indicated that they often react more positively to upward comparisons than to downward ones, but these studies do not clearly indicate that patients actively seek upward comparisons, for the reasons mentioned earlier, and none of the studies of cancer patients' selections suggested that they seek upward comparisons. It is important to recognize, however, that very few studies have been conducted that were designed to address the question of whether cancer patients seek upward comparisons. We suspect that such studies would support Taylor and Lobel's (1989) prediction of upward comparisons under threat. Upward comparisons provide useful information, goals to strive for, and inspiring examples. Hence, our perspective as well predicts that cancer patients will seek upward information (specifically, when they fear that they may decline on the dimension, or when they hope to improve on the dimension). Our conclusion that there is little evidence that cancer patients seek upward comparisons, then, would be phrased more aptly as "there is little such evidence—yet."

Our third conclusion is that most of the evidence that cancer patients react more favorably to upward contacts than to downward contacts involved the dimension of general physical condition, on which downward comparisons are often threatening. This evidence supports our reconciliation perspective, which holds that people find downward comparisons threatening when they fear that they can worsen on the dimension. Similarly, our perspective predicts that people with cancer would find upward comparisons aversive if the upward targets involve superiority that they themselves can never hope to achieve. For example, the average patient may avoid comparisons with others who had smaller tumors to begin with, or who have happier marriages, or who can cope by taking a cruise around the world. We argue, then, that studies of cancer patients' reactions to comparison contacts would yield a more balanced view—more evidence of favorable reactions to downward comparisons and unfavorable reactions to upward comparisons—if they do not involve primarily the dimension of general physical condition. Indeed, the Wood et al. (1985) study suggested that cancer patients felt fortunate and pleased when they contrasted themselves against downward targets on a variety of dimensions other than physical condition.

Our reconciliation perspective has been useful, then, in understanding the contradictory findings in this literature. However, this review of the evidence also raises several issues that need to be addressed through further research. First, as discussed before, is the question of when self-enhancement needs override improvement needs, which would determine when downward and upward comparisons are preferred. In the case of cancer, it seems likely that emotion-regulation and self-enhancement needs predominate around the time of diagnosis and in the case of a recurrence. Taylor (1983) has argued that after a stressful event, unpleasant, intense emotions must be reduced before the individual can engage in active problem solving. In support of this reasoning, Wood et al. (1985) found that respondents made more downward comparisons the closer in time they were to their diagnosis (see Taylor et al., in press, for more discussion of the role of temporal factors in upward and downward comparisons).

Also badly needed are studies that include measures of the construct that is central to our proposed reconciliation, namely the expectation of whether one will improve or decline on the dimension of comparison. Also very enlightening would be data collection concerning mediators and moderators of these perceptions, such as respondents' perceptions of the controllability of the dimension (Major et al., 1991) and the degree to which respondents identify versus contrast themselves with the comparison target (Collins, 1996; Buunk & Ybema, chapter 12, this volume).

This review also revealed a critical gap in our perspective as well as in much of the prior work on upward and downward comparisons: We did not anticipate the importance of comparisons with similar others. Recall that in the Molleman et al. (1986) study, respondents preferred to interact with others who were similar to themselves, and rated others who were similar as the most informative. In addition, Taylor and Dakof (1988) found that cancer patients, in their interactions with other cancer patients, seemed to experience as most helpful "the special kind of understanding that one gets from sharing a similar experience" (p. 110). Perhaps if we researchers did not focus solely on upward and downward comparisons, we would find that similar comparisons are the most preferred. We should not be surprised by this possibility; Festinger (1954) would not have been, nor would have Wills (1981), who predicted that people under threat make comparisons with similar others—what he called *shared fate* comparisons—as well as downward comparisons. In addition, Wood et al. (1985) acknowledged that, despite their respondents' emphasis on downward comparisons, when one looks beyond the specific dimension of comparison to the larger context of comparison targets' attributes, respondents were virtually always comparing themselves with similar others—namely, others who had cancer.

The question should be, then, under what conditions do upward, downward, or similar comparisons occur? It is interesting to note that the evidence for similar comparisons has come primarily from studies involving affiliation (Molleman et al., 1986; Taylor & Dakof, 1988). Perhaps when one interacts with others, it is especially important to avoid the drawbacks of both upward and downward comparisons. Indeed, in general we have much more confidence that our reconciliation perspective holds for information seeking than for affiliation seeking. Affiliation measures are weak indices of social comparison because they are especially vulnerable to interfering motivations and alternative interpretations (Wood, 1996), and Buunk (1994) argued that people under stress prefer information over affiliation as a means of making social comparisons.

More generally, our review points to many methodological weaknesses in the research on cancer patients' social comparisons. Virtually all of the measures involved interviews or questionnaires of unknown reliability and validity. Some of the problems of self-report may be avoided through the use of daily diaries of social comparisons, as Wheeler and Miyake (1992) used, rather than global interview questions (see Wood, 1996). Self-report studies also could be supplemented by studies that incorporate methods used in the laboratory. DeVellis et al. (1990), for example, provided an opportunity for arthritis patients to choose from different types of social information.

Finally, another large gap in this literature on cancer patients' social comparisons is that it has focused almost exclusively on coping—on what types of comparisons patients make to boost their spirits, and what impact comparisons have on patients' feelings and adjustment. Very little attention has been paid to the role of social comparisons in cancer patients' health behaviors. As has been mentioned before but has been underemphasized, upward comparisons may not only be inspiring, but instructive (Taylor & Lobel, 1989). For example, many people may make comparisons with fellow survivors who have made healthy lifestyle changes to learn how they too can implement such changes. Broadening our focus beyond coping to health behaviors would provide a more complete picture of cancer patients' social comparisons.

## ACKNOWLEDGMENTS

We thank Bram Buunk, Meg Gerrard, Rick Gibbons, Shelley Taylor, Howard Tennen, Ladd Wheeler, and Jan Fekke Ybema for their very helpful comments on this chapter. Work on this article was supported by a grant from the Social Sciences and Humanities Research Council of Canada to Joanne Wood. Joanne Wood, who wrote some of this chapter while on sabbatical at the University of Amsterdam, thanks the Vakgroep Sociale Psychologie and the Dutch Science Foundation (Nederlandse Organisatie voor Wetenschappenlijk Onderzoek) for providing resources and support.

## REFERENCES

Brickman, P., & Bulman, R. J. (1977). Pleasure and pain in social comparison. In J. M. Suls & R. L. Miller (Eds.), *Social comparison processes: Theoretical and empirical perspectives* (pp. 149–186). Washington, DC: Hemisphere.

Buunk, B. P. (1994). Social comparison processes under stress: Towards an integration of classic and recent perspectives. In W. Stroebe & M. Hewstone (Eds.), *European review of social psychology* (Vol. 5, pp. 211–241). Chichester: Wiley.

Buunk, B. P., Collins, R. L., Taylor, S. E., Van Yperen, N. W., & Dakof, G. A. (1990). The affective consequences of social comparison: Either direction has its ups and downs. *Journal of Personality and Social Psychology, 59,* 1238–1249.

Collins, R. L. (1996). For better or worse: The impact of upward social comparisons on self-evaluations. *Psychological Bulletin, 119,* 51–69.

Collins, R. L., Dakof, G., & Taylor, S. E. (1988). *Social comparison and adjustment to a threatening event.* Unpublished manuscript.

Conway, M., & Ross, M. (1984). Getting what you want by revising what you had. *Journal of Personality and Social Psychology, 47,* 738–748.

DeVellis, R., Holt, K., Renner, B., Blalock, S., Blanchard, L., Cook, H., Koltz, M., Mikow, V., & Harring, K. (1990). The relationship of social comparison to rheumatoid arthritis symptoms and affect. *Basic and Applied Social Psychology, 11,* 1–8.

Festinger, L. (1954). A theory of social comparison processes. *Human Relations, 7,* 117–140.

Gerrard, M., Gibbons, F. X., & Sharp, J. (1985, August). *Social comparison in a self help group for bulimics.* Paper presented at the annual meeting of the American Psychological Association, Los Angeles, CA.

Gibbons, F. X., & Gerrard, M. (1991). Downward comparison and coping with threat. In

J. Suls & T. A. Wills (Eds.), *Social comparison: Contemporary theory and research* (pp. 317–345). Hillsdale, NJ: Lawrence Erlbaum Associates.

Gibbons, F. X., Gerrard, M., Lando, H. A., & McGovern, P. G. (1991). Social comparison and smoking cessation: The role of the "typical smoker." *Journal of Experimental Social Psychology, 27,* 239–258.

Haney, C. A. (1984). Psychosocial factors in the management of patients with cancer. In C. L. Cooper (Ed.), *Psychosocial stress and cancer* (pp. 201–227). New York: Wiley.

Hemphill, K. J., & Lehman, D. R. (1991). Social comparisons and their affective consequences: The importance of comparison dimension and individual difference variables. *Journal of Social and Clinical Psychology, 10,* 372–394.

Jenkins, R. A., & Pergament, K. I. (1988). Cognitive appraisals in cancer patients. *Social Science and Medicine, 26,* 625–633.

Lazarus, R. S., & Folkman, S. (1984). *Stress, appraisal and coping.* New York: Springer.

Major, B., Testa, M., & Bylsma, W. H. (1991). Responses to upward and downward social comparisons: The impact of esteem-relevance and perceived control. In J. Suls & T. A. Wills (Eds.), *Social comparison processes: Contemporary theory and research* (pp. 237–259). Hillsdale, NJ: Lawrence Erlbaum Associates.

Miller, R. L., & Suls, J. M. (1977). Affiliation preferences as a function of attitude and ability similarity. In J. M. Suls & R. L. Miller (Eds.), *Social comparison processes: Theoretical and empirical perspectives* (pp. 103–124). Washington, DC: Hemisphere.

Molleman, E., Pruyn, J., & van Knippenberg, A. (1986). Social comparison processes among cancer patients. *British Journal of Social Psychology, 25,* 1–13.

Nosanchuk, T. A., & Erickson, B. H. (1985). How high is up? Calibrating social comparison in the real world. *Journal of Personality and Social Psychology, 48,* 624–634.

Pyszczynski, T., Greenberg, J., & LaPrelle, J. (1985). Social comparison after success and failure: Biased search for information consistent with a self-serving conclusion. *Journal of Experimental Social Psychology, 21,* 195–211.

Reis, H. T., & Wheeler, L. (1991). Studying social interaction with the Rochester Interaction Record. In M. P. Zanna (Ed.), *Advances in experimental social psychology* (pp. 269–318). San Diego: Academic Press.

Rofé, Y. (1984). Stress affiliation: A utility theory. *Psychological Review, 91,* 235–250.

Taylor, S. E. (1983). Adjustment to threatening events. *American Psychologist, 38,* 1161–1173.

Taylor, S. E., Aspinwall, L. G., Guiliano, T. A., Dakof, G. A., & Reardon, K. K. (1993). Storytelling and coping with stressful events. *Journal of Applied Social Psychology, 23,* 703–733.

Taylor, S. E., & Brown, J. D. (1988). Illusion and well-being: A social psychological perspective on mental health. *Psychological Bulletin, 103,* 193–210.

Taylor, S. E., Buunk, B. P., Collins, R. L., & Reed, G. M. (1992). Social comparison and affiliation under threat. In L. Montada, S.-H. Filipp, & M. J. Lerner (Eds.), *Life crisis and experiences of loss in adulthood* (pp. 213–228). Hillsdale, NJ: Lawrence Erlbaum Associates.

Taylor, S. E., & Dakof, G. A. (1988). Social support and the cancer patient. In S. Spacapan & S. Oskamp (Eds.), *The social psychology of health: The Claremont symposium on applied social psychology* (pp. 95–116). Newberry Park, CA: Sage.

Taylor, S. E., Lichtman, R. R., & Wood, J. V. (1984). Attributions, beliefs in control, and adjustment to breast cancer. *Journal of Personality and Social Psychology, 46,* 489–502.

Taylor, S. E., & Lobel, M. (1989). Social comparison activity under threat: Downward evaluation and upward contacts. *Psychological Review, 96,* 569–575.

Taylor, S. E., Wayment, H. A., & Carrillo, M. (in press). Social comparison, self-regulation, and motivation. In R. M. Sorrentino & E. T. Higgins (Eds.), *Handbook of motivation and cognition.* New York: Guilford.

Taylor, S. E., Wood, J. V., & Lichtman, R. R. (1983). It could be worse: Selective evaluation

as a response to victimization. *Journal of Social Issues, 39,* 19–40.
Testa, M., & Major, B. (1988, April). *Affective and behavioral consequences of social comparison.* Paper presented at the annual meeting of the Eastern Psychological Association, Buffalo, NY.
Thompson, S. C. (1985). Finding positive meaning in a stressful event and coping. *Basic and Applied Social Psychology, 6,* 279–295.
van den Borne, H. W., & Pruyn, J. F. A. (1985). *Lotgenotencontact bij kankerpatienten* [Support groups of cancer patients]. Maastricht: van Gorcum Assen.
van den Borne, H. W., Pruyn, J. F. A., & van Dam-de Mey, K. (1986). Self-help in cancer patients: A review of studies on the effects of contacts between fellow-patients. *Patient Education and Counselling, 8,* 367–385.
van den Borne, H. W., Pruyn, J. F. A., & van den Heuvel, W. J. A. (1987). Effects of contacts between cancer patients on their psychosocial problems. *Patient Education and Counselling, 9,* 33–51.
VanderZee, K. I., Buunk, B. P., DeRuiter, J. H., Tempelaar, R., VanSonderen, E., & Sanderman, R. (in press). Social comparison and the subjective well-being of cancer patients. *Basic and Applied Social Psychology.*
Wheeler, L., & Miyake, K. (1992). Social comparison in everyday life. *Journal of Personality and Social Psychology, 62,* 760–773.
Wills, T. A. (1981). Downward comparison principles in social psychology. *Psychological Bulletin, 90,* 245–271.
Wood, J. V. (1989). Theory and research concerning social comparisons of personal attributes. *Psychological Bulletin, 106,* 231–248.
Wood, J. V. (1996). What is social comparison and how should we study it? *Personality and Social Psychology Bulletin, 22,* 520–637.
Wood, J. V., Giordano-Beech, M., Taylor, K. L., Michela, J. L., & Gaus, V. (1994). Strategies of social comparison among people with low self-esteem: Self-protection and self-enhancement. *Journal of Personality and Social Psychology, 67,* 713–731.
Wood, J. V., & Taylor, K. L. (1991). Serving self-relevant goals through social comparison. In J. Suls & T. A. Wills (Eds.), *Social comparison: Contemporary theory and research* (pp. 23–49). Hillsdale, NJ: Lawrence Erlbaum Associates.
Wood, J. V., Taylor, S. E., & Lichtman, R. R. (1985). Social comparison in adjustment to breast cancer. *Journal of Personality and Social Psychology, 49,* 1169–1183.
Wortman, C. B., & Dunkel-Schetter, C. (1979). Interpersonal relationships and cancer: A theoretical analysis. *Journal of Social Issues, 35,* 120–155.
Ybema, J. F. (1994). *Up and down: Affective responses to social comparison.* Capelle a/d IJssel: Labyrint Publication.

# CHAPTER 11

# Social Comparisons and Subjective Well-Being

Ed Diener
*University of Illinois at Champaign/Urbana*

Frank Fujita
*Indiana University South Bend*

Subjective well-being comprises people's evaluations—both affective and cognitive—of their lives. It includes facets such as whether individuals are joyful or sad, satisfied with their lives versus despairing, and satisfied versus dissatisfied with their health. Thus, subjective well-being encompasses global happiness and unhappiness, as well as satisfaction with specific domains such as health. Those who study this topic consider the full range of well-being, which varies from depression and despair to elation and consummate life satisfaction. Subjective well-being is relevant to the health area not only because it is an integral component of mental health but also because satisfaction with one's physical health is a component of subjective well-being.

It is often assumed that social comparison has an impact on subjective well-being because people may evaluate their lives by comparing their current circumstances to a standard determined by the level of other people. That is, if people's lives compare favorably to a socially derived standard they will be satisfied and experience positive emotions. If the social comparison process results in an unfavorable match, the literature predicts that the person will be dissatisfied and suffer from unpleasant emotions such as sadness and anxiety. Thus, the core of the social comparison idea is that satisfaction with life, health, and other domains does not depend solely on a person's absolute standing (e.g., whether he or she is vigorous and without infirmities), but also on the standing of other people with whom he or she might compare. Parducci (1995) maintained that all human judgments are relative to the frame of reference in which they are made, and one possible context for satisfaction judgments may be the standing of others in that domain. Therefore, context models such as Parducci's suggest that where people stand in relation to others will influence their health satisfaction.

In this chapter, we contrast two approaches to social comparison that differ in the way social comparison targets are selected. In the first approach, the *forced comparison* conception, comparison targets are the people who live in our local environment. The comparisons are imposed or compelled by our situation in that we look to others who are salient simply because they are in close proximity to us. As is seen here, the idea that environmentally imposed comparisons strongly influence our long-term satisfaction judgments has received little empirical support. The coping approach to social comparison, the one emphasized in most of the chapters of this book, is one in which the person takes a much more active role, consciously selecting comparison targets from a wide array of available others in order to meet varying goals (Wood, 1985).

The coping approach focuses social comparison away from the actual social situation and the environment to internal factors such as personality and flexible cognitive strategies. Whereas the forced comparison approach grants priority to the social environment, the coping approach emphasizes people's flexibility in using social information. As we demonstrate, the coping approach, very different from the forced comparison model, is the one now emphasized in the health domain. We argue that to the extent that people employ social comparison as a flexible coping strategy in the health domain as well as other areas, the effects of imposed social comparisons diminish or disappear. The coping model appears to be more accurate primarily because people are so flexible in natural settings in the information they use to determine their satisfaction. In addition, the coping model recognizes the substantial individual differences that exist in the choice of comparison targets.

## SUPPORTIVE EVIDENCE FOR THE IMPACT OF SOCIAL COMPARISON ON SUBJECTIVE WELL-BEING

Although Festinger's (1954) original social comparison theory was concerned with accurate self-evaluation rather than with subjective well-being per se, others saw the obvious relevance of the theory to happiness. Merton and Kitt (1950) foreshadowed later work in their theory of relative deprivation. They pointed out that in World War II, more educated soldiers had a better chance of promotion but were less satisfied with their opportunities for advancement. Merton and Kitt explained this paradox by examining the career success of people with whom educated and uneducated soldiers were most likely to compare.

Relative deprivation work (e.g., Buunk & Ybema, chapter 12, this volume; Crosby, 1976; Olson, Herman, & Zanna, 1986) is based on the idea that resentment and perceived discrimination depend on comparison to other persons or groups rather than to absolute standards.

Easterlin (1974) also drew heavily on ideas of social comparison in interpreting the influence of money on happiness. He reviewed evidence showing that within nations people's finances correlate with their reported well-being, but that richer nations show no greater happiness than poorer ones. Easterlin explained this pattern by hypothesizing that social comparisons are likely to occur within nations but not between nations. Thus, people's wealth correlates with their subjective well-being in within-nation studies because people compare to others in that society, and those who are better off financially tend to be happier. Between different countries, however, Easterlin maintained that people are unlikely to make comparisons. Because the average person's wealth within nations is the modal comparison standard, nations do not differ in subjective well-being. Thus, Easterlin's approach was congruent with the "hedonic treadmill" idea (Brickman & Campbell, 1971) that states that the average person is doomed to hedonic neutrality. If other people serve as the standard for happiness and satisfaction, half of the people likely will be below the standard and half of the people likely will be above the standard. Therefore, although some individuals will be happy, the overall distribution of subjective well-being will be centered at the affective neutral point.

Other evidence supported the idea that people's satisfaction due to wealth might be based on social comparisons. Duncan (1975) found that the satisfaction of Detroit housewives with their standard of living did not increase from 1955 to 1971, despite the fact that real income increased substantially. The social comparison interpretation of these findings is that people's standards increased as the wealth of those around them increased. A similar interpretation can be placed on data showing that happiness levels in the United States, France, and Japan have not changed since World War II despite rapid economic growth in these societies. Thus, greatly increased purchasing power (even after controlling inflation; Samuelson, 1995) brought no greater satisfaction, possibly because the social comparison standard inevitably moved upward as national income increased.

Kapteyn (Kapteyn & Wansbeek, 1982; Kapteyn, Wansbeek, & Buyze, 1980) maintained that one's welfare function for money, the amount of utility or well-being gained from one's income, depends both on one's past income and on the income of one's reference group. Instead of comparison with people in one's immediate vicinity, Kapteyn stressed the comparison with an individual's "reference group," a concept discussed in Festinger's (1954) seminal article. Kapteyn's approach depended on asking people about the levels of income they considered satisfactory. People with higher levels of income reported that they "required" greater amounts of wealth to be satisfied or to meet their "minimum needs." Kapteyn interpreted these findings as due to the fact that each income group compares to its own reference group, and therefore greater wealth is required for "needs" and satisfaction as one climbs the income ladder. Thus, the hopeful idea that a society could increase its happiness by increasing its wealth might be futile.

In 1985, Alex Michalos advanced the Multiple Discrepancies Theory of satisfaction that maintained that satisfaction is due to a comparison of one's lot with a number of standards, including social comparisons, and comparisons with one's past and with one's own needs. Emmons and Diener (1985) examined several of these discrepancies and found that social comparisons were in most cases the strongest predictors of satisfaction. They found large standardized beta weights for social comparison when it and other variables were used to predict satisfaction with one's friends and one's love life, as well as with the sum of all domains. Indeed, in 21 of 22 comparisons, Emmons and Diener found that social comparison was a stronger predictor of satisfaction than either aspirations or the change from one's past. They wrote that "Social comparison was found to be the major predictor of satisfaction across most domains" (p. 164). As is seen here, the findings of Emmons and Diener probably indicate that satisfied people seek out and find positive social comparisons rather than that people are happy when they are immersed in a situation of unfortunate others.

In 1991, Michalos published an analyses of a worldwide sample of college students, that examined the "comparison gap," the distance between oneself and others. Michalos found that this was one of the strongest correlates of life satisfaction and happiness. The social comparison measure in these studies was based on asking subjects how they compared to other college students, and it was this measure that correlated highly with satisfaction. In the health domain, Michalos (1993) discovered that comparison to others correlated the most highly of any predictor with health satisfaction and was the second strongest predictor when entered in a regression equation. Indeed, social comparison was a significant predictor of satisfaction with health in every nation studied (Michalos, 1993).

Most of the early research was correlational, examining the covariation of reports of comparisons with reports of well-being. The conclusions were supported, however, by laboratory experiments. Strack, Schwarz, and their colleagues demonstrated in an ingenious series of studies that people use immediate comparison information to make satisfaction judgments. Strack, Schwarz, Chassein, Kern, and Wagner (1990), for example, found that the presence of a disabled person in the room in which participants completed a satisfaction questionnaire led them to report higher subjective well-being. The social comparison effect was heightened when the natural salience of the comparison target was raised by the physical orientation of the participants. This study indicates that temporary changes in subjective well-being can be induced by immediate social comparison stimuli.

Schwarz, Hippler, Deutsch, and Strack (1985) also demonstrated that because the response alternatives available to respondents on questionnaires can provide information about the typical distribution of this characteristic in the population, they can serve as social comparison knowledge. Respondents inferred that they watched more television than others when given response alternatives that reflected few hours of television viewing and therefore in this condition reported less satisfaction with the variety of their leisure-time activities. Apparently, respondents inferred from the response alternative that they watched relatively more television than others and therefore were less pleased with their recreation. In a similar paradigm, Schwarz and Scheuring (1988) found that people use social comparison information to evaluate their sex lives. In the health domain, Schwarz and Scheuring (1992; described in Schwarz, Mathiowetz, & Belli, 1995) asked respondents about the frequency with which they experienced 17 physical symptoms, and gave them either low frequency or high frequency response alternatives. Not surprisingly, people reported more frequent symptoms on the high frequency response scales, suggesting that respondents use the response alternatives as a frame of reference to estimate the frequency of their own symptoms. More surprising, however, is the fact that the respondents with the high frequency scale reported greater health satisfaction—even though they reported more symptoms—presumably because they seemed to experience fewer symptoms compared to others.

Smith, Diener, and Weddell (1989) found that in evaluating satisfaction with imagined grades respondents were highly influenced by the grade distribution of the class. Furthermore, the satisfaction judgments followed Parducci's (1984) range-frequency model of judgments. Thus, the conclusions of the correlational work are supported by experimentation in which people's satisfaction responses are influenced by immediately available social comparison information.

The theory of imposed social comparison and subjective well-being appeared to be a promising scientific model in its simplicity. People examined their own levels of health, physical attractiveness, and other characteristics. By comparing their own characteristics to those of people around them, people could easily judge their level of satisfaction in each domain. Taken to its logical conclusion, the social comparison approach suggested that global happiness, as well as satisfaction in particular domains such as health, arose because one was either better or worse off than salient others. At the applied level the approach was disheartening because it indicated that neutrality was the human lot, and that achieving true satisfaction was a phantom for at least half of humanity. As we will see, however, empirical evidence soon cast doubt on the forced social comparison approach to long-term satisfaction.

## DISCONFIRMING EVIDENCE

Despite the evidence in support of the influence of social comparisons on subjective well-being, negative evidence also appeared. For example, Freedman (1978) reported that people who thought that they were either more sexually active or less sexually active than others were equally satisfied with their sex lives. He wrote, "people who lead a reasonably active sex life do not seem to be affected much by their estimates of what others are doing" (p. 63). In other words, it is likely that we have internal standards for some characteristics, and therefore our satisfaction with these traits does not depend much on what others are doing. The internal standards may set one's sexual desires at a certain level, and therefore the fact that others are having either more or less sex does not seem relevant to one's satisfaction.

In addition, it now seems likely that when people "compare" themselves to others, they are often reporting how they feel about their own standing on a trait rather than making an actual comparison. A finding that is suggestive in this regard is that if people rate themselves higher on a trait, they also rate others higher on that trait. In a recent study of 20 personal characteristics (e.g., health and physical attractiveness), we asked respondents to rate the persons with whom they most often compared themselves. We found that of the 20 characteristics, respondents were most satisfied with how "nice" they were, yet also rated their comparison other as highest on this very same trait! Furthermore, for those characteristics for which the comparison others were rated highly, the respondents were most satisfied ($r = .69$, $p < .001$)! Although compatible with an upward comparison model (discussed later), these data do not support the idea that we are most dissatisfied in areas where others are relatively better off. These results are more compatible with assimilation or group identity effects in which the individual identifies with similar others, rather than with a contrast approach to social comparison (see Buunk & Ybema, chapter 12, this volume). In the health domain we found that respondents were more satisfied if they rated the average university student as healthier in absolute terms ($r = .28, p < .01$) than those respondents who did not rate the average other as healthy. Similarly, if respondents were satisfied, they were more likely to rate the most-compared other as healthier ($r = .25, p < .05$). In other words, we found that if we think others are healthier, we are more satisfied with our own health! Of course people who think that others are healthier may think that they themselves are still healthier. As we will see, however, the ratings of others do not add anything beyond self-ratings to the prediction of satisfaction.

Another revealing finding is that those domains that are vaguest are the domains in which respondents are most likely to report being superior to their comparison others. What follows then is that in those domains in which respondents rate themselves highly, they are also very likely to rate their comparison others highly ($r = .85, p < .001$), and at the very same time report that they are better off relative to their comparison others in these domains ($r = .85, p < .001$)! In a similar vein, the findings of Dunning, Meyerowitz, and Holzberg (1989) suggested that people are more likely to report themselves as superior to others for traits that are ambiguous. These findings suggest that in vague domains people will project a good feeling about themselves into their reports of comparison, whereas in a concrete domain it is harder to do this. It is likely that some domains are so vague that positive ratings can be made about every judgment in them, including both self-judgments and self-other comparison ratings. Thus, the fact that the reported social comparison gap correlates with satisfaction appears to have little to do with an actual comparison to others, who may also be seen as better off by satisfied people. This is consistent with Wood's (1996; Wood & VanderZee, chapter 10, this volume) suggestion that what are called *comparative ratings* are often not based on social comparisons at all.

How do we interpret the findings of Emmons and Diener (1985) and Michalos (1993) showing that respondent's reported satisfaction correlates with the gap they perceive between themselves and others? Wright (1985) suggested the possibility that comparisons of this type correlate with satisfaction because of the role of one's own endowment in such comparisons, with the role of others being negligible. In addition to asking people to rate their health compared to others, Wright asked them to assess their health in absolute terms and to rate the average health of the population. The correlation of the comparison gap with satisfaction was eliminated when the subject's own level was controlled. Thus, the level of other people was not important in determining an individual's health satisfaction. Further, confirming the findings we report above, the correlation between one's own health satisfaction and one's assessment of the health of average others was strongly and significantly positive ($r = .41$, $p < .01$), running counter to the forced social comparison prediction.

Wright suggested that reports of how one compares to others contains both self-information and information about others, but that the self-evaluation component carries all of the predictive power for satisfaction, the role of others having little or no weight. In Table 11.1 we present correlations that speak to the issue of whether the comparison to others contributes independently to satisfaction beyond the effects of the self-rating. The correlations shown are between satisfaction in 20 domains and respondents' comparisons to others. At the University of Illinois, 107 students reported their satisfaction in the domains, how they compared to others in these domains, and their self and other ratings in these domains. Two comparison targets were used—the person to whom one most often compares (correlations outside of parentheses) and the average University of Illinois student (correlations in parentheses).

TABLE 11.1
Correlations of Satisfaction and Gaps

| | | | *Calculated Gap* | |
|---|---|---|---|---|
| | *Reported Gap* | *Calculated Gap* | *Partial Self* | *Partial Other* |
| Health | .55 (.74) | .41 (.50) | −.17 (−.27) | .74 (.76) |
| Library Skills | .40 (.63) | .44 (.08) | −.06 (−.06) | .65 (.73) |
| Nice | .36 (.58) | .20 (.53) | −.14 (.19) | .58 (.62) |
| Housing | .34 (.53) | .29 (.52) | −.20 (−.16) | .62 (.73) |
| Simplicity | .49 (.52) | .21 (.33) | −.12 (−.03) | .45 (.46) |
| GPA | .31 (.53) | .31 (.35) | −.23 (−.30) | .64 (.66) |
| Physical attractiveness | .46 (.68) | .40 (.65) | −.10 (.18) | .67 (.69) |
| Artistic | .68 (.72) | .47 (.67) | −.02 (.04) | .75 (.75) |
| Humility | .48 (.47) | .06 (.20) | −.25 (−.20) | .39 (.42) |
| Broadminded | .53 (.65) | .32 (.45) | −.02 (.01) | .60 (.62) |
| Cool | .41 (.47) | .27 (.45) | −.06 (.10) | .50 (.52) |
| Empathy | .35 (.45) | .40 (.46) | .09 (−.02) | .63 (.46) |
| Number of friends | .39 (.51) | .34 (.28) | −.10 (−.24) | .55 (.59) |
| Initiative | .37 (.57) | .34 (.41) | .08 (.02) | .55 (.56) |
| Volunteer activities | .32 (.51) | .29 (.40) | −.01 (.01) | .52 (.54) |
| Understanding | .36 (.51) | .29 (.46) | −.07 (.00) | .62 (.66) |
| Morality | .37 (.41) | .29 (.31) | .05 (−.19) | .50 (.56) |
| Spelling ability | .61 (.74) | −.03 (.00) | −.24 (−.19) | .05 (.05) |
| Procastination | .13 (−.06) | .30 (.41) | −.12 (.08) | .50 (.51) |
| Handwriting ability | .61 (.74) | .49 (.65) | −.02 (.06) | .71 (.72) |

*Note.* $n = 107$. Correlations outside of parentheses are for comparison with the most-compared other, and correlations in parentheses are based on correlations with the average University of Illinois student.

Column 2 of Table 11.1 presents the correlation between the reported self–other gap and satisfaction. As can be seen, the gaps in most cases correlated moderately to highly with satisfaction. It can also be seen that the comparison to the average student usually correlated more highly with satisfaction than the comparison with the most-compared other. Procrastination is an anomalous finding perhaps because participants were confused about scoring directions when saying whether they were above or below others on this undesirable characteristic.

Data on the calculated gap, column 3, represent the correlation between satisfaction in the domains and the gap we calculated based on subtracting the other-rating from the self-rating. It can be seen that, although these correlations tend to be smaller than those for directly reported gaps, they are mostly of moderate size. Columns 4 and 5 are quite revealing, however, in showing why the gaps correlate with satisfaction. In column 5, the calculated gap and satisfaction correlation is shown with the other score partialled out. What is immediately apparent is that these correlations are almost all higher than the zero-order gap correlations. This indicates that the primary contribution of the other to satisfaction via the gap rating is to add random error variance that lowers the prediction of satisfaction. Although gap ratings predict satisfaction, this is certainly not due to the rating of others.

In contrast, when the self-rating is partialled from the gap and satisfaction relation, the correlations drop to near zero, indicating that the self-component causes the correlation between the gap and satisfaction. The fact that many of these correlations are slightly negative indicates that the gap predicts satisfaction inversely (high gap, low satisfaction) once the self-rating is removed. This implies that a high rating of others covaries weakly with satisfaction. These data strongly suggest that the perceptions of others do not predict satisfaction, and that gap ratings correlate with satisfaction only because of the self-component. Although it might be argued that the perception of others is already implicit in the self-rating, the forced comparison data we present later cast doubt on this alternative as well. When one examines the partial correlations based on the directly reported gaps, once again the other reports seem to have no effect on satisfaction. As before, there is a tendency for the partial correlations to be higher than the zero-order correlations, indicating that respondents' perceptions of others (either the average student or the person to whom one compares most often) do not contribute to satisfaction.

The implications of these findings for health satisfaction are several. First, the gap between one's self-perceived health and the health of the most-compared to other or of the average other correlated with one's health satisfaction. These correlations are substantial regardless of whether the self–other gap is reported by the respondent or is calculated based on his or her self and other health ratings. When one partials out the influence of the rating of others' health from the calculated gap, however, the correlation with subjective well-being climbs substantially! This suggests that the rating of others serves as a suppressor variable in predicting health satisfaction. It also suggests that people's perception of their own health is the reason that the self–other gap predicts health satisfaction.

In a related study we collected objective evidence on participants' standings in several domains. We measured subjects' income (parental report of family income), grade point average (from transcripts), physical attractiveness (rated from pictures), and friendships (as reported by informants). The average correlation between these positive attributes was only .03, indicating that among college students our list of objectively good things do not go together. In contrast, the subjects' reports of how they compared to others in these domains averaged .26, and was statistically significant in all cases. Because participants' objective standing in the domains did not correlate, but the comparison judgments did, it appears that some global personality factor such as neuroticism might influence respondents' comparison judgments; their actual standing across domains cannot account for the convergence of comparison judgments.

The data given here suggest that the level of others does not automatically influence one's satisfaction, and indicate clearly that obtaining self-reports of comparison gaps is not a strong method for assessing the effects of social comparison. Indeed, we found that the perceptions of others usually correlate positively with a person's satisfaction. It is possible that comparison judgments may be caused by feelings of satisfaction, in a reverse order of causation, as suggested by Fox and Kahneman (1992). It is also likely that they derive in part from personality and from mood. Although "comparison" judgments may to some extent be influenced by comparing oneself to others, they seem to correlate with satisfaction primarily because of factors that influence the self-rating.

What of Easterlin's analysis of income and subjective well-being? Veenhoven (1991) reviewed the evidence contained in the Easterlin study and concluded that the earlier analyses were faulty. For example, Easterlin concluded that there were not substantial differences between countries in subjective well-being. Veenhoven found, however, that the nations ranged over a large part of the response scales. He also found that the correlations across nations between mean income and mean subjective well-being in the Easterlin samples were .51 and .59. Thus, the substantial national differences in subjective well-being correlate strongly with income. Although Easterlin's analysis is compatible with the idea that the primary benefit of money is in terms of status within one's society, the large differences in happiness between rich and poor nations in subjective well-being cannot be explained by reference to status differences. Finally, Veenhoven pointed out that although happiness has not increased with increasing income in the United States, this is because the United States has for the last 50 years been above the threshold at which basic needs are met. Thus, Easterlin's conclusions were in some cases questioned and in other cases interpreted in an alternate way.

Veenhoven's analysis of national differences in income replicates in the domain of health. When people on different continents were asked about their satisfaction with their health (Gallup, 1976–1977), the following percentages reported being *highly satisfied:* North America, 63%; Western Europe, 51%; Latin America, 48%; Africa, 33%; and the Far East, 18%. If people simply compared themselves in terms of health to others within their locale or nation, we would not expect large differences between regions. Instead, we find large variations that to some extent map onto absolute differences in health.

## SITUATIONALLY IMPOSED COMPARISONS

The data just discussed cast doubt on the influence of forced comparisons on subjective well-being. What about evidence on imposed social comparisons in which we examine the direct influence of surrounding others on reports on subjective well-being? People are constantly around others, and these other people may be objectively superior or inferior on any given characteristic. The forced comparison hypothesis is that others who are nearby serve as the primary standards against which to judge one's own standing because the information they provide is so accessible and salient. The social comparison standards are "forced" because the targets of comparison are in the target person's field of perception. If the comparisons to forced targets are favorable, the model suggests that the person is satisfied, and if they are unfavorable, dissatisfied. Although there might be both superior and inferior others in the environment with whom a person might compare, the idea of forced comparison is that people automatically compare with those around them. Thus, if a person is relatively inferior relative to local others, the person will be exposed to a greater number of superior people and will compare more frequently with them. As we review later, the coping model posits that a person may compare with either inferior or superior other people, even if they are not represented equally in the person's surroundings.

Forced comparisons provide us with a methodology in addition to reports of comparison gaps to assess the impact of the social environment on SWB. In the correlational gap approach reviewed earlier, one finds that people's ratings of other people usually do not correlate inversely with satisfaction. One might argue, however, that people's self-assessment is influenced by the level of others, and thus that social comparison has its effects earlier in the causal chain than is implied by our analysis of self–other discrepancies. In other words, a person's self-rating may contain implicit information about how he or she stands relative to others. One way to explore whether one's self-assessment is based on the influence of other people in the surrounding environment is to analyze the situational effects of forced comparison. If imposed comparisons influence satisfaction indirectly by affecting the self-rating, people in inferior and superior social environments ought to show these effects in their satisfaction ratings. In addition, one might argue that the correlational studies are all based on reports of perceptions, and do not directly assess the impact of others. For example, the influence of others might be unconscious and not captured by respondents' reports of other people's level. Therefore, if we assess the objective standing of people in one's environment, we can determine whether their level directly or indirectly influences respondents' satisfaction. Thus, to test the imposed comparison model rigorously, we must examine the subjective well-being of people with a similar level of a characteristic who live in areas that are either better or worse off on that characteristic. The imposed comparison data are complementary to the reported gap data in that they do not rely on reports of comparisons, but instead depend on objective discrepancies between the target person and others in her environment.

Fujita's (1993) study of imposed comparisons among roommates is noteworthy because the comparison targets were randomly assigned in a natural setting. Thus, Fujita's study provides a naturalistic experiment of the long-term effects of social comparison. Fujita examined respondents' satisfaction with their academic achievement, physical attractiveness, and social relationships. He obtained objective measures of the target's standing and roommate's standing in each of these domains. Fujita found that subjects' objective academic achievement (grade point average, or GPA) influenced their satisfaction in this domain, and their objective frequency of social relationships influenced their satisfaction in that domain. Neither the objective standing nor the perceived standing of their roommate, however, had an influence on their satisfaction in any of the three domains. Thus, a roommate who was randomly assigned to participants for the semester had virtually no influence on their satisfaction with important domains. One might argue that roommates did not compare to their roommate but instead compared to the average other student or to other specific individuals. The income data reviewed next, however, suggests that the comparisons are not made within a geographical area.

Diener, Sandvik, Seidlitz, and Diener (1993) studied people of varying levels of income who lived in either richer or poorer communities in the United States. The theory of forced comparisons suggests that those with similar incomes living in poorer areas will have higher subjective well-being, and those living in wealthier areas will have lower subjective well-being. Although Diener et al. found that wealthier individuals were somewhat happier, they uncovered no influence on subjective well-being of the wealth of the geographical area in which respondents lived.

Diener, Diener, and Diener (1995) examined income and social comparison at the national level, hypothesizing that nations that are surrounded by poorer societies would express more subjective well-being and nations surrounded by wealthier societies would express less of this quality. In fact, they found an opposite pattern: Nations with rich neighbors reported higher subjective well-being and those with poor neighbors reported lower subjective well-being. When the income of the target nation was controlled, the influence of the wealth of the neighboring nation remained in the opposite direction to that predicted by social comparison but was nonsignificant.

Diener et al. also analyzed whether income-skewing within societies leads to differences in subjective well-being between nations. Based on Parducci's (1984) range-frequency model, we predicted that nations that have income distributions that are less positively skewed ought to have higher subjective well-being because there are fewer extremely rich individuals with whom to compare. We found, however, that income skewing did not correlate with the subjective well-being of nations. We also examined whether the standard deviations of incomes in nations were correlated with the standard deviation of subjective well-being in nations. The reasoning was that if income is a cause of well-being, and social comparison affects the impact of well-being, there ought to be more spread in subjective well-being in nations where income has a larger range. We found a nonsignificant correlation between spread on these two types of measures, as did Veenhoven (1991) in a similar analysis.

Another method of studying forced comparisons is to examine personal characteristics that differ in vagueness versus concreteness (Dunning, Meyerowitz, & Holzberg, 1989), and in their public versus private nature. Comparisons are not imposed in areas that are vague or that are private—the person can imagine anything she likes. For characteristics that are public and concrete, however, the person is exposed to actual information about the characteristics of others. In Fig. 11.1 we show the correlations between the ratings of others and one's satisfaction ratings for selected domains that are rated as either more public or more private, and as either more concrete or vaguer. These data are based on the same 107 college students reported on in Table 11.1. As can be seen, the correlations are positive, and in some cases significantly so—again showing that one's ratings of comparison others do not covary inversely with satisfaction. More germane to the forced comparison idea, we did not find that the correlations were inverse in concrete and public areas where comparison information would be forced on the rater. We did find, however, that participants reported making more frequent comparisons in the concrete than in the vague areas (4.62 vs. 3.48 on a 7-point frequency of comparison scale). Thus, although people report more frequently comparing themselves to others in concrete domains, this does not seem to affect their satisfaction ratings in a way that the forced social comparison model predicts. Even in concrete, public domains, if people are satisfied they tend to see their comparison others as better off than do people who are dissatisfied.

In a daily diary study we examined the forced comparison of other people's social lives to see if they influenced respondents' satisfaction with their own social lives. We asked participants about their moods and their objective social relationships (e.g., going on a date, time spent talking to friends) each day, as well as about how their relationships compared to those of others that day. Individuals were in a class, and were to report how their relationships each day compared to others in the class that day. This analysis showed that the comparison judgment was correlated with one's own moods as well as with one's objective frequency of social relationships that day, but that the objective social relationships of others that day did not predict the comparison judgments. In other words, "comparison judgments" (with others in the

| Concrete nature of domain | | Public nature of domain | | | |
|---|---|---|---|---|---|
| | | Private | | Public | |
| | Vague | Empathy | .13 | Nice | .25** |
| | | Intuitive | .16 | Cool | .20* |
| | Concrete | Grade point average | .31** | Physically attractive | .18 |
| | | Procrastination | .18 | Number of friends | .26** |

FIG. 11.1. Correlations of characteristic satisfaction and most-compared other ratings for various characteristics. $^{*}p < .05$. $^{**}p < .01$.

class) were not based on the actual social relationships of others in the class. In fact, the objective social relationships of others correlated positively, not inversely, with one's comparative judgment. These data indicate that respondents in this case formed their social comparison judgments based on their moods and on their own behavior, without actual reference to the behavior of others. On days in which subjects were in a good mood, they thought they compared favorably to others, but simultaneously rated others as having better social relationships too! Although it might be argued that subjects did not really know much about the social relationships that day of other people in the class, the point is that they made "comparison judgments" that were not influenced by what others were doing. Thus, again we have evidence that reports of "social comparisons" can reflect mood and self information rather than actual comparative information. Although respondents rated their social life that day better if they were involved in more social activities, the "comparison" judgment was unaffected by the actual social lives of others.

How can it be that social comparisons often do not influence satisfaction? One reason is that people may use other information besides social comparison in order to evaluate their satisfaction with life domains. For example, Johnson et al. (1995) asked people what kinds of things they would think about in answering whether "your health is excellent, very good, good, fair, or poor." On average, about 7% of respondents said they would compare their health to that of others, whereas 67% said they would consider whether they had health problems, and 46% said they would consider their health-related behaviors. In our laboratory we asked respondents what they had considered when answering the five items of the Satisfaction with Life Scale, once again, only about 7% mentioned a comparison of their life to that of others. Thus, information other than the functioning of others may be much more relevant to making natural satisfaction judgments when social comparison information has not been primed.

## PREDICTED NEUTRALITY OF SUBJECTIVE WELL-BEING

If people base their satisfaction on both upward and downward comparisons of themselves to others in their environment, a corollary is that people ought on average to be neutral in terms of subjective well-being. For example, on average, people in different regions of the world and different nations ought to be neutral in happiness (Easterlin, 1974). This follows from the imposed social comparison idea because about half of the people ought to be above the mean (and be satisfied) and about half should be below the local mean (and be dissatisfied), at least when the attribute is approximately normally distributed (see Parducci, 1995). In fact, most people in most regions report being happy and satisfied (Diener & Diener, 1996) and this conclusion is supported by cognitive evidence (Matlin & Stang, 1978; Taylor & Brown, 1988) as well as nonself-report data (Diener & Diener, 1996). Furthermore, even very disadvantaged U.S. groups report positive levels of subjective well-being (Diener & Diener, 1996). Therefore, the corollary that subjective well-being is inevitably neutral that is implicit in the idea of imposed social comparisons is incorrect.

The finding that most people are happy is consistent with data showing that most people also think they compare favorably to others. Headey and Wearing (1988) described the "sense of relative superiority," meaning that most people think they are above average on most traits. For example, when comparing themselves to their peers, 60% of high school students rate themselves above average in athletic skill, 70% rate themselves above average in leadership, and 85% report that they are above average in their social relationships (cited in Dunning, Meyerowitz, & Holzberg, 1989). Fujita has found similar data in that 71% of college students reported possessing above average grades, whereas only 8% reported that their grades were below average compared to the average U.S. college student. In other domains more respondents admitted being average, but many more nevertheless thought they were above average than thought they were below average: physical attractiveness, 46% versus 10%; finances, 53% versus 12%; and number of friends, 48% versus 14%. Interestingly, Alicke et al. (1995) show that the better-than-average effect is strongest when people compare themselves to a vague, "average" other rather than to a specific other person. The data on sense of relative superiority suggest that global social comparison reports are often based more strongly on positivity bias (Taylor & Brown, 1988) than on actual comparisons of one's objective characteristics with those of others. The Alicke et al. findings support this contention in that people seem to automatically assume superiority when "comparing" themselves to vague targets, but do not do so when comparing themselves to specific others.

In summary, we find three converging lines of evidence suggesting that social comparison may not influence satisfaction ratings. First, we find that the perception of others does not predict satisfaction. Furthermore, the prediction from gap ratings to satisfaction seems to depend exclusively on the self-perception component of the gap rather than on the perceptions of others. Second, we find that forced comparisons in one's environment usually do not influence long-term satisfaction. And finally, we find that corollaries of the forced comparison idea such as the neutrality of subjective well-being are not upheld by the evidence.

## WHY CONFLICTING EVIDENCE?

If so much evidence refutes the idea that imposed social comparisons influence long-term levels of subjective well-being, why was the initial evidence positive? In the first place, some of the initial evidence that purportedly supported the influence of imposed social comparisons was based on post-hoc explanations of data in situations where alternative explanations were readily available. In many of these situations, social comparison theory could have predicted any outcome that occurred. If military police were unhappy with their promotion possibilities, it was because they compared to the Air Corp where there were so many more promotions. If military police were no less happy with their promotions, it was because they compared to other military police. If they were satisfied with their promotions, it was because they compared to some other more disadvantaged group. If Blacks are less happy than Whites, it is because they compare themselves to Whites. If they are no less happy, it is because they compare themselves to their own reference group. If nations differ in satisfaction with income, it is because they compare to America and Switzerland. If nations do not differ in financial satisfaction, it is because people compare within their nations. Thus, early "evidence" for the effect of social comparison on subjective well-being was often of a post hoc nature.

A second reason that early evidence supported the impact of social comparison on subjective well-being was that it was based on reports of comparison gaps—a reported distance between the self and others. As discussed earlier, such reports are likely to result from mood and personality, as well as one's own self-standing on the characteristic. The standing of others seems not to inversely influence one's comparative judgments. Correlations of perceived gaps between the self and others with subjective well-being are no longer convincing evidence that comparisons cause satisfaction.

Finally, comparisons that are induced in the laboratory seem sometimes to influence satisfaction judgments that are made immediately in that setting. The ease with which such factors are introduced, however, also indicates that other factors can easily become salient at other times, and suggests that in natural settings people may rely on so many different types of information that social comparisons may not carry much long-term weight. When natural situations have been examined where the level of surrounding people's social circumstances differed, it was found that long-term subjective well-being judgments were not affected by the social environment. It may be that long-term subjective well-being is not usually influenced by subjective well-being because people habituate to comparison others, because so many factors influence satisfaction in a domain that single factors take on relatively little significance, or because usually there are such a variety of people to whom one may choose to compare.

## THE COPING PERSONALITY MODEL

In contrast to the imposed comparison idea, many social comparison theorists emphasize an adjustment and coping view of social comparison. Although most social comparison researchers construed people as active in seeking social information from the very beginning of this line of inquiry, more recently there has been a strong emphasis on strategies such as avoiding comparisons and constructing comparison targets (e.g., Wood, 1989). People are seen as actively selecting certain comparison targets (who may be people who are either better or worse off) not just to evaluate themselves but also to enhance their moods or to motivate themselves in terms of coping behaviors. In other cases people may avoid making social comparisons altogether in order to cope. For example, Gibbons, Benbow, and Gerrard (1994) found that students whose academic performance was poor lowered the amount of social comparison in which they engaged. In the social comparison coping model, the comparison process is not seen as one in which people carefully evaluate themselves, make an objective evaluation of others, and then calculate a comparison judgment. Instead, social comparison, when it does occur, is seen as constructed by the person for strategic reasons. Rather than information imposed on the individual, social comparison is now defined as the social information to which the person chooses to attend (DeVellis et al., 1990). A number of other chapters in this volume, most notably those by Wood and VanderZee (chapter 10), Wills (chapter 6), and Tennen and Affleck (chapter 9), reflect this perspective.

In most forms of the social comparison coping model, the individual's self-perceptions are seen as biased. People select targets carefully or even invent imaginary social comparison targets. Although the objective social world may place constraints on such constructed comparisons, most of the variance occurs in the imagination and flexible strategies of the "comparer." Brown and Dutton (1995) wrote that people "compare themselves with others when they think it will make them feel good, but shy away from comparing with others when they think it will make them feel bad" (p. 1292). This hedonic model has been expanded to include strategic comparisons that can help one cope by learning new behaviors, giving one hope, and so forth.

In contrast to the forced comparison model, social comparison data indicate that "referent others with whom persons might wish to compare are quite diverse and unconstrained" (Kruglanski & Mayseless, 1990, p. 204). As is manifest from many chapters in the present volume, social comparison researchers now support the idea that people take an active role in the comparison process—selecting targets, avoiding comparisons, and actively inferring comparisons. As Kruglanski and Mayseless wrote: "Thus, comparison tendencies appear to be highly fluid and contingent on the overall psychological context affecting human judgment" (p. 206). The idea that social comparison is a fluid and strategic process is also consistent with the finding that there are varied motives for comparing to others. Helgeson and Michelson (1995) found that social comparisons may be motivated by self-evaluation but are also prompted by the desire to form a common bond and the desires for self-improvement, for self-enhancement, and for altruism. Thus, social comparisons do not inevitably lead to objective self-assessments made on the basis of contrasting oneself with others.

The limitations of the forced comparison model are brought into clear focus by the work of Buunk, Collins, Taylor, VanYperen, and Dakof (1990). These researchers note that the directionality of comparison is an uncertain indicator of its impact on subjective well-being. The forced comparison model assumes that comparisons to superior others result in feelings of dissatisfaction, whereas downward comparisons (Wills, 1981) result in feelings of positive well-being. However, Buunk et al. showed that upward comparisons can have both positive and negative hedonic effects. One may feel inferior, or one may hope of becoming like the superior other. A downward comparison may make one feel superior, but can also make one think that things could get worse for oneself. Buunk et al. concluded that comparison direction is not automatically linked to affect as was often assumed in the literature. The conclusion of Buunk et al. that "a comparison can produce either positive or negative feelings about oneself, independent of its direction" (p. 1238) seems to sever the direct tie between the imposed social environment and subjective well-being. In a similar vein, Pelham and Wachsmuth (1995) demonstrated that some upward social comparisons produce assimilation effects, so that people may feel similar to a desirable other rather than contrast themselves with the target person.

In the coping model, constructed comparisons are just one of many ways that a person can cope with his or her situation. People can also adjust their goals and goal importance to coincide with their resources and successes (e.g., Diener & Fujita, 1995; Gibbons, Benbow, & Gerrard, 1994). For example, people who are not athletic can focus their goals in the academic sphere and denigrate the importance of sports. If they start to suffer unfavorable comparisons in academia, they may decide to focus on a career in another field such as sales. In addition, individuals can seek help from others, pray, or increase their effort. People can focus on the future or past, on ideals or on concrete details, and can otherwise adjust their cognitions and behavior to maximize their outcomes. Thus, there are numerous ways of coping with difficult circumstances; strategic comparisons are just one method.

In the coping approach, accurate self-evaluation, the cornerstone of early social comparison theory, is seen as only one motive among many. For example, Sirgy (1986) described three major self-related motives: self-knowledge, self-esteem, and self-consistency. The latter two motives may often work in opposite directions from the desire for accurate self-knowledge. Furthermore, in the coping approach there are many standards that are important to judging satisfaction besides the level of other people. For example, in judging satisfaction, people may use standards based on feelings of deservingness, on past experience, on expectations, or on their ideals (Sirgy et al., 1995). Thus, in the coping approach, social comparisons do not automatically influence satisfaction because people may use other standards, and motives other than accurate self-knowledge may lead people to compare themselves only to selected other people. Furthermore, in the coping model unfavorable comparisons may result in processes that reduce stress such as further information seeking or self-concept compartmentalization (Sirgy, 1990). Through such processes, people may seek to keep their esteem and satisfaction intact despite unfavorable information.

Predictions that upward comparisons would lead to dissatisfaction and that downward social comparisons would lead to satisfaction were based on the idea of contrast—the person views herself as different from the comparison other. In the social comparison literature, the idea of "reference groups" has been prominent. Many authors have suggested that reference groups of similar others were the people with whom people would be most likely to compare. However, people are also likely to identify with these groups. If a person identifies with other people in the reference group, their successes may make her feel good, and their failures may make her feel bad. This effect was shown by Brown, Novick, and Kelley (1992) in that contrast effects occurred when others were dissimilar but assimilation effects occurred when others were perceived as similar. Thus, a forced comparison model built on contrast effects with comparison others is oversimplified. People may identify with similar others and in-group members, and in this case, social comparisons may produce effects that are opposite to those typically assumed in the forced comparison approach.

In contrast to the forced comparison approach, Wood (1985, 1989) suggested that comparison targets might even be constructed in one's imagination. Taylor and Lobel (1989) discuss how cancer patients sometimes invented downward comparison targets in an effort to adjust better to their condition. With the recognition that comparison others can be imaginary, the field is remote from the concept of situationally forced comparisons.

An emphasis on personality effects in social comparison accompanies the focus on coping (e.g., Allan & Gilbert, 1995). The type of comparison one makes may depend on one's personality (e.g., Baumeister, Tice, & Hutton, 1989), and people with low subjective well-being tend to make more unfavorable comparisons with others (e.g., Gilbert & Trower, 1990; Swallow & Kuiper, 1988). Swallow and Kuiper (1993) showed that nondepressed people used a self-protective downward comparison strategy, whereas dysphoric individuals did not. People with high self-esteem compare less to inferior others when they succeed (Wood, Giordano-Beech, Taylor, Michela, & Gaus, 1994). Fujita (1995) found a tendency of neurotics to compare themselves more frequently to others in a variety of domains, and VanderZee, Buunk, and Sanderman (1996) found that neurotics more often make upward comparisons. In a similar vein, Swallow and Kuiper (1990) found that mildly depressed persons showed a relatively strong interest in social comparison. Thus, making positive or negative comparisons, or making any comparisons at all, may often be a function of one's personality. A related topic is envy, a state in which people resent others who are perceived to have what they do not have (Smith, Parrott, Diener, Hoyle, & Kim, 1995). In this case, a predisposition to feelings of inferiority and hostility may figure prominently in the social comparisons that are made. McFarland and Miller (1994) found that optimists tend to make more positive comparisons as the size of the group grows. Optimists could more easily find a downward comparison target in a large group, and therefore were more likely to make a self-enhancing comparison when they were in large groups. In contrast, pessimists made more negative comparisons in larger groups. Although pessimists might find it hard to find an upward comparison target in a small group, they are more likely to find someone better off than they are in a large group. In other words, people with different personalities select differing targets with whom to compare as the availability of comparison targets changes. It also appears that people with different personalities focus either up or down when making social comparisons.

The coping model of social comparison indicates that people may gain inspiration from comparing upward, or may identify with a superior person. At the same time, unhappy people usually compare socially more and are likely to make comparisons that add to their dysphoria. People do not always obtain satisfaction by downward comparison, but may become discouraged by looking at unfortunate others. Finally, comparisons may not be computed accurately and may even be made with imaginary others. It is much more difficult to make simple predictions about levels of well-being from the coping approach than from the forced comparison model. As the model has come to reflect the complexity of actual coping, the simple situational approach has lost its force. Situational factors are seen as less powerful, and cognitive and personality factors have come to the fore.

An interesting question for future research is whether strategic comparisons have a causal influence on subjective well-being once global personality variables such as neuroticism and self-esteem are controlled. In such research, measurement error should be controlled through the use of multiple measures and latent trait analyses. A related research question is the degree to which the effects of global personality traits are mediated by social comparison processes. One important question is whether coping models of social comparison are completely descriptive and whether they can make predictions. The critical question, however, is whether selected comparisons influence subjective well-being or only follow from personality and subjective well-being.

## DO IMPOSED SOCIAL COMPARISONS EVER MATTER?

The evidence reviewed above indicates that imposed social comparisons often have little or no long-term impact on subjective well-being. This does not mean that social comparisons cannot have a long-term causal effect. For one thing, the social and cultural environment is likely, at least in part, to provide the information on which people base their goals. Thus, the social environment might influence subjective well-being by providing goals that differ in difficulty. Furthermore, social information from various sources may influence a person's self-evaluations. Social feedback of many different types (e.g., criticism from others, learning about a new product from others) might add together to influence subjective well-being. Following this line of reasoning, a "total environment" that greatly narrows the information that a person possesses might influence subjective well-being. In a provocative set of studies Marsh (1987; Marsh & Parker, 1984) explored the "big-fish-little-pond" effect. He found that students' academic self-concepts depended on the type of school in which they were enrolled. If students were enrolled in a high ability school, one in which the average standardized ability level of students was distinguished, they were likely to think less of their own academic abilities (controlling for ability level) than were students in low ability schools. Goethals and Darley (1987) vividly describe how a variety of social forces in the classroom can act in unison to shape a child's conception of his or her mental abilities. The teacher emphasizes the importance of doing well on class assignments, and children know how they and others are doing. The child has little other information by which to evaluate his or her performance, and grade rank-ordering occurs constantly. Comparative evaluations are often emphasized rather than progress or task mastery. In such a setting, social comparison may be so pervasive, and alternative sources of information so few, that comparative judgments become central to making satisfaction judgments. This description suggests that under some circumstances the imposed environment can influence a person's self-concept and probably his satisfaction as well.

Why are Marsh's findings on self-concept at odds with other data on imposed environmental influences on satisfaction? Perhaps lower schools more nearly approximate "total environments" (strongly controlling the information that the individual receives about the distribution of academic abilities, and also emphasizing feedback that has primarily a comparative meaning) than the environments examined in other forced comparison studies. For example, in the case of health, comparative information seems less relevant than in the case of school grades. People can determine if they are healthy (they feel energetic and have an absence of symptoms and pains) without any comparison to others, and physicians rarely make comparative judgments in assessing people's health.

An alternative explanation of why social comparison influences self-concept in the school studies is that satisfaction judgments are less subject to imposed environmental effects than are self-concept ratings. Individuals may be more influenced by their social surroundings in determining their ability level, for example, than in deciding their satisfaction with this ability. People may be motivated by hedonic reasons to be satisfied with their characteristics, and may use coping strategies such as downplaying the importance of an area to keep satisfaction high. Self-concept ratings may be less influenced by social comparison than satisfaction ratings because people can invoke an additional layer of protective cognitions (e.g., emphasizing other standards, downplaying the importance of the area) in determining their satisfaction. Exploration of these alternatives is important to shed light on when imposed comparisons might influence subjective well-being.

What we do know, however, is that social comparisons that are imposed by the natural social environment often do not influence long-term subjective well-being as was once thought. It appears that cognitive coping mechanisms are too flexible, hedonic seeking capacities too successful, and possible comparison others too diverse for imposed social comparisons to be the important and omnipresent influences on subjective well-being envisioned by Easterlin. In addition, processes such as attributions (e.g., "I must be really ill if I am living here with all these sick people"), "birds of a feather flock together" (Pelham & Wachsmuth, 1995), identity formation, and hedonic motivation may operate in opposite directions from the contrast form of social comparison.

Another interesting demonstration of social comparison influences is offered by the perception-of-risk studies reported by Klein and Weinstein (chapter 12, this volume). In these studies, subjects use social comparison information that they are given directly. In this case, subjects have no option of avoiding such information or selectively choosing comparison targets. The findings of Klein and Weinstein suggest that social comparison information will be used, at least in the short-term, when the situation is constrained so that they cannot avoid this information. A future challenge obviously is to determine under what circumstances personality and coping processes predominate, and in what situations imposed social information is likely to influence subjective well-being.

## CONCLUSIONS

People may use social comparisons in a flexible and strategic way to cope with situations and enhance their subjective well-being. The flexibility of the cognitive system means that only in special circumstances might the environment force a satisfaction standard on an individual for a long period of time. In addition to carefully choosing comparison others, people can base their satisfaction on alternative standards such as their own goals, culturally prescribed ideals, physiological drive states, the ease of thinking of counterfactual situations (Miller & Prentice, 1996), their past levels of achievement, affective reactions, and so forth. Furthermore, in many domains such as health, standards other than social comparison may be most relevant to a person's goals. Miller and Prentice hypothesized that victims of illness generate alternative worlds, and it is to these worlds rather than to other people that these individuals compare their outcomes.

Imposed social comparisons are unlikely to have long-term effects except possibly in the situation where a total environment imposes a standard that is adopted by virtually everyone. In this instance, social comparison and cultural norms may be indistinguishable, and the individual might be unable to avoid such standards even with adaptive cognitive coping mechanisms. In most situations, however, it appears that flexible coping can overcome imposed social information, as is evidenced by the coping behavior of cancer patients reviewed in this volume. What of our intuitions that we sometimes make comparisons that harm or benefit our moods? Although this undoubtedly occurs, it now appears that imposed social comparisons often have only short-term effects on mood and momentary satisfaction, and usually do not have a long-lasting influence on subjective well-being.

One intriguing idea is that imposed social comparisons and comparisons selected by the individual might work together. People may be below average in a distribution but still select people who are below them with whom to compare. Nevertheless, the imposed environment may place some constraints on the availability of comparison others. Thus, examining the availability of comparison targets in combination with who is selected in natural settings is a promising avenue of future research. Another important avenue for future research is to determine how social comparison standards interact with other standards such as one's past, one's goals, and one's ideals in creating levels of subjective well-being. Of particular interest is how social information influences these other standards.

In determining how social comparisons influence subjective well-being, several interesting questions confront researchers. To the question of whether social comparisons can influence one's current mood, laboratory studies yield an unequivocal yes. Regarding the question of whether the social surrounding automatically imposes comparison standards that cause a person's well-being, the answer seems to be no. Nevertheless, there are likely to be situations where the social environment does force information on the person that can influence subjective well-being, but the determinants of when this is likely to occur are unknown. One likely possibility is that social information can influence satisfaction when it influences a person's goals. Finally, there is the question of whether the person's actively chosen comparison others can affect subjective well-being. Although the data are promising, the case for the causal influence of these comparisons is not yet strong.

## ACKNOWLEDGMENTS

We extend thanks to Joanne Wood, Richard Smith, M. Joseph Sirgy, Bram Buunk, Howard Leventhal, and Frederick X. Gibbons for their helpful comments on this chapter.

## REFERENCES


Alicke, M. D., Klotz, M. L., Breitenbecher, D. L., Yurak, T. J., & Vredenburg, D. S. (1995). Personal contact, individuation, and the better-than-average effect. *Journal of Personality and Social Psychology, 68,* 804–825.

Allan, S., & Gilbert, P. (1995). A social comparison scale: Psychometric properties and relationship to psychopathology. *Personality and Individual Differences, 19,* 293–299.

Baumeister, R. F., Tice, D. M., & Hutton, D. G. (1989). Self-presentational motivations and personality differences in self-esteem. *Journal of Personality, 57,* 547–579.

Brickman, P., & Campbell, D. T. (1971). Hedonic relativism and planning the good society. In M. H. Appley (Ed.), *Adaptation level theory: A symposium* (pp. 287–302). New York: Academic Press.

Brown, J. D., & Dutton, K. A. (1995). Truth and consequences: The costs and benefits of accurate self-knowledge. *Personality and Social Psychology Bulletin, 21,* 1288–1296.

Brown, J. D., Novick, N. J., & Kelley, A. (1992). When Gulliver travels: Social context, psychological closeness, and self-appraisals. *Journal of Personality and Social Psychology, 62,* 717–727.

Buunk, B. P., Collins, R. L., Taylor, S. E., Van Yperen, N. W., & Dakof, G. A. (1990). The affective consequences of social comparison: Either direction has its up and downs. *Journal of Personality and Social Psychology, 59,* 1238–1249.

Crosby, F. (1976). A model of egoistical relative deprivation. *Psychological Review, 83,* 85–113.

DeVellis, R. F., Holt, K., Renner, B. R., Blalock, S. J., Blanchard, L. W., Cook, H. L., Klotz, M. L., Mikow, V., & Harring, K. (1990). The relationship of social comparison to rheumatoid arthritis symptoms and affect. *Basic and Applied Social Psychology, 11,* 1–18.

Diener, E., & Diener, C. (1996). Most people are happy. *Psychological Science, 7,* 181–185.

Diener, E., Diener, M., & Diener, C. (1995). Factors predicting the subjective well-being of nations. *Journal of Personality and Social Psychology, 69,* 851–864.

Diener, E., & Fujita, F. (1995). Resources, personal strivings, and subjective well-being: A nomothetic and ideographic approach. *Journal of Personality and Social Psychology, 68,* 926–935.

Diener, E., Sandvik, E., Seidlitz, L., & Diener, M. (1993). The relationship between income and subjective well-being: Relative or absolute? *Social Indicators Research, 28,* 195–223.

Duncan, O. D. (1975). Does money buy satisfaction? *Social Indicators Research, 2,* 267–274.

Dunning, D., Meyerowitz, J. A., & Holzberg, A. D. (1989). Ambiguity and self-evaluation: The role of idiosyncratic trait definitions in self-serving assessments of ability. *Journal of Personality and Social Psychology, 57,* 1082–1090.

Easterlin, R. A. (1974). Does economic growth improve the human lot? Some empirical evidence. In D. Reder (Ed.), *Nations and households in economic growth* (pp. 89–125). New York: Academic Press.

Emmons, R. A., & Diener, E. (1985). Factors predicting satisfaction judgments: A comparative examination. *Social Indicators Research, 16,* 157–167.

Festinger, L. (1954). A theory of social comparison processes. *Human Relations, 7,* 117–140.

Fox, C. R., & Kahneman, D. (1992). Correlations, causes and heuristics in surveys of life satisfaction. *Social Indicators Research, 27,* 221–234.

Freedman, J. (1978). *Happy people.* New York: Harcourt Brace Jovanovich.

Fujita, F. (1993). *The effects of naturalistic social comparison on satisfaction with life domains.* Unpublished doctoral dissertation, University of Illinois, Urbana-Champaign.

Fujita, F. (1995, October). *There are two kinds of people in the world: Those who engage in social comparison and those who do not.* Paper presented at the University of Illinois, Urbana-Champaign.

Gallup, G. (1976–1977). Human needs and satisfactions: A global survey. *Public Opinion Quarterly, 40,* 459–467.

Gibbons, F. X., Benbow, C. P., & Gerrard, M. (1994). From top dog to bottom half: Social comparison strategies in response to poor performance. *Journal of Personality and Social Psychology, 67,* 638–652.

Gilbert, P., & Trower, P. (1990). The evolution and manifestation of social anxiety. In W. R. Crozier (Ed.), *Shyness and embarrassment: Perspectives from social psychology* (pp. 144–177). Cambridge, UK: Cambridge University Press.

Goethals, G. R., & Darley, J. M. (1987). Social comparison theory: Self-evaluation and group life. In B. Mullen & G. R. Goethals (Eds.), *Theories of group behavior* (pp. 21–47). New York: Springer-Verlag.

Headey, B., & Wearing, A. (1988). The sense of relative superiority–Central to well-being. *Social Indicators Research, 20,* 497–516.

Helgeson, V. S., & Michelson, K. D. (1995). Motives for social comparison. *Personality and Social Psychology Bulletin, 21,* 1200–1209.

Johnson, T. P., O'Rourke, D., Chavez, N., Sudman, S., Warnecke, R., Lacey, L., & Horm, J. (1995, April). *Social cognition and responses to survey questions among culturally diverse populations.* Paper presented at the International Conference on Survey Measurement and Process Quality, Bristol, England.

Kapteyn, A., & Wansbeek, T. (1982). Empirical evidence on preference formation. *Journal of Economic Psychology, 2,* 137–154.

Kapteyn, A., Wansbeek, T. J., & Buyze, J. (1980). The dynamics of preference formation. *Journal of Economic Behavior and Organization, 1,* 123–157.

Kruglanski, A. W., & Mayseless, O. (1990). Classic and current social comparison research: Expanding the perspective. *Psychological Bulletin, 108,* 195–208.

Marsh, H. W. (1987). The big-fish-little-pond effect on academic self-concept. *Journal of Educational Psychology, 79,* 280–295.

Marsh, H. W., & Parker, J. W. (1984). Determinants of student self-concept: Is it better to be a relatively large fish in a small pond even if you don't learn to swim as well? *Journal of Personality and Social Psychology, 47,* 213–231.

Matlin, M. W., & Stang, D. J. (1978). *The Pollyanna Principle: Selectivity in language, memory, and thought.* Cambridge, MA: Schenkman.

McFarland, C., & Miller, D. T. (1994). The framing of relative performance feedback: Seeing the glass as half empty or half full. *Journal of Personality and Social Psychology, 66,* 1061–1073.

Merton, R. K., & Kitt, A. S. (1950). Contributions to the theory of reference group behavior. In R. K. Merton & P. F. Lazarsfeld (Eds.), *Continuities in social research: Studies in the scope and method of "the American soldier"* (pp. 40–105). Glencoe, IL: Free Press.

Michalos, A. C. (1985). Multiple discrepancies theory (MDT). *Social Indicators Research, 16,* 347–413.

Michalos, A. C. (1991). *Global report on student well-being. Vol. I: Life satisfaction and happiness.* New York: Springer-Verlag.

Michalos, A. C. (1993). *Global report on student well-being. Vol. IV: Religion, education, recreation, and health.* New York: Springer-Verlag.

Miller, D. T., & Prentice, D. A. (1996). The construction of social norms and standards. In E. T. Higgins & A. W. Kruglanski (Eds.), *Social psychology: Handbook of basic principles* (pp. 799–829). New York: Guilford.

Olson, J. M., Herman, C. P., & Zanna, M. P. (Eds.). (1986). *Relative deprivation and social comparison: The Ontario symposium.* Hillsdale, NJ: Lawrence Erlbaum Associates.

Parducci, A. (1984). Value judgments: Toward a relational theory of happiness. In R. Eister (Ed.), *Attitudinal judgment* (pp. 3-21). New York: Springer.

Parducci, A. (1995). *Happiness, pleasure, and judgment: The contextual theory and its applica-*

*tions.* Mahwah, NJ: Lawrence Erlbaum Associates.

Pelham, B. W., & Wachsmuth, J. D. (1995). The waxing and waning of the social self: Assimilation and contrast in social comparison. *Journal of Personality and Social Psychology, 69,* 825–838.

Samuelson, R. J. (1995). *The good life and its discontents.* New York: Random House.

Schwarz, N., Hippler, H. J., Deutsch, B., & Strack, F. (1985). Response scales: Effects of category range on reported behavior and comparative judgments. *Public Opinion Quarterly, 49,* 388–395.

Schwarz, N., Mathiowetz, N., & Belli, R. F. (1996). *Assessing satisfaction with health and health care: Cognitive and communicative processes.* In R. Warnecke (Ed.), *Health survey research method* (pp. 21–24). Hyattsville, MD: National Center for Health Statistics (DHHS Publication No. PHS 96-103).

Schwarz, N., & Scheuring, B. (1988). Judgments of relationship satisfaction: Inter- and intraindividual comparisons as a function of questionnaire structure. *European Journal of Social Psychology, 18,* 485–496.

Schwarz, N., & Scheuring, B. (1992). Selbstberichtete Verhaltens- und Symptomhaufigkeiten: Was Befragte aus Anworthvorgaben des Fragebogens lernen. *Zeitschrift fur Klinische Psychologie, 22,* 197–208.

Sirgy, M. J. (1986). *Self-congruity: Toward a theory of personality and cybernetics.* New York: Praeger.

Sirgy, M. J. (1990). Self-cybernetics: Toward an integrated model of self-concept processes. *Systems Research, 7,* 19–32.

Sirgy, M. J., Cole, D., Kosenko, R., Meadow, H. L., Rahtz, D., Cicic, M., Jin, G. X., Yarsuvat, D., Blenkhorn, D. L., & Nagpal, N. (1995). A life satisfaction measure: Additional validational data for the congruity of life satisfaction measure. *Social Indicators Research, 34,* 237–259.

Smith, R. H., Diener, E., & Wedell, D. (1989). The range-frequency model of happiness applied to temporal and social comparisons. *Journal of Personality and Social Psychology, 56,* 317–325.

Smith, R., Parrot, G., Diener, E., Hoyle, R. H., & Kim, S. H. (1995). *Dispositional envy.* Manuscript in preparation.

Strack, F., Schwarz, N., Chassein, B., Kern, D., & Wagner, D. (1990). The salience of comparison standards and the activation of social norms: Consequences for judgements of happiness and their communication. *British Journal of Social Psychology, 29,* 303–314.

Swallow, S. R., & Kuiper, N. A. (1988). Social comparison and negative self evaluation: An application to depression. *Clinical Psychology Review, 8,* 55–76.

Swallow, S. R., & Kuiper, N. A. (1990). Mild depression, dysfunctional cognitions, and interest in social comparison information. *Journal of Social & Clinical Psychology, 9,* 289–302.

Swallow, S. R., & Kuiper, N. A. (1993). Social comparison in dysphoria and nondysphoria: Differences in target similarity and specificity. *Cognitive Therapy and Research, 17,* 103–122.

Taylor, S. E., & Brown, J. D. (1988). Illusion and well-being: A social psychological perspective on mental health. *Psychological Bulletin, 103,* 193–210.

Taylor, S. E., & Lobel, M. (1989). Social comparison activity under threat: Downward evaluation and upward contacts. *Psychological Review, 96,* 569–575.

VanderZee, K. I., Buunk, B. P., & Sanderman, R. (1996). The relationship between social comparison processes and personality. *Personality and Individual Differences, 22,* 551–565.

Veenhoven, R. (1991). Is happiness relative? *Social Indicators Research, 24,* 1–34.

Wills, T. A. (1981). Downward comparison principles in social psychology. *Psychological Bulletin, 90,* 245–271.

Wood, J. V. (1985). Social comparison in adjustment to breast cancer. *Dissertation Abstracts*

*International,* March, Volume 45 (9-B), 3090–3091.

Wood, J. V. (1989). Theory and research concerning social comparisons of personal attributes. *Psychological Bulletin, 106,* 231–248.

Wood, J. V. (1996). What is social comparison and how should we study it? *Personality and Social Psychology Bulletin, 22,* 520–537.

Wood, J. V., Giordano-Beech, M., Taylor, K. L., Michela, J. L., & Gaus, V. (1994). Strategies of social comparison among people with low self-esteem: Self-protection and self-enhancement. *Journal of Personality and Social Psychology, 67,* 713–731.

Wright, S. J. (1985). Health satisfaction: A detailed test of the multiple discrepancies theory model. *Social Indicators Research, 17,* 299–313.

# CHAPTER 12

# Social Comparisons and Occupational Stress: The Identification–Contrast Model

Bram P. Buunk
Jan F. Ybema
*University of Groningen*

Work plays a very important symbolic role in the lives of most people in our society. Being employed not only entails making a living but implies that one is part of a social network and participates in society as a whole. Even more important, the work sphere is the main area of life in which people may attain prestige, recognition, and self-esteem. Precisely because of this central place of work in life, work can be very frustrating and upsetting when people do not obtain the goals they have set for themselves. There is an extensive literature showing that the work situation can contain a variety of stressors, including lack of career prospects, lack of control, time pressure, role ambiguity, uncertainty about the future, and interpersonal conflicts (see, e.g., Cooper & Payne, 1988; Karasek & Theorell, 1990), and that the impact of such stressors on well-being can be rather serious. Job stress may affect mental health and may lead to burnout, depression, and psychosomatic complaints (e.g., Fletcher, 1988; Schaufeli & Buunk, 1986; Warr, 1987). It may affect physical health, in particular coronary heart disease (e.g., Marmot, 1994; Siegrist & Peter, 1994), and may in general lead to sick leaves and disability (e.g., Kompier et al., 1990).

Most work-related stress is caused by social factors. Although this is not always made explicit, many of the factors that make a situation at work stressful are social in nature. It can be assumed that in general, people in social groups try to fulfill two major needs: first, the need for a sense of belonging, the wish to be part of a group in which one feels safe and accepted, and the establishment of positive emotional bonds with others. We refer to this as the need for *connectedness*. The second major need—and the one on which this chapter focuses—is *status*. The need for status is conceived here rather broadly, encompassing the striving for positive self-esteem by performing well on certain dimensions, winning competitions with others, and seeking appreciation and prestige from others. Depression and the physiological changes that accompany it have in general been linked to a loss either of connectedness or status or both (Gilbert, 1988). Most potential stressors at work imply a threat to the fulfillment of one or both of these needs. For instance, interpersonal conflicts threaten people's ability to satisfy their need for connectedness by forming harmonious bonds with their co-workers. Lack of career prospects make it difficult to attain higher status and more prestige. A role conflict may interfere with maintaining a smooth relationship with co-workers, thus frustrating the connectedness need, and it may threaten one's reputation as a competent person, interfering with fulfillment of the status need. And, of course, loss of a job due either to forced unemployment or disability, seriously threatens the needs both for connectedness and for status. In fact, in our society losing one's job usually implies a serious loss in postive emotional bonds, appreciation from others, and concomitantly, self-esteem.

In this chapter we examine first how occupational stress, and in particular, uncertainty, instigates a desire to obtain social comparison information, for example, information about what similar others feel and think, and a desire for contact with such others. This type of comparison refers in particular back to the work of Schachter (1959), and, as we show, may lead to adapting one's stress responses to those of other group members. Next we examine comparison choice: with whom do individuals want to affiliate and about whom do they want to learn more? With respect to this issue, we point to a number of contradictory findings in the literature. To reconcile such findings, we present our identification-contrast model, which maintains that individuals prefer to identify upward but to contrast themselves downward. We outline the way stress may activate a coping process through which individuals aim to restore their self-esteem by identifying with others better off and by finding ways to feel that they are doing—at least in some ways—better than others. Although we focus primarily on the work setting, we think our identification-contrast model has a broader scope, applying to social comparison processes as they occur in a variety of other settings, and most notably in health-related situations.

## SOCIAL COMPARISONS IN RESPONSE TO STRESS AND UNCERTAINTY

The need for connectedness implies that humans are extremely social animals, who tend to seek support from others and to use others' responses to decide how to respond themselves to new and threatening situations. Young children look for their mother for guidance when confronted with a new stimulus, and adults seek out the company of others when faced with danger and threat. Such tendencies are not coincidental, but reflect adaptive evolutionary strategies. Shaver and Klinnert (1982) and Cottrell and Epley (1977) reviewed many studies among human beings and other primates that show that adults in these species, when confronted with a stressful stimulus, experience less distress when they are with familiar others. Within social psychology, Schachter (1959) was probably the first to suggest that fear enhances affiliative tendencies owing especially to the uncertainty inherent in many stressful situations. Schachter suggested that fear of an electric shock induces a desire for social comparison because individuals confronted with such a new and threatening situation feel a need to know what the most appropriate response is. According to Schachter (1959), "the emotions or feelings, like the opinions and abilities, require social evaluation when the emotion producing situation is ambiguous or uninterpretable in terms of past experience" (p. 129). Several experiments following Schachter's paradigm showed that affiliative needs are indeed aroused when individuals feel uncertain about how to feel and react (e.g., Gerard, 1963; Gerard & Rabbie, 1961), or when the source of their arousal was unknown (Mills & Mintz, 1972). Moreover, Singer and Shockley (1965) showed that individuals who received no information about how others had done on an ability test, and as a result were uncertain about their standing on the ability dimension, preferred to affiliate with others more than did individuals who had received such norm information.

Remarkably, although uncertainty is considered to be a characteristic aspect of stressful events (e.g., Lazarus & Folkman, 1984), little research has been done to determine whether uncertainty about one's feelings, beliefs, and responses fosters the need for affiliation among individuals experiencing stress in occupational settings (Buunk, 1994). Nursing is a profession in which uncertainty is rather common (e.g., McGrath, Reid, & Boore, 1989). For example, nurses may wonder if they are too involved with patients or not involved enough, they may feel uncertain how to deal with patients' varying problems, including appeals for help and expressions of anxiety, and they may experience uncertainties about whether they are doing things correctly. Cherniss (1980) considered "doubts about competence" to be a major source of stress that can lead to burnout in human services professionals, particularly in the early stages of their careers. In the same vein, Gray-Toft and Anderson (1981) found that "inadequate preparation" and "uncertainty concerning treatment" were among the most severe stressors in nursing.

Buunk, Schaufeli, and Ybema (1994) examined the role of social comparison in coping with uncertainty in a sample of registered nurses from various health care institutions. With respect to the measurement of the desire for social comparison, it was assumed that individuals would be interested in comparing their work-related feelings and the way they responded to various situations at work with those of similar others. Such an interest can be met, for instance, by observing others, by reading about how others are doing, or by trying to assess how others behave and react (e.g., Taylor & Lobel, 1989). But who are these similar others? Some authors have suggested that in this context similarity should reside primarily in personality characteristics (Miller & Zimbardo, 1966) or in level of emotional intensity (Dabbs & Helmreich, 1966). But both the experimental literature on stress and affiliation and field research on social comparison information (e.g., DeVellis et al., 1990; Molleman, Pruyn, & Van Knippenberg, 1986) generally emphasize situational similarity, that is, comparison with others facing the same stress is focused on. In line with this operationalization, the desire for social comparison was operationalized as interest in how others in a similar situation think and feel. To see whether uncertainty had an effect on this desire that was independent of an effect of distress in general, the study included the burnout scale of Maslach and Jackson (1982), which consists of three dimensions: *emotional exhaustion* (i.e., the depletion or draining of emotional resources), *depersonalization* (a negative, callous, and cynical attitude toward the recipients of one's care), and *reduced personal accomplishment* (the tendency to evaluate oneself negatively with regard to one's accomplishments at work). The results showed that emotional exhaustion and uncertainty made additive and independent contributions to the desire for social comparison. Depersonalization and reduced personal accomplishment were not independently related to this desire (Buunk et al., 1994). Why would people want to compare their emotional distress rather than their opinions (depersonalization) and abilities (reduced personal accomplishment)? It is possible that comparisons on the last two dimensions are likely to put one in a bad light, and people may be unlikely to share with others that they feel they are not doing well. For example, if a nurse confides to other nurses that he has ceased to regard his patients as human beings, this would be sure to elicit some sort of negative and perhaps critical reaction. Thus, comparisons on these dimensions might lead to a lowering of one's status.

In a study by Buunk (1995) among individuals affected by the Netherlands Disablement Insurance Act, the association between social comparison needs and uncertainty was explored again. In the early 1990s in The Netherlands, around 900,000 individuals were receiving disability payments under this act. Since the mid-1970s, mental health problems have become the cause for disablement among an increasing percentage of new cases. Recently, people have become increasingly aware that the system has to be changed, and various proposals have been put forward to limit the number of people who are diagnosed as disabled for work. In mid-1991, a new law was proposed by the government that suggested making payments under the Disablement Insurance Act dependent on the person's duration of employment, and freezing payments for those under 50 who were then receiving disability payments. This proposal generated extensive public discussion and various forms of political protest, as well as frustration and uncertainty about their financial future among those currently falling under the act. The research by Buunk (1995) was conducted in precisely this period, thus offering a unique opportunity to examine social comparison processes under stress and uncertainty. Not only was the desire for social comparison information assessed—that is, the desire to obtain information about the feelings and opinions of other individuals receiving disability payments—but also the desire for affiliation, focusing on the desire to discuss one's viewpoints with others in a similar situation. Although both social comparison measures were highly correlated, the desire for social comparison information was in general stronger than the desire for affiliation. Apparently, individuals under stress like to know how others are doing but are more or less reluctant to engage in a direct interaction in which they have to share their experiences with another person because this might be painful (see Brickman & Bulman, 1977). Furthermore, the results clearly showed that uncertainty and frustration, but not health problems, were related to both indices of social comparison. Thus, in this sample, not health problems, but psychological distress was related to a desire for affiliation and for comparison information.

## EFFECTS OF SOCIAL COMPARISON AND AFFILIATION UNDER STRESS

Affiliating with others when one is faced with stress and uncertainty will not necessarily lead to a decrease in stress. Even when one feels connected with supportive others, stress may increase rather than decrease. For example, a study by Buunk, Janssen, and VanYperen (1989) showed that in a number of high stressor work units, strongly supportive relationships with colleagues were related to a higher prevalence of stress symptoms. One of the explanations for this finding was that in supportive relationships people communicate with each other a lot, and this may lead to the aggravation of stress. Research on group polarization would suggest that individuals who engage in a discussion of certain work problems in a group in which a negative view of these problems predominates will have developed a more negative view after the discussion. Social comparison processes and new arguments provided by the other group members both seem to play a role in such situations (Myers & Lamm, 1976). Thus, through a process of information exchange and social comparison, persons may become more convinced of the fact that their situation is bad, develop negative feelings such as anger or fear and, consequently, become distressed. In line with this reasoning, Geurts, Buunk, and Schaufeli (1994b) found that blue collar employees who experienced health complaints and communicated about work problems with their colleagues tended to attribute their health complaints to the work situation. This attribution was associated with the perception of being worse off than others outside the company, which affected sick leaves; we discuss this later in greater detail.

Other individuals may not only influence the perception of stressors, and thereby stress reactions, but may also have a direct influence on these reactions by acting as models showing certain symptoms that others then imitate. The classical experiments of Schachter and Singer (1962) showed that artificially induced arousal makes it more likely that people will imitate the reactions of others who are in the same situation. In a similar vein, Pennebaker and his colleagues (Pennebaker & Brittingham, 1982; Skelton & Pennebaker, 1982) have, in a series of experiments, shown that various physical symptoms, including scratching, coughing, and flu symptoms may be adopted from others. Skelton and Pennebaker (1982) suggested that persons under stress may develop hypotheses about having certain diseases, begin examining themselves for symptoms, and thus, through self-fulfilling prophecies, develop psychosomatic complaints. Sullins (1991) showed that social comparison (observing another individual about to undergo the same experiment) induced mood convergence even in the absence of verbal communication. Moreover, negative moods appeared to be more contagious than positive moods, suggesting that stress symptoms would be likely candidates for social influence. Suls, Leventhal, and Martin (chapter 7, this volume) describe how social comparisons may lead to the adoption of symptoms from others. As they note, case studies on mass psychogenic illness in organizations illustrate that through a process of behavioral contagion in cohesive groups, fairly severe physical symptoms, including fainting and nausea, may be spread to others within minutes or hours (Colligan, 1985). Again, being closely connected to others may increase rather than decrease stress.

Although mass psychogenic illness involves the short-term development of symptoms, some recent studies suggest that also the longer-term development of professional burnout may be affected by the perception of similiar symptoms in co-workers. Edelwich and Brodsky (1980, p. 25) noted that burnout in human services is like "staph infection in hospitals: it gets around. It spreads from clients to staff, from one staff member to another, and from staff back to clients. Perhaps it should be called 'staff infection'." And indeed, Miller, Stiff, and Ellis (1988) found some evidence for contagion as a precursor to burnout among human service workers. In a similar vein, Golembiewski and Munzenrider (1988) describe two large-scale studies showing that between 70% and 86% of the employees classified as burn-out were in work groups at least 50% of whose membership were in the most extreme phases of burnout. These investigators conclude that work groups have a tendency to develop homogeneous levels of burnout. Finally, Buunk and Schaufeli (1993) found that nurses who had a strong desire for social comparison expressed a higher level of emotional exhaustion when they perceived that many of their colleagues showed burnout symptoms. The fact that this interaction effect was observed only with respect to emotional exhaustion and not with regard to depersonalization or personal accomplishment supports the validity of the emotional contagion explanation. Of course, it must be noted that none of the studies quoted shows unequivocally that among nurses with a high need for social comparison burnout is caused by the perception of burnout in others. It is also possible that, as the literature on false consensus (e.g., Goethals, 1986) and social projection (e.g., Miller, Gross, & Holtz, 1991) would suggest, these nurses project their burnout onto others as a way of validating the fact that they are burned out themselves. Whatever the precise mechanism, the perception that others have similar symptoms may act to support the persistence of one's own burnout symptoms, and it seems likely that this applies to a variety of health problems.

## DIRECTION OF AFFILIATION AND INFORMATION SEEKING UNDER STRESS

Do individuals faced with occupational stress and uncertainty prefer information about, and affiliation with, others doing worse or others doing better than they are doing themselves? Or do they prefer lateral comparisons? Taylor and Lobel (1989) argued that individuals under stress avoid contact with and information about persons who are doing worse, and that these stressed people prefer to affiliate with and learn more about persons who are doing better. According to Taylor and

Lobel, such contact may provide a person with valuable information for potential long-term survival and successful coping and may constitute a method for meeting emotional needs by providing hope, motivation and inspiration and by increasing morale. As also noted by Wood and VanderZee (chapter 10, this volume), not all evidence is directly compatible with this model, and we present the identification–contrast model to reconcile the Taylor and Lobel model with a number of contradictory findings.

A number of studies conducted outside organizational settings are in line with the assumptions of Taylor and Lobel (1989). In some early studies, an aversion to contact with worse-off others had been found, particularly among those under stress (e.g., Gerard, 1963; Rabbie, 1963), and there is also more direct evidence for an enhanced upward-information preference under stress. An early experiment by Thornton and Arrowood (1966) showed that when confronted with a threat, most individuals belonging to the worst-off group preferred to seek out others who were better off rather than worse off than they were themselves. Miller and Suls (1977) found that the tendency to choose partners who possess at least somewhat higher ability than oneself was particularly strong in subjects who had received feedback that they had performed at an average or below average level. In addition, Wheeler and Miyake (1992) found that respondents compared upward when they felt bad, and downward when they felt good. Finally, some studies suggest that the upward drive is particularly activated in situations were there is some need or motivation to do better (cf. Nosanchuck & Erickson, 1985; Ybema & Buunk, 1993).

Nevertheless, there is also a body of field and experimental research that indicates that when under threat, individuals prefer downward comparison information. For example, a study by DeVellis et al. (1991) showed that arthritis patients more often preferred to read about another patient who had worse arthritis than they had, supposedly because this would make them feel better. In their research on support groups, Gibbons and Gerrard (1991) found evidence that subjects with fairly serious problems such as eating disorders and smoking preferred groups that included others who had more serious problems than they had themselves. Pyszczynski, Greenberg, and LaPrelle (1985) found that subjects who had failed a test requested more information on the performance of other subjects, when they expected this to reveal that most others performed poorly than when they expected it to reveal that most others had performed well. Those who had succeeded showed little interest in this additional information, regardless of their expectancies as to what it would reveal. In a similar vein, Swallow and Kuiper

(1993) found more downward preferences among individuals evaluating their performance as poor than among those evaluating their performance as well, a pattern that was especially pronounced among nondysphoric subjects. Friend and Gilbert (1973) showed that individuals threatened by failure on a test were more inclined to avoid information about better off others than individuals who had done well.

When examining current theorizing on social comparison under stress and the available evidence three more or less competing hypotheses can be formulated. The *self-enhancement* hypothesis proposed by Wills (1981) would suggest that individuals under stress will prefer information about and affiliation with others doing worse. The *self-improvement* hypothesis as put forward by Taylor and Lobel (1989) would predict that those under more stress feel a stronger need to learn from others and therefore feel a relatively stronger interest in information about and contact with others doing better, despite the fact that such comparisons might be painful. The *self-protection* hypothesis would predict that although those under stress would prefer upward comparisons, this preference would be reduced by the fact that confrontation with others doing better would be more painful for such individuals. Therefore, individuals under stress would prefer comparisons with others who perform slightly better rather than with others performing much better than oneself. In a study testing these last two hypotheses in particular, Buunk et al. (1994) asked nurses to what extent they wanted to learn more about and affiliate with others who were more competent and experienced than they were themselves. Most preferred lateral or upward comparisons, and virtually nobody was interested in social comparison with others less competent or less experienced. Unlike the result that would be predicted by Wills (1981), even those under stress generally preferred upward comparisons. However, evidence was found for self-protection among those under stress: nurses who scored high in emotional exhaustion and in reduced personal accomplishment (see page 362) preferred relatively less upward information. Apparently, those high in stress prefer information about others doing better, provided that these others are not doing too well.

## THE DRIVE TO PERCEIVED SUPERIORITY: THE IDENTIFICATION–CONTRAST MODEL

How is the clear preference for upward comparisons, even among those under stress in the study of Buunk et al. (1994), compatible with the findings of studies such as those by DeVellis et al. (1991), Pyszczynski et al. (1985), and Swallow and Kuiper (1993) who found evidence for a preference for downward comparisons among those who failed? And why is the upward preference, contrary to what Taylor and Lobel (1989) would predict, not especially enhanced among those under stress but rather lowered? The social comparison literature is plagued by such discrepant findings, and various authors have aimed to provide syntheses of these contradictions, for instance by pointing to the different measures that have been used (Taylor & Lobel, 1989), and by illuminating the different motives that social comparisons may serve (Wood, 1989). We would like to suggest that many discrepant findings in the social comparison literature can be understood from the perspective of our *identification–contrast model.* This model expands that presented in our article on "either direction has its ups and downs" (Buunk, Collins, Taylor, VanYperen, & Dakof, 1990), and borrows elements from a number of other models in the social comparison field, most notably those of Taylor and Lobel (1989), Mettee and Smith (1977), Tesser (1988), and the original work of Heider (1958) on responses to the lot of the other. Our model holds that people are in general motivated to identify themselves with others doing better, that is, to focus on the similarities between themselves and the better-off other, to recognize things of themselves in the other, and to regard the others' position as similar or attainable for themselves. Whereas upward identification will evoke positive affect, identification with worse-off others may be painful, and may therefore be avoided. Even more so, individuals are motivated to contrast themselves with others doing worse, that is, to focus on differences with the comparison other and on their own superiority.

The identification–contrast model links such social comparison perspectives to evolutionary psychology. As noted by Gilbert, Price, and Allan (1995), because of the adaptive value of adequately sizing up one's competitors, the need to compare self with others is phylogenetically very old, biologically very powerful, and recognizable in many respects. The identification–contrast model assumes that human beings compete with each other for status and prestige in groups. Individuals have a deeply rooted tendency to try to find ways in which they can attract attention and appreciation from others, and can develop what has been referred to as "social attention holding potential" (Gilbert, 1990). Moreover, human beings try to reach a state in which they feel that they are in some respects more attractive and talented than other group members. From an evolutionary perspective, this search for symbolic dominance over others is the translation of the physical struggle among primates for social dominance in a group. As noted by Barkow (1989), human beings have evolved a strong desire to develop positive self-esteem by assigning themselves symbolic prestige and status in their reference group. Such a reference group need not actually be present and may even be cognitively constructed: "With human self-esteem . . . others not only need not be physically present, they need not have physical existence" (p. 191). In the course of evolution, humans have developed the potential for self-deception and cognitive distortions in building a positive self-concept. Evolutionary psychology provides a different perspective on the drive upward in the theory of Festinger (1954), and views this drive as an inherent part of the evolution of human beings into a species that, in part, uses symbolic, internal means to attain prestige in a social group.

The identification–contrast model assumes that human beings are strongly motivated to develop and maintain a self-concept according to which they are at least on some important dimensions doing better than most others in their chosen reference group (cf. Tesser, 1988). Cognitive processes such as selective memory, differential availability of information, and biased information processing may partly explain how this motivation is satisfied. We assume that when individuals are confronted with a stressful event, their sense of relative superiority is violated, and they have a need to re-establish such a self-perception. This upward drive leads to an asymmetry in the perception of upward and downward comparison information. Early studies on performance and ability information showed that individuals preferred upward comparisons in part to confirm that they were similar to the better-off other (Wheeler, 1966; see also Mettee & Smith, 1977). As we found in our studies, and as other researchers have reported (e.g., DeVellis et al., 1991), even individuals under stress have a very strong resistance to acknowledging the superiority of others but find it quite easy to admit that others are inferior to them. In general, and probably also when under stress, individuals are keen on avoiding identification with worse-off others, and will try to contrast themselves with these others. However, they will—as much as reality permits—try to identify with others doing better and see these others as similar to themselves. When individuals identify with a comparison target, they focus on the similarities between themselves and the target, which means that they may regard the position of the other as their own future. On the other hand, when individuals contrast themselves, they focus on differences and may regard the other's position as a standard for themselves. By identifying with others doing better, individuals attain a number of things; for example, the feeling of belonging to the best in their reference group, the vicarious or actual attention that is bestowed on the high status others, the alliance of such others, and the potential of self-improvement by learning from others who are doing better (cf. Gilbert, 1990). Thus, identification may fulfill the earlier mentioned need for connectedness as well as the need for status.

The identification–contrast model assumes that for individuals under stress there is no general preference for downward or upward comparisons and that neither direction of comparison in itself leads to positive or negative affect. Rather, such preferences and consequences depend on the extent to which a particular social comparison can be construed as supporting a positive self-concept. When individuals confronted with a threat seek out comparison information, and when they are confronted with such information, they will prefer upward comparisons when these comparisons offer the opportunity for identification rather than contrast with the comparison other. In contrast, a downward comparison will be more attractive when it offers the opportunity for contrast and not for identification. Indeed, Aspinwall (chapter 5, this volume) has argued that downward comparisons will be particularly threatening and upward comparisons stimulating when they imply that one could become like the comparison other; that is, when there is a high identification with that other. In addition, the argument of Gibbons and Gerrard (chapter 2, this volume) that individuals distance themselves from prototypical others who show health risk behavior as a way of coping with health threats is in line with our suggestion that people may cognitively manufacture a contrast with worse-off others. It must be emphasized, however, that downward comparison is not always more beneficial when it offers the opportunity for contrast rather than for identification. Sometimes people under stress may derive some benefit from identifying with downward targets through a "shared stress" mechanism ("I'm not the only one with such problems"; cf. Gibbons & Gerrard, 1991). This type of downward identification implies a feeling of relief that others are facing the same problems and does not exclude the possibility of simultaneously deriving inspiration and motivation from identification with a superior model, provided that upward contrast can be avoided (Bandura, 1982; Helgeson & Taylor, 1993).

Whether individuals will identify or contrast themselves with others will depend in part on the goals they pursue and the phase of skill acquisition that they have reached (Brickman & Bulman, 1977; Ruble & Frey, 1991; Trope, 1986). For instance, when individuals are learning a skill, upward comparisons are very adaptive for they may help them to master this skill (Butler, 1992). Because individuals know they are still in the learning stage, they can easily discount the fact that others are doing better. Social information about others doing better may then provide these individuals with an obtainable goal for themselves, and they are likely to identify with these upward targets. Under such conditions, information about others doing worse is rather irrelevant. On the other hand, when individuals have arrived at a more or less stable level they are more likely to use social information to evaluate the level of their skills. Under these conditions, individuals may primarily contrast themselves with both upward and downward targets to obtain an accurate appraisal of their ability.

Furthermore, a number of factors in the kind of information that individuals may obtain in social comparison may determine whether social comparisons will result in identification or contrast. First, when information about the *scores* of others is obtained, most subjects may have a better opportunity to contrast themselves with these others, whereas *vivid information* about or *contact* with others in a similar situation may more often evoke identification with them. Indeed, most studies in which individuals preferred downward comparison information after failure (e.g., Pyszczynski et al., 1985; Swallow & Kuiper, 1993) offered only the opportunity to obtain information about test scores (see also Wood & VanderZee, chapter 10, this volume, for an alternative explanation). In studies that focused on actual contact, more evidence was found that people under stress avoid others who are doing worse (e.g., Rabbie, 1963; Molleman et al., 1986). The relatively less upward—but still upward—comparison preference among burned out nurses found in the Buunk et al. (1994) study can be understood from this perspective: downward comparisons might entail the risk of identification, whereas a too highly upward choice might entail a risk of contrast.

The second factor that may moderate the upward comparison preferences is closely related to the first, and concerns the *comparison mode,* that is, affiliation versus information seeking. Brickman and Bulman (1977, Experiment 2) have documented that individuals are inclined to avoid exchanging comparison information under conditions in which they are clearly inferior to their partner. When one can obtain information about others without having to disclose one's own standing on a dimension, the advantages may compensate for the disadvantage of upward contrast. However, affiliation with mutual exchange of positions might imply a direct contrast between oneself and the other and a concomitant lowering of status, not just because one may perceive oneself as inferior but, in particular, because the other may actually not accord one prestige and esteem. Various experimental studies have indeed shown that the tendency to compare upward is stronger when the comparison can be made privately than when one anticipates actual contact with the comparison other (although in the last case the comparison may still be upward; see, e.g., Wilson & Benner, 1971; Ybema & Buunk, 1993). Smith and Insko (1987) found that people more often chose the highest ranking other when only the other's score and test material were obtained than when they affiliated and talked with the other subject. It can therefore be argued that, because information seeking does not require people to reveal their inferiority to the other and does not imply the risk of the other looking down on them, seeking out upward information when under stress would be relatively less threatening for those facing stress at work than upward affiliation. Indeed, in line with this reasoning, both in the study among nurses (Buunk et al., 1994) and in the study among individuals facing work-related disability (Buunk, 1995), information seeking was more upwardly directed than affiliation.

Another factor that, according to the identification–contrast model, may affect upward comparison preferences is the *comparison dimension.* Identification with a better-off other is more likely, and upward comparisons will be more often preferred as a dimension offers more opportunities for self-improvement, is more controllable, and can more easily be cognitively distorted (cf. VanYperen, 1992). In such a case, one can more easily recognize oneself in the other, and see the other as similar. In line with this reasoning, in the study among nurses, comparisons were more upward on the *experience* dimension than on the *competence* dimension; that is, individuals preferred more often to compare with others more experienced than with others more competent (Buunk et al., 1994). A direct confrontation with a more competent other may make contrast with such an individual unavoidable, and may make one feel inferior. A better performance of another who clearly has more experience, will be seen as something one can attain oneself. Moreover, it is not only less threatening but also more useful to compare with someone more experienced than with someone more competent, as one can more easily identify with them and learn from the former person. In a similar vein, in the study among those facing work-related disability, a distinction was made between two comparison dimensions; *problem severity,* the severity of the problems one has to deal with, and *coping adequacy,* the efficacy of one's coping with the situation (cf. Gibbons & Gerrard, 1991). Preferences were more strongly upward on the coping than on the problem severity dimension (Buunk, 1995). Identification with someone who is coping better is easier than with someone who is facing less serious problems than oneself because the coping dimension is more susceptible than the problem severity dimension to perceptual and cognitive distortion, and because coping adequacy may be thought easier to change and more controllable (cf. Major, Testa, & Bylsma, 1991). Moreover, contact with others who have less serious problems is more likely to instill feelings of envy and increased awareness of the problems one is facing.

Although the studies of the nurses and the disabled provided indirect support for part of the identification–contrast model, the evidence was mainly correlational. Moreover, no direct evidence was provided for the role of identification. The role of this variable was examined in a field experiment by Ybema and Buunk (1995) in which disabled individuals were presented with a fictitious interview with another disabled individual. Disabled individuals and others facing work-related stress are often confronted with such forced comparisons. They may meet someone in a similar situation, may read about such an individual, or may hear others tell stories about a disabled person. Usually such comparison others will be perceived either as doing worse or as doing better than oneself (for similar paradigms, see for instance, Aspinwall & Taylor, 1993; Brewer & Weber, 1994; Gibbons & Gerrard, 1989). In the Ybema and Buunk study, before presenting the bogus interview fragment with someone doing better or worse than oneself, perceived control was assessed as a continuous variable. Ybema and Buunk argued that for those feeling in control of their situation, identification with an individual doing better would be easier and would evoke more positive affect. The results showed indeed that upward comparisons evoked more positive affective consequences than downward comparisons but only among those feeling in control of their situation. Downward comparison generated more negative affect than upward comparison, regardless of the level of perceived control. Furthermore, the higher in perceived control that subjects were the more they identified with a person doing better. As would be predicted by the identification–contrast model, identification mediated between perceived control and a positive affective response to the social comparison information, only among those confronted with an upward comparison. Thus, this study provides evidence that upward comparisons are positively valued because they offer the opportunity for identification.

In a similar field experiment among secretaries (Study 3, Ybema, 1994), subjects who regarded relative performances as controllable by effort experienced more positive affect following upward comparison than following downward comparison. This was not the case for subjects who were led to believe that effort could not explain these relative performances. In line with the correlational evidence by Buunk (1995), these findings suggest that upward comparisons are more positively interpreted when they are on a controllable dimension and thus offer the opportunity for identification than when they are seen as due to the effort of the other. In another experiment, Ybema (1994, Study 4) examined the affective consequences of social comparison of academic stress by presenting college students with a part of a fictitious interview with another student. This interview contained upward or downward social comparison information about academic success in which attribution to either effort or ability was induced. The results showed effects only for subjects high in academic stress. For these subjects, upward comparison generated more positive affect than downward comparison when the target's academic performance was attributed to effort. This suggests that subjects high in stress identified upward when they saw the target's superior performance as attainable by increased effort. In contrast, downward comparison generated more positive affect than upward comparison when the target's performance was attributed to ability. This indicates that when differences in stable ability were salient, subjects seemed primarily to contrast themselves with the comparison target.

An important implication of the identification–contrast model is that, in line with what evolutionary psychology would predict, individuals have a "wired in" tendency to develop a positive self-concept by attaining a subjective feeling of doing better than others on relevant dimensions. Therefore, individuals who are able to attain this feeling by identifying themselves with better-off others and by contrasting themselves with worse-off others will exhibit higher levels of adjustment and mental health (cf. Gilbert, 1990; Taylor & Brown, 1988). Although it is difficult to unravel whether mental health leads to a sense of superiority or vice versa, both variables are closely related (Heady & Wearing, 1988). This implies that probably especially for those high in self-esteem the feeling of superiority is shaken when facing a failure or a threat, which will invoke a strong tendency to restore the feeling of superiority by contrasting oneself with others doing worse (cf. Tesser, 1988). Indeed, there is evidence that those high in self-esteem engage in more derogation of others after failure than those low in self-esteem (Brown & Gallagher, 1992; Gibbons & Boney-McCoy, 1991). Furthermore, the finding that neurotics (VanderZee, Buunk, & Sanderman, 1996), depressed individuals (Swallow & Kuiper, 1987) and Type-A individuals (Yuen & Kuiper, 1992) compare more upward, probably means that these individuals contrast themselves with others doing better (derogating themselves), and feel that the "grass is always greener at the other side". Finally, it must be emphasized that, as we outline later, the most powerful way of contrasting oneself with others doing worse is by cognitively constructing comparison dimensions and comparison others in such a way that one looks better than others on important dimensions (e.g., Wood, Taylor, & Lichtman, 1985). Individuals attempt to construe reality in such a way that they are doing better than others, and when such a representation is not possible, well-being may be threatened (cf. Taylor & Brown, 1988).

## SOCIAL COMPARISONS AND SEEKING STATUS AND PRESTIGE: CONTRASTING ONESELF WITH OTHERS

As we have outlined, work is a major area in which individuals in our society try to attain prestige and status and build positive self-esteem (Brockner, 1987). These goals can be achieved, for example, in intergroup comparisons with other work units and with other organizations, as well as in interpersonal comparisons. The inability to reach and maintain a perception of superiority in comparison with other individuals or groups on important dimensions may lead to a deterioration of health. In competitive situations, contrast with relevant others is especially salient, and identification with them is reduced (Mettee & Smith, 1977). Indeed, whether one succeeds or fails to reach a good position depends largely on the worse or better qualities of one's competitors. Therefore, especially on work-related dimensions the possibility of being able to contrast oneself downward with others by finding or creating dimensions on which one is doing better than others in one's reference group seems very important for one's well-being. Similarly, a forced contrast with a colleague doing better may have negative effects on psychological health. In fact, there are clear links between one's increase or loss in status and physiological parameters. For example, among human beings, increase of status by academic graduation and success in non-physical competitive games such as chess can lead to increases in testosterone (Gilbert et al., 1995; Kemper, 1990). Animal research shows that the position in the dominance hierarchy may have physiological consequences, and that high and low status animals can be distinguished in terms of a number of neurochemical and neuroendocrine differences (Gilbert, 1988; Gilbert et al., 1995). Rank changes often cause physiological changes (Kemper, 1990). For instance, studies among captive vervets showed that dominant males had a relatively high level of serotonin, a neurotransmitter, that fell sharply when they were isolated from the group and thus removed from their position, and that rose sharply when they became dominant again (see Barkow, 1989). Research among rats in The Netherlands by Koolhaas and his colleagues (e.g., Korte, Smit, Bouws, & Koolhaas, 1990) shows that losing a battle with another rat generates much more stress than winning a battle, as indicated by parameters such as heart rate, blood pressure and levels of corticosterone, adrenaline, and noradrenaline. More important, such changes after a single social battle often lead to long-term physiological and behavioral changes, including an animal analog of depression (Gilbert, 1988). Often, for many days after the loss the normal day–night rhythm in heart rate, body temperature, and activity remained disturbed.

In a similar vein, losing an actual or symbolic social struggle for status at work may lead to permanent depression and health damage. Individuals may lose competition with others for a valued position, may not attain what they desire, or may be unable to find dimensions on which they feel superior to others. Such events may often lead to feelings of relative deprivation, and affect well-being of many employees seriously because self-enhancing perceptions are widespread in organizations. For instance, Meyer (1980) found that most people felt they performed better than about 75% of others with the same job. Only very few people considered themselves less than average. No less than 80% of the higher professionals and managers felt they belonged to the best 10% of people with the same job as they had. A likely interpretation of these findings is that most participants in this study engaged predominantly in downward contrasts, and thus assumed themselves to be quite high in the hierarchy. It is not difficult to imagine that individuals seeing themselves in this way may feel aggrieved when others are promoted and they are not. This will be particularly the case when one feels one obtains less than one is entitled to. As Major (1994) outlined in detail, social comparisons play a role in determining how fair and just the outcomes that one obtained are perceived to be.

Despite the apparent potential impact of social comparison processes at work, there is little empirical research assessing the health consequences of such processes. Many studies have examined the role of social comparisons with respect to perceptions of organizational fairness, feelings of entitlement, and outcome satisfaction (e.g., Ambrose, Harland, & Kulik, 1991; Cropanzano & Greenberg, in press; DeCarufel, 1979; Dornstein, 1988; Jackson, Gardner, & Sullivan, 1992; Major, McFarlin, & Gagnon, 1984), but little research has been conducted on the effects of these processes on mental and physical health. Although it does not deal directly with social comparisons, interesting work of Siegrist and his colleagues (e.g., Siegrist & Peter, 1994) provides one relevant exception. These researchers have shown that a variable that they label *low status control* is an important precursor of coronary risk factors. Low status control refers to an imbalance between high effort spent at work (as expressed in competition or sustained anger) and poor reward in terms of long-term expectations of status in terms of promotion prospects and job stability. In a study among blue-collar workers, no less than 48% of coronary risk subjects, but only 13% of the remaining group were characterized by low status control. In terms of social comparisons, these individuals attached a high value to being better than others (as manifested in their competitiveness), but felt at the same time that they would not be able to attain the status and prestige they felt they deserved.

In a number of other studies, particularly among blue-collar workers, it has been found that upward comparisons in the form of pay inequity may be accompanied by occupational stress (McKenna, 1987), and may lead to absenteeism (Dittrich & Carrell, 1979; Hendrix & Spencer, 1989). In a prospective study in two metal factories in The Netherlands, Geurts, Buunk, and Schaufeli (1994a) used objectively recorded number of sick leaves, and asked blue-collar workers how well off they thought they were in comparison to others within the company in terms of eleven different job aspects such as physical safety, autonomy and freedom, promotion prospects, and social atmosphere. In addition, the study assessed one's personal norm with respect to the conditions under which absenteeism was justified. LISREL analyses showed that in both samples feeling worse off than others led to a relatively high number of sick leaves through a tolerant personal absence norm. Thus, these data seem to suggest that sickness behavior can be fostered by unfavorable social comparisons at work—that is, by upward contrast (see also Geurtz, Schaufeli, & Buunk, 1993).

Health problems due to unfavorable social comparisons may occur even more among professional men, especially around the age of 40, when the attainments in terms of one's career become an issue, and when it may become obvious that certain aspirations cannot be realized. Professionals may become concerned about the likelihood of attaining their career goals in future, and may see that similar others have accomplished more. Career-oriented individuals usually monitor their own progress closely in comparison to similar others, and feelings of failure and lack of accomplishment are likely to occur when they perceive that similar others have attained a higher status (cf. Suls, 1986). In addition, they may experience a feeling of entitlement that has been built up as a consequence of high investments during the preceding career, accompanied by the fear that such feelings are violated due to the fact that only a few can reach the highest positions. Such perceptions will be particularly manifest as the opportunities to change jobs decrease as one gets older. Buunk and Janssen (1992) examined this situation in terms of *relative deprivation*. Combining models of Crosby (1976) and Folger (1986, 1987), Buunk and Janssen (1992) argued that relative deprivation involves an active cognitive process in which the current situation is evaluated against upward criteria, showing that all criteria distinguished in the models of Folger and Crosby constitute aspects of the same underlying latent construct. These criteria include unfavorable social comparisons, strong feelings of entitlement, weak justification of the present situation, and little likelihood of amelioration. In a study among a representative sample of professional men, Buunk and Janssen (1992) found that relative deprivation operationalized in this way correlated strongly with depression in the mid-career group (35–45 years of age), more so than in the early career group (25–35 years of age), and much more so than in the late career group (45–55 years of age). Furthermore, although relative deprivation was associated with dissatisfaction in all age groups, it was only during midcareer that it correlated significantly with health complaints. Presumably, younger people still feel they have a chance to attain what they want, whereas older people may have accepted their situation.

Although not attaining one's career goals may be rather stressful, those who have lost a job probably face the worst threat in terms of loss of prestige, status, and self-esteem. Not only will they often contrast themselves in upward comparisons with their former colleagues, but when comparing themselves with their past, they may feel deprived in a variety of ways (a temporal comparison process, cf. Albert, 1977). They often experience changes in lifestyle, in environmental pressures and supports, and in general health (Warr, 1987), and are deprived of several psychological benefits of paid work, for example, earning one's living, enjoying personal status and identity, having a structured daily schedule, having contacts with people outside the family, and pursuing goals and purposes beyond one's own (Jahoda, 1982). Next to the loss of these psychological values of paid work, unemployment is likely to result in a severely reduced income that may affect well-being through subjectively appraised financial strain and life-style deprivation (Whelan, 1992). In addition, loss of a job may result in strains and conflict in one's relations with close others and thus threaten one's sense of connectedness (e.g., Madge, 1983; Thomas, McCabe, & Berry, 1980). Thus, many people who move into unemployment feel uncertain about their future (Payne, Warr, & Hartley, 1984), feel threatened in their self-esteem (Warr & Jackson, 1983), and experience a significant drop in well-being (Jahoda, 1982; Warr, 1987). Under these conditions, social comparisons may become especially salient. Indeed, a study by Walker and Mann (1987) among unemployed subjects showed that feelings of relative deprivation were related to stress symptoms. In a similar vein, Ybema, Buunk, and Heesink (1996) showed that the more stress individuals facing a loss of work experienced, the more negative affect both upward and downward comparisons generated. In line with the identification–contrast model, especially in downward comparison, these feelings of negative affect were mediated by identification with the downward comparison other.

As noted previously, from the perspective of the identification–contrast model, and in line with evolutionary psychology (Barkow, 1989), individuals who experience a potential loss of their self-esteem, status and prestige, will try to find or create comparison others and comparison dimensions that will give them a feeling of doing better than at least some others on at least some dimensions (VanYperen, 1992), for example by cognitively constructing prototypical others (Taylor, Buunk, & Aspinwall, 1990). As Goethals, Messick, and Allison (1991) noted, "people wish to perceive themselves as superior to others, and they will in fact construct perceptions of themselves and social reality that support this wish to the maximum degree that physical and social reality permit" (p. 163). Such downward contrast is one of the various active cognitive attempts to make one's situation psychologically more livable. Indeed, Taylor, Wood, and Lichtman (1983) examined downward comparisons under stress from the wider perspective of *selective evaluation*, arguing that individuals under threat are inclined to selectively evaluate themselves in ways that are self-enhancing. Based on interviews with breast cancer patients, Taylor et al. proposed five mechanisms of selective evaluation: (a) downward comparisons with less fortunate others (e.g., "there are others still worse off"); (b) selectively focusing on attributes that make one appear advantaged (e.g., "the cancer could have spread all over"); (c) the creation of hypothetical worse worlds (e.g., "I could have been dead"); (d) construing benefit from the victimizing event (e.g., "I enjoy life much more now"); and (e) the manufacturing of normative standards of adjustment that make one appear to be coping very well (e.g., "I am doing very well under the circumstances").

In the research project among individuals falling under the Disablement Insurance Act, Buunk and Ybema (1995) examined selective evaluation processes, basing their work primarily on studies by Taylor et al. and Wills (1987). Buunk and Ybema identified six major strategies of selective evaluation: (a) construing benefits of the disability, (b) downward comparison, (c) devaluing former dimensions (e.g., "think that working hard is not all there is"), (d) imagining "worse worlds," (e) positive framing (e.g., "try to view problems in a positive way"), and (f) creating new dimensions of evaluation. In line with the self-enhancement motive, downward comparisons were more prevalent among those experiencing stress. This indicates that regaining self-esteem is a major motive for contrasting oneself downward under stress (cf. Wills, 1981). Longitudinal data showed that over a period of one year, when controlling for level of stress and general evaluation at Time 1, subjects evaluated their situation significantly more positively at Time 2 when they had engaged in imagining that things could have been worse ("worse worlds"), and in creating new dimensions of evaluation at Time 1. This study showed that selective evaluation does not alter stress per se but does change the way individuals feel about their stress, that is, how they evaluate their own situation even if they face serious problems.

## CONCLUSION

Job stress and loss of work may seriously affect one's well-being, as such situations usually imply a threat to important social needs—the needs for connectedness, status, prestige and self-esteem. Over the past decade, researchers focused on the various cognitive and behavioral ways in which individuals may cope with such stressors and strains at work, and with the actual and potential loss of work (e.g., Edwards, 1988). However, until recently, little attention has been paid to the role of social comparisons in coping with job-related stress. By linking the social comparison literature, especially as it concerns health and coping, to the literature on stress at work, the present chapter offers evidence that various types of job-related stress are accompanied by affiliative needs and by a desire to obtain information about how others in similar circumstances feel and respond. In line with Festinger's (1954) social comparison theory and subsequent research using the fear and affiliation paradigm (e.g., Gerard, 1963; Mills & Mintz, 1972), the need for social comparison is especially elevated among individuals who feel uncertain about their own feelings, attitudes, and responses.

In general, it seems that, contrary to what Wills (1981) would predict, people under occupational stress also prefer upward comparisons. Although the upward preference is in line with Taylor and Lobel's (1989) model, their model cannot explain why the preference for upward comparisons is reduced among those under stress. To reconcile such discrepant findings and theories, we have suggested the identification–contrast model, that builds in part on existing models like Taylor and Lobel's as well as on a quite different literature, that of evolutionary psychology. The identification–contrast model assumes that individuals compete for status and prestige and have a strong desire to identify upward and contrast downward to be able to achieve and maintain a perception of themselves as doing better than others on dimensions they consider important. It also postulates that upward identification and downward contrast are especially characteristic of individuals with high self-esteem and positive mental health. Although the identification–contrast model has thus far not been tested directly, many existing findings are in line with this model. For instance, individuals appear to have a stronger desire for upward information than for upward affiliation, to compare more upward on controllable, cognitively malleable dimensions such as coping adequacy, to identify more with upward others the more control they perceive over their situation, to derive more positive affect from upward comparisons than from downward comparisons, to feel threatened when they perceive others are doing better, and to employ various cognitive strategies that allow them to achieve a sense of relative superiority. In fact, characteristic of many forms of occupational stress is that individuals come to view themselves as inferior to others, which instigates various attempts to restore their sense of relative superiority.

It has to be emphasized that the proposed identification–contrast model is compatible with Festinger's (1954) "drive upward," with downward comparison theory (Wills, 1981), and with the motive of self-improvement emphasized by Wood (1989) and Major et al. (1991). In fact, our model sheds a new light on the meaning of the drive upward in Festinger's (1954) original theory that has generated considerable confusion (Latané, 1966). In our view, this drive refers to the strong and general motive to achieve a moderate superiority in comparison with others on relevant dimensions, and to the resistance to acknowledging the superiority of others on relevant dimensions. When the sense of relative superiority is threatened for individuals under stress, self-enhancement as meant by Wills (1981) and self-improvement as meant by Wood (1989) can be met in a process of identification with others doing better, and of contrasting oneself with others doing worse. Thus, it can be expected that when individuals are asked how well they are doing, they will exhibit downward contrast by saying "better than others," but when they are asked about whom they want to learn more and with whom they identify, they will show a preference for upward comparisons by referring to others doing better.

The cognitive distortions individuals are willing to make to achieve and maintain a sense of relative superiority may be more in line with Festinger's ideas than often is assumed. As Gruder (1977) and Goethals et al. (1991) suggested, Festinger clearly considered the psychologically important stake people have in the outcome of comparisons. "The subjective feelings of correctness in one's opinions, and the subjective evaluation of the adequacy of one's performance on important abilities are some of the satisfactions that persons attain in the course of these associations with other people" (Festinger, 1954, pp. 135–136). Given the role of cognitive distortion in social comparison, Goethals et al. (1991) suggested that Festinger would have devised a different social comparison theory if he had done so after rather than before developing cognitive dissonance theory and would have incorporated elements from cognitive dissonance theory emphasizing that "people construct social reality in ways that support self-enhancing appraisals of their opinions and abilities and seek out information that bolsters positive appraisals while avoiding or distorting information that threatens them" (p. 153). Hopefully, the present chapter further helps in illuminating the continuity in research on social comparisons over the past forty years, and in suggesting the role of identification and contrast as basic processes underlying social comparison, particularly under threat.

## ACKNOWLEDGMENTS

The authors thank Lisa Aspinwall, Meg Gerrard, Rick Gibbons, Paul Gilbert, Nico VanYperen, and Karen VanderZee for their helpful comments on earlier versions of this chapter.

## REFERENCES

Albert, S. (1977). Temporal comparison theory. *Psychological Review, 84,* 485–503.

Ambrose, M. I., Harland, L. K., & Kulik, C. T. (1991). Influence of social comparison on perceptions of organizational fairness. *Journal of Applied Psychology, 76,* 239–246.

Aspinwall, L. G., & Taylor, S. E. (1993). Effects of social comparison direction, threat, and self-esteem on affect, self-evaluation, and expected success. *Journal of Personality and Social Psychology, 64,* 708–722.

Bandura (1982). Self-efficacy mechanism in human agency. *American Psychologist, 37,* 122–147.

Barkow, J. H. (1989). *Darwin, sex, and status. Biological approaches to mind and culture.* Toronto: University of Toronto Press.

Brewer, M. B., & Weber, J. G. (1994). Self-evaluation effects of interpersonal versus intergroup comparison. *Journal of Personality and Social Psychology, 66,* 268–275.

Brickman, P., & Bulman, R. J. (1977). Pleasure and pain in social comparison. In J. M. Suls & R. L. Miller (Eds.), *Social comparison processes: Theoretical and empirical perspectives* (pp. 149–186). Washington, DC: Hemisphere.

Brockner, (1987). *Self-esteem at work. Research, theory, and practice.* Lexington, MA: Lexington Books.

Brown, J. D., & Gallagher, F. M. (1992). Coming to terms with failure: Private self-enhancement and public self-effacement. *Journal of Experimental Social Psychology, 28,* 3–22.

Butler, R. (1992). What young people want to know when: Effects of mastery and ability goals of interest in different kinds of social comparison. *Journal of Personality and Social Psychology, 62,* 934–943.

Buunk, B. P. (1994). Social comparison processes under stress: Towards an integration of classic and recent perspectives. In W. Stroebe & M. Hewstone (Eds.), *European review of social psychology* (Vol. 5, pp. 211–241). Chichester: Wiley.

Buunk, B. P. (1995). Comparison direction and comparison dimension among disabled individuals: Towards a refined conceptualization of social comparison under stress. *Personality and Social Psychology Bulletin, 21,* 316–330.

Buunk, B. P., Collins, R. L., Taylor, S. E., VanYperen, N. W., & Dakof, G. A. (1990). The affective consequences of social comparison: Either direction has its ups and downs. *Journal of Personality and Social Psychology, 59,* 1238–1249.

Buunk, B. P., & Janssen, P. P. M. (1992). Relative deprivation, and mental health among men in midlife. *Journal of Vocational Behavior, 40,* 338–350.

Buunk, B. P., Janssen, P. P. M., & VanYperen, N. W. (1989). Stress and affiliation reconsidered: The effects of social support in stressful and non-stressful work units. *Social Behaviour, 4,* 155–171.

Buunk, B. P., & Schaufeli, W. B. (1993). Professional burnout: A perspective from social comparison theory. In W. B. Schaufeli, C. Maslach, & T. Marek (Eds.), *Professional burnout: Recent developments in theory and research* (pp. 53–69). Washington, DC: Taylor & Francis.

Buunk, B. P., Schaufeli, W. B., & Ybema, J. F. (1994). Burnout, uncertainty and the desire for social comparison among nurses. *Journal of Applied Social Psychology, 24,* 1701–1718.

Buunk, B. P., & Ybema, J. F. (1995). Selective evaluation and coping with stress: Making one's situation cognitively more livable. *Journal of Applied Social Psychology, 25,* 1499–1517.

Cherniss, C. (1980). *Staff burnout: Job stress in the human services.* Beverly Hills: Sage.

Colligan, M. (1985). An apparent case of mass psychogenic illness in an aluminum assembly plant. In C. L. Cooper & M. J. Smith (Eds.), *Job stress and blue collar work* (pp. 171–181). Chichester: Wiley.

Cooper, C. L., & Payne, R. (1988, Eds.). *Causes, coping and consequences of stress at work.* Chichester: Wiley.

Cottrell, N. B., & Epley, S. W. (1977). Affiliation, social comparison, and socially mediated stress reduction. In J. M. Suls & R. L. Miller (Eds.), *Social comparison processes: Theoretical and empirical perspectives* (pp. 43–68). Washington, DC: Hemisphere.

Cropanzano, R., & Greenberg, J. (in press). Progress in organizational justice: Tunneling through the maze. In C. L. Cooper & I. T. Robertson (Eds.), *International review of industrial and organizational psychology: 1997.* New York: Wiley.

Crosby, F. (1976). A model of egoistical relative deprivation. *Psychological Review, 83,* 85–113.

Dabbs, J. M., & Helmreich, R. L. (1966). Fear, anxiety and affiliation following a role-played accident. *Journal of Social Psychology, 24,* 143–153.

DeCarufel, A. C. (1979). Factors affecting the evaluation of improvement: The role of normative standards and allocator resources. *Journal of Personality and Social Psychology, 37,* 847–857.

DeVellis, R. F., Blalock, S. J., Holt, K., Renner, B. R., Blanchard, L. W., & Klotz, M. L. (1991). Arthritis patients' reactions to unavoidable social comparisons. *Personality and Social Psychology Bulletin, 17,* 392–399.

DeVellis, R. F., Holt, K., Renner, B. R., Blalock, S. J., Blanchard, L. W., Cook, H. L., Klotz, M. L., Mikov, V., & Harring, K. (1990). The relationship of social comparison to rheumatoid arthritis symptoms and affect. *Basic and Applied Social Psychology, 11,* 1–18.

Dittrich, J. E., & Carrell, M. R. (1979). Organization equity perceptions, employee job satisfaction, and departmental absence and turnover rates. *Organizational Behavior and Human Performance, 24,* 29–40.

Dornstein, M. (1988). Wage reference groups and their determinants: A study of blue-collar and white-collar employees in Israel. *Journal of Occupational Psychology, 61,* 221–235.

Edelwich, J., & Brodsky, A. (1980). *Burn-out: Stages of disillusionment in the helping professions.* New York: Human Sciences Press.

Edwards, J. R. (1988). The determinants and consequences of coping with stress. In C. L. Cooper & R. Payne (Eds.), *Causes, coping and consequences of stress at work* (pp. 233–263). Chichester: Wiley.

Festinger, L. (1954). A theory of social comparison processes. *Human Relations, 7,* 117–140.

Fletcher, B. (1988). The epidemiology of occupational stress. In C. L. Cooper & R. Payne

(Eds.), *Causes, coping and consequences of stress at work* (pp. 3-53). Chichester: Wiley.

Folger, R. (1986). Rethinking equity theory: A referent cognitions model. In H. W. Bierhoff, R. L. Cohen, & J. Greenberg (Eds.), *Justice in social relations* (pp. 145-162). New York: Plenum Press.

Folger, R. (1987). Reformulating the preconditions of resentment: A referent cognitions model. In J. C. Masters & W. P. Smith (Eds.), *Social comparison, social justice, and relative deprivation: Theoretical, empirical, and policy perspectives* (pp. 183-215). Hillsdale, NJ: Lawrence Erlbaum Associates.

Friend, R. M., & Gilbert, J. (1973). Threat and fear of negative evaluation as determinants of locus of social comparison. *Journal of Personality, 41,* 328-340.

Gerard, H. B. (1963). Emotional uncertainty and social comparison. *Journal of Abnormal and Social Psychology, 66,* 568-573.

Gerard, H. B., & Rabbie, J. M. (1961). Fear and social comparison. *Journal of Abnormal and Social Psychology, 62,* 586-592.

Geurts, S. A., Schaufeli, W. B., & Buunk, B. P. (1993). Social comparison, inequity, and absenteeism among bus drivers. *European Work and Organizational Psychologist, 3,* 191-203.

Geurts, S. A., Buunk, B. P,. & Schaufeli, W. B. (1994a). Social comparison and absenteeism: A structural modeling approach. *Journal of Applied Social Psychology, 24,* 1871-1890.

Geurts, S. A., Buunk, B. P,. & Schaufeli, W. B. (1994b). Health complaints, social comparisons and absenteeism. *Work and Stress, 8,* 220-234.

Gibbons, F. X., & Boney McCoy, S. (1991). Self-esteem, similarity, and reactions to active versus passive downward comparison. *Journal of Personality and Social Psychology, 60,* 414-424.

Gibbons, F. X., & Gerrard, M. (1989). Effects of upward and downward social comparison on mood states. *Journal of Social and Clinical Psychology, 8,* 14-31.

Gibbons, F. X., & Gerrard, M. (1991). Downward comparison and coping with threat. In J. M. Suls & T. A. Wills (Eds.), *Social comparison: Contemporary theory and research* (pp. 317-345). Hillsdale, NJ: Lawrence Erlbaum Associates.

Gilbert, P. (1988). Psychobiological interaction in depression. In S. Fisher & J. Reason (Eds.), *Handbook of life stress, cognition and health* (pp. 559-580). Chichester: Wiley.

Gilbert, P. (1990). Changes: rank, status and mood. In S. Fisher & C. L. Cooper (Eds.), *On the move: the psychology of change and transition* (pp. 33-52). Chichester: Wiley.

Gilbert, P., Price, J., & Allan, S. (1995). Social comparison, social attractiveness and evolution: How might they be related? *New Ideas in Psychology, 13,* 149-165.

Goethals, G. R. (1986). Fabricating and ignoring social reality: Self-serving estimates of consensus. In J. M. Olson, C. Peter Herman, & M. P. Zanna (Eds.), *Relative deprivation and social comparison: The Ontario Symposium* (Vol. 4, pp. 135-158). Hillsdale, NJ: Lawrence Erlbaum Associates.

Goethals, G. R., Messick, D. M., & Allison, S. T. (1991). The uniqueness bias: Studies of constructive social comparison. In J. M. Suls & T. A. Wills (Eds.), *Social comparison: Contemporary theory and research* (pp. 317-345). Hillsdale, NJ: Lawrence Erlbaum Associates.

Golembiewski, R. T., & Munzenrider, R. F. (1988). *Phases of burnout: Developments in concepts and applications.* New York: Praeger.

Gray-Toft, P. A., & Anderson, J. G. (1981). Stress among hospital nursing staff: Its causes and effects. *Social Science and Medicine, 15a,* 639-647.

Gruder, C. L. (1977). Choice of comparison person in evaluating oneself. In J. M. Suls & R. L. Miller (Eds.), *Social comparison processes: Theoretical and empirical perspectives* (pp.

21–41). Washington, DC: Hemisphere.

Heady, B., & Wearing, A. (1988). The sense of relative superiority–central to well-being. *Social Indicators Research, 20,* 497–516.

Heider, F. (1958). *The Psychology of Interpersonal Relations.* New York: Wiley.

Helgeson, V. S., & Taylor, S. E. (1993). Social comparisons and adjustment among cardiac patients. *Journal of Applied Social Psychology, 23,* 1171–1195.

Hendrix, W. H., & Spencer, B. A. (1989). Development and test of multivariate model of absenteeism. *Psychological Reports, 64,* 923–938.

Jackson, L. A., Gardner, P. D., & Sullivan, L. A. (1992). Explaining gender differences in self-pay expectations: Social comparison standards and perceptions of fair pay. *Journal of Applied Psychology, 77,* 651–663.

Jahoda, M. (1982). *Employment and unemployment.* Cambridge, UK: Cambridge University Press.

Karasek, R., & Theorell, T. (1990). *Healthy work: Stress, productivity, and the reconstruction of working life.* New York: Basic Books.

Kemper, T. D. (1990). *Social structure and testosterone: Explorations of the socio-bio-social chain.* New Brunswick, NJ: Rutgers University Press.

Kompier, M., Mulders, H., Meijman, T. F., Boersma, M., Groen, G., & Bullinga, R. (1990). Absence behaviour, turnover and disability: A study among city bus drivers in the Netherlands. *Work and Stress, 4,* 83–89.

Korte, S. M., Smit, J., Bouws, G. A., & Koolhaas, J. M., et al. (1990). Behavioral and neuroendocrine responses to psychosocial stress in male rats: the effect of the 5-HT 1A agonist ipsapirone. *Hormones and Behavior, 24,* 554–567.

Latané, B. (1966). Studies in social comparison: Introduction and overview. *Journal of Experimental Social Psychology, 2, Supplement 1,* 1–5.

Lazarus, R. S., & Folkman, S. (1984). *Stress, appraisal, and coping.* New York: Springer.

Madge, N. (1983). Unemployment and its effects on children. *Journal of Child Psychology and Psychiatry, 24,* 311–19.

Major, B. (1994). From social inequality to personal entitlement: The role of social comparisons, legitimacy appraisals, and group membership. *Advances in Experimental Social Psychology, 26,* 293–356.

Major, B., McFarlin, D. B., & Gagnon, D. (1984). Overworked and underpaid: On the nature of gender differences in personal entitlement. *Journal of Personality and Social Psychology, 47*(6), 1399–1412.

Major, B., Testa, M., & Bylsma, W. H. (1991). Responses to upward and downward social comparisons: The impact of esteem-relevance and perceived control. In J. M. Suls & T. A. Wills (Eds.), *Social comparison: Contemporary theory and research* (pp. 237–260). Hillsdale, NJ: Lawrence Erlbaum Associates.

Marmot, M. (1994). Work and other factors influencing coronary health and sickness absence. *Work and Stress, 8,* 191–201.

Maslach, C., & Jackson, S. E. (1982). Burnout in health professions: A social psychological analysis. In G. S. Sanders & J. Suls (Eds.), *Social Psychology of Health and Illness* (pp. 227–251). Hillsdale, NJ: Lawrence Erlbaum Associates.

McGrath, A., Reid, N., & Boore, J. (1989). Occupational stress in nursing. *International Journal of Nursing Studies, 3,* 3–31.

McKenna, J. F. (1987). Equity/inequity, stress and employee commitment in a health care setting. *Stress Medicine, 3,* 71–74.

Mettee, D. R., & Smith, G. (1977). Social comparison and interpersonal attraction: The case for dissimilarity. In J. M. Suls & R. L. Miller (Eds.), *Social comparison processes: Theoretical and empirical perspectives* (pp. 21–41). Washington, DC: Hemisphere.

Meyer, H. H. (1980). Self-appraisal and job performance. *Personnel Psychology, 33,* 291–295.

Miller, R. L., & Suls, J. M. (1977). Affiliation preferences as a function of attitude and ability similarity. In J. M. Suls & R. L. Miller (Eds.), *Social comparison processes: Theoretical and empirical perspectives* (pp. 21–41). Washington, DC: Hemisphere.

Miller, N., Gross, S., & Holtz, R. (1991). Social projection and attitudinal certainty. In J. M. Suls & T. A. Wills (Eds.), *Social comparison: Contemporary theory and research* (pp. 177–209). Hillsdale, NJ: Lawrence Erlbaum Associates.

Miller, K. I., Stiff, J. B., & Ellis, B. H. (1988). Communication and empathy as precursors to burnout among human service workers. *Communication Monographs, 55,* 250–265.

Miller, N., & Zimbardo, P. (1966). Motives for fear induced affiliation: Emotional comparison or interpersonal similarity? *Journal of Personality, 34,* 481–503.

Mills, J., & Mintz, P. M. (1972). Effect of unexplained arousal on affiliation. *Journal of Personality and Social Psychology, 24,* 11–14.

Molleman, E., Pruyn, J., & van Knippenberg, A. (1986). Social comparison processes among cancer patients. *British Journal of Social Psychology, 25,* 1–13.

Myers, D. G., & Lamm, H. (1976). The group polarization phenomenon. *Psychological Bulletin, 83,* 602–627.

Nosanchuck, T. A., & Erickson, B. H. (1985). How high is up? Calibrating social comparison in the real world. *Journal of Personality and Social Psychology, 48,* 624–634.

Payne, R. L., Warr, P. B., & Hartley, J. (1984). Social class and the experience of unemployment. *Sociology of Health and Illness, 6,* 152–174.

Pennebaker, J. W., & Brittingham, G. L. (1982). Environmental and sensory cues affecting the perception of physical symptoms. In A. Baum & J. E. Singer (Eds.), *Advances in environmental psychology* (Vol. 4, pp. 115–130). Hillsdale, NJ: Lawrence Erlbaum Associates.

Pyszczynski, T., Greenberg, J., & LaPrelle, J. (1985). Social comparison after success and failure: Biased search for information consistent with a self-serving conclusion. *Journal of Experimental Social Psychology, 21,* 195–211.

Rabbie, J. M. (1963). Differential preference for companionship under threat. *Journal of Abnormal and Social Psychology, 67,* 643–648.

Ruble, D. N., & Frey, K. S. (1991). Changing patterns of comparative behavior as skills are acquired: A functional model of self-evaluation. In J. M. Suls & T. A. Wills (Eds.), *Social comparison: Contemporary theory and research* (pp. 79–113). Hillsdale, NJ: Lawrence Erlbaum Associates.

Schachter, S. (1959). *The psychology of affiliation.* Stanford, CA: Stanford University Press.

Schachter, S., & Singer, J. E. (1962). Cognitive, social, and physiological determinants of emotional state. *Psychological Review, 69,* 379–399.

Schaufeli, W. B., & Buunk, B. P. (1996). Professional burnout. In M. J. Schabracq, J. A. M. Winnubst, & C. L. Cooper (Eds.), *Handbook of work and health psychology* (pp. 311-346). New York: Wiley.

Shaver, P., & Klinnert, M. (1982). Schachter's theories of affiliation and emotion: implications of developmental research. In L. Wheeler (Ed.), *Review of personality and social psychology* (Vol. 3, pp. 37–72). Beverly Hills, CA: Sage.

Siegrist, J., & Peter, R. (1994). Job stressors and coping characteristics in work-related disease: issues of validity. *Work and Stress, 8,* 130–140.

Singer, J. E., & Shockley, V. L. (1965). Ability and affiliation. *Journal of Personality and Social Psychology, 1,* 95–100.

Skelton, J. A., & Pennebaker, J. W. (1982). The psychology of physical symptoms and sensations. In G. S. Sanders & J. Suls (Eds.), *Social psychology of health and illness* (pp. 99–128). Hillsdale, NJ: Lawrence Erlbaum Associates.

Smith, R. H., & Inkso, C. A. (1987). Social comparison choice during ability evaluation: The effects of comparison publicity, performance feedback, and self-esteem. *Personality and Social Psychology Bulletin, 13,* 111–122.

Sullins, E. S. (1991). Emotional contagion revisited: Effects of social comparison and expressive style on mood convergence. *Personality and Social Psychology Bulletin, 17,* 166–174.

Suls, J. (1986). Comparison processes in relative deprivation: a life span analysis. In J. M. Olson, C. P. Herman, & M. P. Zanna (Eds.), *Relative deprivation and social comparison* (pp. 95–116). Hillsdale, NJ: Lawrence Erlbaum Associates.

Swallow, S. R., & Kuiper, N. A. (1987). The effects of depression and cognitive vulnerability to depression on judgments of similarity between self and other. *Motivation and Emotion, 11,* 157–167.

Swallow, S. R., & Kuiper, N. A. (1993). Social comparison in dysphoria and nondysphoria: Differences in target similarity and specificity. *Cognitive Therapy and Research, 17,* 103–122.

Taylor, S. E., & Brown, J. D. (1988). Illusion as well-being: A social psychological perspective on mental health. *Psychological Bulletin, 103,* 193–210.

Taylor, S. E., Buunk, B. P., & Aspinwall, L. G. (1990). Social comparison, stress, and coping. *Personality and Social Psychology Bulletin, 16,* 74–89.

Taylor, S. E., & Lobel, M. (1989). Social comparison activity under threat: Downward evaluation and upward contacts. *Psychological Review, 96,* 569–575.

Taylor, S. E., Wood, J. V., & Lichtman, R. R. (1983). It could be worse: Selective evaluation as a response to victimization. *Journal of Social Issues, 39,* 19–40.

Tesser, A. (1988). Towards a self-evaluation maintenance model of social behavior. In L. Berkowitz (Ed.), *Advances in experimental social psychology* (Vol. 21, pp. 181–227). San Diego: Academic Press.

Thomas, L. E., McCabe, E., & Berry, J. E. (1980). Unemployment and family stress: A reassessment. *Family Relations, 29,* 517–24.

Thornton, D. A., & Arrowood, A. J. (1966). Self-evaluation, self-enhancement, and the locus of social comparison. *Journal of Experimental Social Psychology, 2, Supplement 1,* 40–48.

Trope, Y. (1986). Self-enhancement and self-assessment in achievement behavior. In R. M. Sorrentino & E. T. Higgins (Eds.), *Handbook of motivation and cognition* (pp. 350–378). Chichester: Wiley.

VanderZee, K., Buunk, B. P., & Sanderman, R. (1995). Social comparison as a mediator between health problems and subjective health evaluations. *British Journal of Social Psychology, 34,* 53–65.

VanderZee, K., Buunk, B. P., & Sanderman, R. (1996). The relationship between social comparison processes and personality. *Personality and Individual Differences, 20,* 551–565.

VanYperen, N. W. (1992). Self-enhancement among major league soccer players: The role of importance and ambiguity on social comparison behavior. *Journal of Applied Social Psychology, 22,* 1186–1198.

Walker, I., & Mann, L. (1987). Unemployment, relative deprivation, and social protest. *Personality and Social Psychology Bulletin, 13,* 275–283.

Warr, P. B. (1987). Workers without a job. In P. B. Warr (Ed.), *Psychology at work* (pp. 335–356). London: Penguin.

Warr, P., & Jackson, P. (1983). Self-esteem and unemployment among young workers. *Le Travail Humain, 46,* 355–366.

Wheeler, L. (1966). Motivation as a determinant of upward comparison. *Journal of Experimental Social Psychology, 2, Supplement 1,* 27–31.

Wheeler, L., & Miyake, K. (1992). Social comparison in everyday life. *Journal of Personality and Social Psychology, 62,* 760–773.

Whelan, C. T. (1992). The role of income, life-style deprivation and financial strain in mediating the impact of unemployment on psychological distress: Evidence from the Republic of Ireland. *Journal of Occupational and Organizational Psychology, 65,* 331–344.

Wills, T. A. (1981). Downward comparison principles in social psychology. *Psychological Bulletin, 90,* 245–271.

Wills, T. A. (1987). Downward comparisons as a coping mechanism. In C. R. Snyder & C. E. Ford (Eds.), *Coping with negative life events: Clinical and social psychological perspectives* (pp. 243–268). New York: Plenum Press.

Wilson, S. R., & Benner, L. A. (1971). The effects of self-esteem and situation upon comparison choices during ability evaluation. *Sociometry, 34,* 381–397.

Wood, J. V. (1989). Theory and research concerning social comparisons of personal attributes. *Psychological Bulletin, 106,* 231–248.

Wood, J. V., Taylor, S. E., & Lichtman, R. R. (1985). Social comparison in adjustment to breast cancer. *Journal of Personality and Social Psychology, 49,* 1169–1183.

Ybema, J. F., & Buunk, B. P. (1993). Aiming at the top: Upward social comparison after failure. *European Journal of Social Psychology, 23,* 627–645.

Ybema, J. F., & Buunk, B. P. (1995). Affective responses to social comparison: A study among disabled individuals. *British Journal of Social Psychology, 34,* 279–292.

Ybema, J. F. (1994). *Up and down: Affective responses to social comparison.* Capelle a/d Yssel: Labyrint Publication.

Ybema, J. F., Buunk, B. P., & Heesink, J. A. M. (1996). Affect and identification in social comparison after loss of work. *Basic and Applied Social Psychology, 18,* 151–169.

Yuen, S. A., & Kuiper, N. A. (1992). Type A and self-evaluations: A social comparison perspective. *Personality and Individual Differences, 13,* 549–562.

# CHAPTER 13

# Social Comparison Processes in Depression

Anthony H. Ahrens
*American University*

Lauren B. Alloy
*Temple University*

Knowing the experiences of others brings both hope and hopelessness. An individual in the early stages of Alzheimer's disease may become despondent on thinking of others who have suffered dementia. After listening to a recording by Heifetz, a young violinist may dream of playing in Carnegie Hall. Hopelessness and hope are central to depression and its absence. This chapter discusses the role of social comparison in hopelessness and depression.

According to the hopelessness theory of depression (Abramson, Metalsky, & Alloy, 1989), hopelessness serves as a proximal, sufficient cause of depression. Hopelessness, in turn, is produced by negative inferences about the self, negative inferences about the consequences of negative events, and stable, global attributions about the causes of negative events. That is, people become hopeless, and thus depressed, when, after negative events occur, they judge that the events imply negative factors about the self, that the consequences of the events will be negative and long-lived, and that the causes of those events will recur in many situations, thus producing other negative future events.

Social comparison information plays a role in determining each of these steps: whether individuals perceive themselves to have experienced a negative event; what the perceived cause of the event is; what an individual infers about the self as a result of the event; and what consequences are believed likely to flow from the event. For instance, a person who has just been promoted might perceive his or her success as a failure if a rival has received a bigger promotion. A person who fails a test may attribute this to his incompetence if others passed the test easily. Alzheimer's patients may compare themselves with others whose dementia is more advanced and infer that the disease will soon have profound consequences for their own functioning. Finally, observing others' successes might lead a person to infer that she or he is worthless, as society accords worth to the most successful.

We need to make two distinctions before we explore the relation of depression to social comparison. First, the causes of depression's onset are, quite possibly, distinct from those of its maintenance and remission (e.g., Abramson et al., 1989; Needles & Abramson, 1990). These causal factors, in turn, may be distinct from the consequences of depression. For example, in the case of social comparison, it may be that comparison to others better off than the self causes negative self-evaluation and depression, that depression might prompt increases in attention to upward social comparison information, and that depression might lead to attempts at recovery that involve focus on downward social comparison information. Different research strategies are called for to examine these different relations (Alloy, Hartlage, & Abramson, 1988). At the least, it is important to establish whether depression preceded social comparison or vice versa. For instance, to test the hypothesis that downward social comparison prompts recovery from depression, it would be helpful to study the social comparison choices of currently depressed individuals to see whether those engaging in downward comparison are more likely to recover. Longitudinal research on the psychosocial processes involved in depression appears to have been on the rise in recent years (e.g., Davila, Hammen, Burge, Paley, & Daley, 1995; Joiner & Metalsky, 1995; Robins, Hayes, Block, Kramer, & Villena, 1995; Robinson, Garber, & Hilsman, 1995). However, most of the research on social comparison and depression has used cross-sectional designs. Differences between depressed and nondepressed individuals in these studies may reflect factors that have caused depressed individuals to become depressed, concomitants of depression, or attempts to recover from depression.

Second, the operational definition of depression varies considerably across the studies described in this chapter. In some cases, depression is equated with negative mood. In others, depression is defined by elevated, but not extreme, scores on the Beck Depression Inventory (BDI; Beck, Ward, Mendelson, Mock, & Erbaugh, 1961), a measure of depressive symptoms. Yet other studies define depression via alternative criteria. There is considerable debate as to whether depression occurs on a continuum, that is, whether processes present in low levels of depression are related to and/or inform us about more severe depression (e.g. Coyne, 1994; Vredenburg, Flett, & Krames, 1993). We believe that sufficient data have not been collected to address whether social comparison processes are continuously or discretely related to depression. However, there is reason to believe that analog depression studies might inform us about more severe depression (e.g., Vredenburg et al., 1993). In this chapter, the term *mildly depressed* is used to refer to subjects classified as depressed by virtue of scoring at least 9 or 10 on the BDI. We indicate other criteria for classification as we report studies.

In examining the relation of social comparison to hopelessness and depression, we begin by examining the processes by which depressed and nondepressed people make social comparisons. Next, we turn to the consequences of these processes for depression, which include the judgments of self and other that arise from social comparison processes and the effect of these judgments on symptoms of depression.

## OPENNESS TO SOCIAL COMPARISON INFORMATION

For social comparison to influence judgments of hope and hopelessness, people must be open to information about others. This openness is determined, in part, by people's motivation for collecting information about others (Webster & Kruglanski, 1994). For instance, those who need to protect their self-esteem might stop searching for information about others once they have enough to support favorable conclusions about the self. In contrast, those motivated by a need for accuracy might stop searching after they had gathered enough information to make reasonably accurate judgments.

Several theorists have suggested that depressed people are characterized by an absence of motivation to protect self-esteem (Abramson & Alloy, 1981; Bibring, 1953; Freud, 1917/1957). In contrast, nondepressed people are believed to be more prone to self-esteem protection. If so, then once nondepressed subjects receive favorable social comparison information, they should stop being open to further information. In contrast, an absence of this need to protect self-esteem should leave depressed people open to more information, as their need for accuracy would not be compromised by their need to protect themselves (for a review of studies on depressive accuracy, see Alloy & Abramson, 1988).

Alternatively, perhaps depressed people are more open to social comparison information because of their tendency to ruminate on negative events (e.g., Morrow & Nolen-Hoeksema, 1990). Nondepressed people are more likely to cope with negative events by distracting themselves from the situation, thus making it quite difficult to gather social comparison information about the event. In contrast, depressed people are more prone to attempt to cope by thinking about the event, which may include seeking information about others' outcomes in the same situations.

Even if depressed subjects are attempting to protect their self- esteem, this is likely to lead to an ongoing openness to social comparison information. This is because, given depressed subjects' negative views of self (e.g., Beck, 1967), it will be more difficult for them to find the favorable, downward, social comparison information that would end a search. Thus, they may continue to look for information about others after nondepressed people would have stopped, having reached favorable conclusions about themselves. Thus a variety of perspectives suggest that depressed people will be more open to social comparison information.

Weary and her colleagues have offered some indirect evidence for the hypothesis that depressed people are more open to social comparison information (Weary, Elbin, & Hill, 1987; Weary, Marsh, & McCormick, 1994). For instance, in one study, subjects were presented with information that others had abilities in "social perceptiveness" that were similar or dissimilar to their own. These bogus "other subjects" had, purportedly, made attributions about the causes of outcomes in stories that were similar or dissimilar to subjects' own attributions for the outcomes (Weary et al., 1994). Subjects were then asked to indicate their preferences for a partner on a task that was supposed to follow. All subjects preferred the similar agreer, that is, the "other subject" who had abilities that were similar to the subject's and who had reached similar conclusions. However, depressed subjects preferred the similar disagreer more than did nondepressed subjects, whereas the nondepressed subjects preferred the dissimilar agreer. The authors argued that the similar disagreer provides more information concerning the construction of possible attributions, whereas someone who is dissimilar but agrees with the subject serves mostly to validate subjects' opinions. Thus, these data suggest depressed subjects are more open to social comparison information that might alter their beliefs about the world. However, the results of this study should be considered tentative as the dependent variable was preference for interacting with a particular partner, rather than the search for social comparison information per se.

Although depressed people are more open to social comparison information when protecting their self-esteem, there is evidence that some depressed people are more inclined to protect their self-esteem than others. This could apply particularly to those depressed subjects who believe that their self-worth is contingent on external events, such as whether they are loved or are successful in their work (Kernis, 1993; Roberts & Monroe, 1994; Rogers, 1961; Swallow & Kuiper, 1988). If, for instance, people believe that their worth is dependent on their being successful at work, it is important for them to find others who are less successful at work. This should be particularly difficult for depressed people. In contrast, if people believe that their worth is intrinsic to their being, it is less important to find others who have fared less well.

Swallow and Kuiper (1990) conducted initial work testing this proposition. Depressed subjects, scoring above 27 on the Center for Epidemiological Studies-Depression Scale (CES-D; Radloff, 1977), and non-depressed subjects, scoring below 16, were divided into those low and high in dysfunctional attitudes, used as a measure of self-worth contingency. Dysfunctional attitudes included items such as "My life is meaningless unless I am loved by everyone." Subjects were asked to imagine they had received either a 48, 68, or 88 on a test, and then were asked if they wanted to look at superior, average, or inferior others. An interaction of depression and self-worth contingency predicted social comparison activity. Those high in depression and self-worth contingency were the most likely to seek information about others, as predicted. Thus, depressed subjects were more open to social comparison information, but this held true only for a subset of depressed subjects.

If self-esteem protection matters, then depression status should affect social comparison activity most strongly when self-esteem is threatened, for instance, after failure. In one study, subjects performed a task in which they attempted to remember sequences of numbers, allegedly measuring a component of intelligence (Swallow & Kuiper 1992). Among subjects who had scored low on the task, depressed subjects sought information about more others than did nondepressed subjects. There were no differences among those subjects who had scored higher on the task.

Openness to social comparison information might depend on the similarity of self to other. If, for instance, people compare themselves to others who are dissimilar, this might provide discounting information so that less strong dispositional attributions would be made for one's own performance (Miller, Turnbull, & McFarland, 1988). That is, a dissimilar other might have performed better due to a situational factor such as practice at the test. Thus one's own failure would reflect a lack of practice rather than a lack of ability.

For instance, in one study, subjects scoring higher or lower in depression symptoms performed an alleged test of "one component of intelligence" (Swallow & Kuiper, 1993). Subjects could choose how many pieces of information they wished to receive about others who had performed the same test as the subjects. For nondepressed subjects, worse performance predicted less information seeking. For depressed subjects, performance was unrelated to amount of information seeking. The authors argued that the nondepressed subjects who had not performed well wanted to avoid finding out that the "other subjects" were similar so as to preserve the possibility to discount. That is, by not seeking information, they might be able to conclude that the others were, for example, far more advanced students who would have had an undue advantage on the test. However, there was no measure of discounting to test this hypothesis. Such discounting might help to prompt the differences in attributions of depressed and nondepressed individuals suggested by hopelessness theory (Abramson et al., 1989).

Openness to social comparison information should lead to a willingness to compare in areas that are more important. Kuiper and McCabe (1985) examined subjects' judgments of the appropriateness of topics for discussion in social interactions. Those who were mildly depressed, scoring 14 or higher on the BDI, or more at risk for depression, as indicated by elevated scores on the Dysfunctional Attitude Scale (Weissman & Beck, 1978), were more likely to indicate that negative self-disclosure topics, such as "things in the past or present that I feel ashamed or guilty about," were appropriate for discussion than were nondepressed, nonvulnerable subjects.

As self-esteem protection becomes less important and improvement of future performance more so, social comparison activity may shift (e.g., Wood & Taylor, 1991). For instance, it seems likely that nondepressed people would be more open to social comparison information, as they would not be truncating their searches for information once favorable information was found. Flett, Vredenburg, Pliner, and Krames (1987) performed two studies in which mildly depressed and nondepressed subjects who had taken a real exam could look at folders that included other subjects' scores. The exams were early enough in the semester that subjects' performance could improve over the course of the semester, and so seeking more information might be helpful. Under these circumstances, hopeful subjects might seek the knowledge that could fulfill their hopes. Hopeless, depressed subjects, on the other hand, would have less reason to look at the performance of others. In these studies, subjects who were less depressed looked at more folders, a sign of being open to, rather than closed to, social information.

In summary, there is some evidence that, particularly after failure or for those with contingent self-worth, depressed people are more open to social comparison information than are nondepressed people. This may depend on the possibility of future performance. However, not all comparison others are equal. We turn next to preferences on the part of depressed and nondepressed people for upward versus downward comparison targets.

## CHOICE OF COMPARISON TARGET

One possible source of hopelessness is the choice of target for comparison. If depressed people are characterized by a lack of self-esteem protection, then relative to nondepressed people they should be more likely to choose comparisons that lead to unfavorable conclusions, and should be more open to information suggesting that they fare less well. In contrast, those who are non-depressed are less likely to be open to all types of social comparison information, as they are motivated to create a favorable view of self. Thus depressed people, relative to those who are not depressed, would make more upward comparisons.

A contrasting view, however, is that depressed individuals may seek out comparison to others who are less fortunate so as to allow them to feel better about themselves. Gibbons (1986) had subjects write about positive or negative events from their own lives. After this, subjects could read stories that varied in how positive or negative they were. Depressed subjects were selected on the basis of scores above 11 on the BDI 2 to 6 weeks prior to participation. Depressed subjects who wrote about negative events chose to look at more negative stories from others, consistent with the hypothesis that depressed people will seek downward comparisons so as to protect their self-esteem.

Research conducted with individuals who have rheumatoid arthritis also suggests that those who are less well off engage in downward comparison (DeVellis et al., 1990). On 6 of 10 self-report items, those subjects with more negative affect (derived from the combination of a depression measure and a self-esteem measure) reported significantly more downward comparison activity. There was no difference, however in their actual choice of examining the folder of a patient who had performed better as opposed to that of someone who was worse off. The authors controlled for self-reported symptom severity, which is likely correlated with depression. This is likely to have made it more difficult to detect depression effects in the choice of folders to examine. However, evidence on whether depressed individuals are more likely to prefer downward comparison is mixed. For instance, Schulz and Decker (1985) found that, for patients with spinal cord injuries, choice of comparison target "to decide how good their life situation was" was not correlated with depression symptoms. Similarly, Heidrich and Ryff (1993) found that older individuals with more depression symptoms engaged in both more upward and more downward comparison on a general measure of social comparison. Both of these studies used the CES-D to measure depression symptoms.

Albright and Henderson (1995) gave students the opportunity to answer questions about their coping with life events in comparison to that of one of three bogus "other students." One of the fictions presented an upward comparison, one a downward comparison, and the third a similar-to-self comparison, based on manner of coping with negative events. Subjects could choose which of the three they wished to compare themselves to. There was no difference between mildly depressed and nondepressed subjects' choice of other.

Some research suggests a preference on the part of *nondepressed,* not depressed, people for downward comparison. For example, in the study by Swallow and Kuiper (1993), subjects could choose to look at the scores of others performing in any of four quartiles. Subjects who were more depressed initially chose more often than less depressed subjects to compare themselves to someone else who had done better on the test. Subjects were allowed to look at more than one other person's score. The average choice of other was predicted by an interaction of depression level and performance. Regardless of depression symptoms, subjects who performed well looked at the scores of others who had done slightly better. Among those who did less well, depressed subjects looked at others who, on average, had performed similarly. Nondepressed subjects, on the other hand, looked at others who had performed less well. This study, then, suggests that depressed subjects are less likely than are nondepressed subjects to choose to compare themselves to those who are worse off.

Wheeler and Miyake (1992) examined social comparisons in a field setting. Subjects recorded their social comparison activity when they were cued at random intervals. Although depression was not measured, positive and negative affect were. When subjects were experiencing more positive affect, and, presumably, less depression, they were more likely to engage in downward comparison.

How might these mixed results be reconciled? One possibility is that they reflect different processes. If those who are depressed sometimes seek more downward social comparison (DeVellis et al., 1990; Gibbons, 1986), sometimes just as much (Albright & Henderson, 1995; Heidrich & Ryff, 1993; Schulz & Decker, 1985), and sometimes less (Swallow & Kuiper, 1993; Wheeler & Miyake, 1992) than do those who are less depressed, perhaps this reflects differences in the degree to which depressed subjects are attempting to recover hope, as opposed to remaining hopeless. If so, direction of social comparison would be predictable from the stage of recovery of subjects (see Aspinwall, chapter 5, this volume). However, this is a post hoc explanation and needs to be investigated in future work.

## USE OF INFORMATION ABOUT COMPARISON OTHERS

In addition to choosing comparison targets, people also need to reconcile mixed, forced, information about the performance of others (Diener & Fujita, chapter 11, this volume; Wood, 1996). Depressed subjects are prone to more negative thought than are nondepressed subjects (Beck, 1967; Haaga, Dyck, & Ernst, 1991). This might manifest itself in social comparison by discounting of downward social comparison information by depressed subjects and of upward comparison information by nondepressed subjects.

To test this, Ahrens (1991) had mildly depressed and nondepressed subjects perform a bogus "spatial abilities" task. He told subjects either that one other subject had performed better than they had, that one had performed worse, or that one had performed better and one worse (mixed information condition). In judging how many other subjects would perform better than they had, depressed subjects in the mixed information condition made judgments just like those given upward comparison information. In contrast, nondepressed subjects in the mixed information condition made judgments just like those given downward comparison information, appearing to be uninfluenced by the upward information.

In a related finding, after receiving mixed social comparison information, subjects who had more depressive symptoms judged that they had performed less well than did those who had fewer symptoms (Swallow & Kuiper, 1993). These results suggest that even if depressed subjects do prefer to compare themselves to others who are worse off, if they receive a mixture of information they may not be able to help but make their judgments based on information about those who have performed better. It seems particularly likely that depressed people will receive mixed information, given their relative openness to social comparison information. This weighting of relatively negative information, in turn, would again prompt the negative inferences about the self and about the consequences of negative events as well as the negative attributions hypothesized to be associated with depression (Abramson et al., 1989).

Indeed, exposure to increasing amounts of combined social comparison information apparently does prompt more negative inferences about the self among those who are mildly depressed than among those who are not. In a study by McFarland and Miller (1994), subjects performed a bogus test of "social perceptiveness," and then were told that they had performed at the 30th or 70th percentile of either 1,000 or 10 subjects. Among those who allegedly scored at the 30th percentile, increasing the sample size led to more negative beliefs about subjects' social perceptiveness for those with more negative orientations (a combination of depression symptoms and pessimism), but tended to have the opposite effect on those with more positive orientations. This suggests that those with a more negative orientation were more likely to weigh information about additional more successful others rather than unsuccessful others.

Cognitive biases are likely not only to affect the combination of information about others, but also the representation, and so the use of information about a single comparison target (e.g., Nisbett & Ross, 1980). Albright and Henderson (1995) had subjects rate themselves and others in terms of how well they had coped with particular life events. Mildly depressed subjects judged others more favorably than was objectively warranted, whereas nondepressed subjects rated the other person accurately. Thus, confronted with a given individual, mildly depressed individuals are likely to hold an inflated view of that person, which would likely prompt more negative social judgments.

Combining these studies, we find that given social comparison information, depressed individuals are more prone to reach more negative conclusions about themselves than are nondepressed individuals. This occurs both because of the way depressed people combine mixed information about multiple others and the way in which they create views of a single other. Perhaps negative depressive social judgments arise not so much from the information that is gathered about others as it does with how that information is interpreted.

## DEPRESSIVES' JUDGMENTS OF SELF RELATIVE TO OTHER

One consequence of the processes described above is that depressed individuals are more likely to judge themselves less favorably than they do others. These results have been reviewed elsewhere (e.g., Ahrens, 1987; Alloy, Albright, & Clements, 1987; Swallow & Kuiper, 1988), and so we just mention a few examples. Martin, Abramson, and Alloy (1984) had subjects judge the degree of control they and others had over a favorable outcome. In particular, subjects attempted to control the onset of a light, and received money based on the number of times the light came on. Mildly depressed subjects were more likely than nondepressed subjects to judge that others would experience more control than they themselves would.

Similar results appear in studies in which subjects judged how likely they were to win at a dice game, depending on whether they threw the dice themselves or if a croupier threw them (Golin, Terrell, & Johnson, 1977; Golin, Terrell, Weitz, & Drost, 1979). Mildly depressed students judged that they were more likely to win if the croupier threw the dice than if they did (Golin et al., 1977). Severely depressed psychiatric patients believed that it did not matter who threw the dice (Golin et al., 1979). In contrast, nondepressed students (Golin et al., 1977) and psychiatric patients (Golin et al., 1979) believed they were more likely to win if they threw the dice themselves than if the croupier threw them.

In another study, subjects were given information, such as Scholastic Aptitude Test (SAT) scores, about hypothetical students and were asked to predict the likelihood that these students would make the Dean's list or be placed on academic probation (Alloy & Ahrens, 1987). Then subjects provided the equivalent information for themselves and made predictions of their own likelihoods. Mildly depressed individuals predicted that they were just as likely to make the Dean's list or be put on academic probation as a similar other, for instance someone who had the same SAT scores. In contrast, nondepressed subjects judged that they were more likely to make the Dean's list and less likely to be put on probation than were similar others.

These differences in judgment of self and other appear early in life. For instance, in one study, mildly depressed and nondepressed children performed an interpersonal problem solving task (Sacco & Graves, 1984). For each of three story sequences, subjects were asked a series of questions assessing such variables as interpersonal sensitivity and means–ends problem solving. Mildly depressed children were more likely to judge that they had performed worse than others. In a similar study (Meyer, Dyck, & Petrinack, 1989), children did sequencing problems modified from the Wechsler Intelligence Scale for Children-Revised (WISC-R; Wechsler, 1974). Both before and after the task, mildly depressed children judged that they would do worse than others. Nondepressed children said that they would perform about equally to others.

There are two limiting conditions on this tendency for negative depressive social comparison. First, depressed persons do not reach negative conclusions about themselves in comparison to all others. For instance, Albright, Alloy, Barch, and Dykman (1993) had subjects rate themselves on depression-relevant (e.g., "I am insecure"), nondepression relevant (e.g., "I am confident") and depression- irrelevant (e.g., "I like mystery novels") items in comparison to the average depressed, average nondepressed, and average general other. Mildly depressed subjects judged themselves more favorably than they did the average depressed other, and so did not judge that they were worse than all groups of others, although they did make less favorable comparisons than did nondepressed subjects.

Second, in a pair of studies, Pelham (1991) had subjects rate themselves relative to college students their own age on such attributes as social competence, athletic ability, and physical attractiveness. After controlling for self-esteem, severely depressed subjects—those scoring above 23 on the BDI—judged their best self-aspect more favorably than did nondepressed subjects. Interestingly, mildly depressed subjects did not show this tendency. Pelham suggested that some severely depressed individuals use positive thinking, in this case favorable judgments of best self-aspects, to overcome their depressions. Thus unfavorable social comparisons may be a symptom, or even cause, of depression, and favorable social comparisons might be a sign of efforts to escape depression. These results should be interpreted with some caution, however, as it is difficult to interpret the meaning of depressive symptoms once self-esteem has been controlled.

In sum, depressed people generally make more negative social comparisons than do nondepressed people. As a result, they are likely to conclude that their experiences are more negative. These conclusions in turn seem to promote the negative inferences and attributions postulated by hopelessness theory.

## CONSEQUENCES OF SOCIAL COMPARISON

We have examined the social comparison activity of depressed and nondepressed individuals. We turn, now, to the consequences of social comparisons for depression.

The lives of both those better off and those worse off than the self can provide information fostering either hope or hopelessness (Buunk, Collins, Taylor, Van Yperen, & Dakof, 1990; Collins, 1996; Hemphill & Lehman, 1991; Taylor & Lobel, 1989). If others have done well, this can provide a road map to success. Absent the map however, successful others just let people know that they are lost. Similarly, the fact that others are not faring well may make people feel better off, by comparison, but might also suggest that the future holds even worse possibilities.

Upward comparison and downward comparison, thus, might both lead to either increased or decreased depression symptoms. What are the factors moderating these outcomes? Hopelessness theory suggests that they would be any variables prompting relatively negative or positive expectations of the future. One such factor is whether there is a chance for future performance. If there is no possibility for future performance, the upward comparison knowledge that people could have done better cannot provide hope that they will perform better in the future (see Aspinwall, chapter 5, this volume). Instead, knowledge that others have done better is likely to foster negative inferences about the self, and, so, hopelessness and depression.

Most research involving depression and social comparison has included only a single performance, and is consistent with this prediction. For instance, Gibbons (1986) found that, following self-disclosure, depressed individuals who received negative information about others were more likely to improve in mood. In a similar study, Gibbons and Boney McCoy (1991) found that the affect of subjects low in self-esteem who had been informed that they had done poorly on a test of social awareness was improved by information that others had done even worse. Given the high correlation of self-esteem and nondepression, this suggests that similar results would have held for depression. In their naturalistic study, described above, Wheeler and Miyake (1992) found that upward comparison predicted increased negativity of affect and downward comparison predicted increased positivity. Major, Sciacchitano, and Crocker (1993) informed men that three either similar or dissimilar others had performed better or worse on a test of their verbal-spatial ability. Subjects who learned that similar others had performed better were more prone to increased depressive affect. Finally, Rosenblatt and Greenberg (1991) had mildly depressed and nondepressed individuals interact with another person who was either mildly depressed or not depressed. Depressed people who interacted with nondepressed others subsequently had more negative affect than any of the other subjects, perhaps because these nondepressed others provided upward comparison targets.

One study has examined the consequences of social comparison activity for depression symptoms when subjects have an opportunity for multiple performances (Gibbons, Blanton, Gerrard, & Eggleston, 1996). Subjects were asked to imagine that they got a test score back and to indicate with whom they would be most interested in comparing. This information was collected during each of subjects' first three semesters in college. Controlling for initial grade point average, comparison level, and depression symptoms, a drop in grades predicted a subsequent choice of more downward targets. This, in turn, predicted subsequently declining grades. The downward shift in comparison targets predicted increased depressive symptoms, both directly and through declining grades. Thus, comparison to more successful others might have helped some students keep their grades, and spirits, lifted, and keeping standards elevated in the aftermath of failure predicts the relative absence of subsequent negative affect (Ahrens & Abramson, 1991).

In a related study, Aspinwall and Taylor (1993) induced a positive or negative mood in either high or low self-esteem subjects, and then forced them to engage in either an upward or downward social comparison. The comparison involved another student who had fared well or badly at the university. As the subjects were far from graduation, there was ample opportunity for them to improve their outcomes after the comparison. This should be the circumstance under which upward comparison would be helpful. Indeed, after negative mood induction, upward comparisons improved the affect of those both high and low in self-esteem. After the positive mood induction, downward comparison led to increased negative affect, particularly for those high in self-esteem. It should be noted that low self-esteem subjects who had had a negative mood induced were helped by downward comparison if they had experienced a setback in the last week. Combined, these studies support the premise that the effects of social comparison on depression will be moderated by the presence of an opportunity for future performance.

Will upward comparison always lead to improved affect when there is a chance for performance in the future? We think that this will depend on the inferences subjects have drawn from the comparison. If subjects look to the other and find a process by which they can subsequently excel, then this should improve affect. If not, upward comparison might lead to more depression, even if there is the possibility of future performance (cf. Aspinwall, chapter 5, this volume; Buunk & Ybema, chapter 12, this volume). Next, we consider some of the factors that might affect the inferences drawn from upward comparison.

If the information is simply the evaluation of the performance of the comparison target (e.g., someone else received a perfect score on a test), this might be quite depressing. In contrast, if the information about the other demonstrates how that person achieved the score, this would provide hope, assuming the steps are replicable. Indeed, modeling by upward comparison targets is central to a variety of effective therapies (Bandura, 1986).

Degree of depressive symptomatology present at the time of comparison likely also will affect the consequences of comparison. Depressed individuals are hypothesized to be more prone to negative inferences about the self (Abramson et al., 1989). Presented with an upward comparison target, then, they are more likely to conclude that, while others can attain such heights, they themselves cannot. In addition, given the motivational deficits of depressed individuals (e.g., Beck, 1967), they may be likely to put in less effort in trying to understand how the comparison target performed so well, and so will be less able to believe that they, too, can do it.

Initial research supports this suggestion. Ybema, Buunk, and Heesink (1996) gave people who had recently lost their jobs in collective dismissals social comparison information about others who were coping either well or poorly with losing their jobs. Those who were more stressed, assessed in part by feelings of depression, identified more with the comparison target coping poorly and less with the comparison target coping well than did those who were less stressed. In addition, high stress subjects experienced less positive and more negative affect than did less stressed subjects. The effect of stress on negative affect was mediated by identification with a comparison target. Extrapolated to depression, this would suggest that depressed people would see possibilities of their own bleak futures when given information about others who do not cope well, and that this would likely lead to maintenance of depression. This study should be interpreted with some caution, however, as depressive symptoms were not assessed directly and there was no interaction of social comparison target and stress in predicting negative affect or positive affect.

Attributions may also moderate the relation of social comparison direction to depression. In particular, hope, and so depression, is likely to depend on the attributions made for discrepancies between self and other (Ybema, 1994). For instance, upward comparison in which success is likely due to effort may be inspiring because it suggests that further effort will prompt future success. In contrast, comparison to others whose success seems due to ability would tend to prompt hopelessness. An initial demonstration suggests that this is the case (Ybema, 1994). Freshmen who had taken a final test received information about an upward or downward comparison other whose outcome was attributed to either effort or ability. Among students high in academic stress, upward comparison led to more positive affect if the other's performance was attributed to effort. In contrast, downward comparison led to more positive affect when it was attributed to ability rather than to effort. As depressed individuals are more prone to attribute their own failures to more stable, global factors than are nondepressed individuals (e.g., Sweeney, Anderson, & Bailey, 1986), this should lead upward comparisons to be relatively uninspiring for depressed people.

Upward comparisons in which others' success seems to be based on effort do seem to inspire subsequent success. For instance, Wilson and Linville (1982) gave students who had not done well in their first year of college information about others who had improved in performance after their first year. Compared to control subjects, those with this information about others who had improved performance subsequently showed improved performance themselves. Perhaps this is because the upward comparison information had provided hope and so reduced the depression associated with academic failure.

Hope is closely tied to control. If individuals perceive control over their destiny they may have hope if they believe they can exert control. Another factor moderating the relation of direction of social comparison to affect is perception of control (see also Wood & VanderZee, chapter 10, this volume). In one study exploring this issue, subjects on disability for a variety of diseases were surveyed about their control over their disease. They were also given information about either an upward or downward comparison target in terms of coping with the disease (Ybema & Buunk, 1995). Positive affect was particularly high following exposure to an upward target for those high in perceived control. Once again, as depressed people tend to believe that they have less control over favorable outcomes than do nondepressed people (Alloy, Clements, & Koenig, 1993), this increase in positive affect should be more likely for those who are nondepressed.

In general, the effect of social comparison on depressive symptoms such as negative affect is moderated by choice of target and ability to repeat performance. If there is no repeated performance, downward comparisons tend to lead to less depression. If there is a possible future performance, upward comparison, at least under some circumstances, leads to less depression. Unfortunately, depressed individuals are more prone to give up (e.g., Hahn-Smith & Agostinelli, 1993), more likely to attribute their own failures to lack of ability (e.g., Sweeney et al., 1986), and more prone to believe positive outcomes to be uncontrollable (e.g., Martin et al., 1984), which suggests that the positive effects of upward comparisons are most likely for nondepressed individuals.

Social comparison is likely to have other consequences as well. For example, research on persistence suggests that the mere fact of social comparison by depressed subjects might be harmful (Hahn-Smith & Agostinelli, 1993). Mildly depressed and nondepressed subjects performing an anagram problem-solving task received either favorable, unfavorable, or no social comparison information. Subsequently, those depressed subjects given any comparison information persisted less than did nondepressed subjects. There were no persistence differences among subjects given no social comparison information.

In addition to its effects on self, social comparison might have effects on others as well. Depressed people seem to seek more reassurance (e.g., Joiner & Metalsky, 1995). Many dimensions on which we wish to seek information (e.g., salary) are considered personal. Swallow and Kuiper (1988) suggested that depressed people, given their motivation to seek comparison information, might be prone to asking others about this sort of sensitive information (see also Kuiper & McCabe, 1985). If so, this might alienate others, leading to the rejection experienced by depressed persons (e.g., Coyne, Burchill, & Stiles, 1990). This, of course, would need to be explored by future research.

## CONCLUSION

In summary, social comparison provides a window for understanding depression and hopelessness. Depressed individuals do make more negative comparisons of self to other than do nondepressed individuals. These might arise from tendencies to interpret social comparison information more negatively, to be more open to social comparison information and to make upward comparisons, although some evidence suggests that depressed people seek downward comparisons so as to cope with their circumstances.

There are several directions open for future research. For instance, much of the research described is cross-sectional. More longitudinal research on these topics would be valuable. For example, does seeking more comparison information lead to more, long-term, depressive symptoms? Does the increased social comparison activity of depressed people over time tend to drive their friends away?

More research needs to be performed on the steps hypothesized to lead from these comparisons to depression. Social comparison information may affect attributions (McArthur, 1972). For example, learning that someone else has a similar problem may make an attribution to the self less likely. In addition, attributions predict subsequent depression (e.g., Dixon & Ahrens, 1992; Metalsky, Halberstadt, & Abramson, 1987; Nolen-Hoeksema, Girgus, & Seligman, 1986). However, no study has examined whether shifts in attributions prompted by social comparison information prompt changes in depression, as suggested by hopelessness theory. Nor have the links from social comparison information to depression through negative inferences about the self and the consequences of negative outcomes been directly tested.

In addition, social comparison is a set of several different processes (e.g., Wood, 1996). We have touched on several of these above, but others have yet to be explored. For instance, we have discussed processes involved in seeking and encountering social comparison information. How does depression play into the construction of social comparison information?

What others do informs us of our own possibilities and realities. This can create optimism and nondepression for those who can look to improved future performance or focus on those who have done less well. However, it can also prompt hopelessness and depression in those who have no future performance and seem drawn to information that others have done better.

## ACKNOWLEDGMENTS

We are grateful to Jim Kulik and Steve Misovich and, especially, Bram Buunk and Rick Gibbons for their extremely helpful comments on previous drafts of this chapter. Lauren Alloy was supported by NIMH Grant MH48216 during preparation of this chapter.

## REFERENCES

Abramson, L. Y., & Alloy, L. B. (1981). Depression, nondepression, and cognitive illusions: A reply to Schwartz. *Journal of Experimental Psychology: General, 110,* 436–447.

Abramson, L. Y., Metalsky, G. I., & Alloy, L. B. (1989). Hopelessness depression: A theory-based subtype of depression. *Psychological Review, 96,* 358–372.

Ahrens, A. H. (1987). Theories of depression: The role of goals and the self-evaluation process. *Cognitive Therapy and Research, 11,* 665–680.

Ahrens, A. H. (1991). Dysphoria and social comparison: Combining information regarding others' performances. *Journal of Social and Clinical Psychology, 10,* 190–205.

Ahrens, A. H., & Abramson, L. Y. (1991). Changes in personal standards and dysphoria: A longitudinal approach. *Cognitive Therapy and Research, 15,* 47–68.

Albright, J. S., Alloy, L. B., Barch, D., & Dykman, B. M. (1993). Social comparison by dysphoric and nondysphoric college students: The grass isn't always greener on the other side. *Cognitive Therapy and Research, 17,* 485–510.

Albright, J. S., & Henderson, M. C. (1995). How real is depressive realism? A question of scales and standards. *Cognitive Therapy and Research, 19,* 589–609.

Alloy, L. B., & Abramson, L. Y. (1988). Depressive realism: Four theoretical perspectives. In L. B. Alloy (Ed.), *Cognitive processes in depression* (pp. 223–265). New York: Guilford.

Alloy, L. B., & Ahrens, A. H. (1987). Depression and pessimism for the future: Biased use of statistically relevant information in predictions for self versus other. *Journal of Personality and Social Psychology, 52,* 366–378.

Alloy, L. B., Albright, J. S., & Clements, C. (1987). Depression, nondepression, and social comparison biases. In J. E. Maddux, C. D. Stoltenberg, & R. Rosenwein (Eds.), *Social processes in clinical and counseling psychology* (pp. 94–112). New York: Springer-Verlag.

Alloy, L. B., Clements, C. M., & Koenig, L. J. (1993). Perceptions of control: Determinants and mechanisms. In G. Weary, F. Gleicher, & K. L. Marsh (Eds.), *Control motivation and social cognition (pp. 33–73). New York: Springer-Verlag.*

Alloy, L. B., Hartlage, S., & Abramson, L. Y. (1988). Testing the cognitive diathesis-stress theories of depression: Issues of research design, conceptualization, and assessment. In L. B. Alloy (Ed.), *Cognitive processes in depression* (pp. 31–73). New York: Guilford.

Aspinwall, L. G. & Taylor, S. E. (1993). Effects of social comparison direction, threat, and self-esteem on affect, self-evaluation, and expected success. *Journal of Personality and Social Psychology, 64,* 708–722.

Bandura, A. (1986). *Social foundations of thought and action: A social cognitive theory.* Englewood Cliffs, NJ: Prentice-Hall.

Beck, A. T. (1967). *Depression: Clinical, experimental, and theoretical aspects.* New York: Harper & Row.

Beck, A. T., Ward, C. H., Mendelson, M., Mock, J., & Erbaugh, J. (1961). An inventory for measuring depression. *Archives of General Psychiatry, 4,* 561–571.

Bibring, E. (1953). The mechanism of depression. In P. Greenacre (Ed.), *Affective disorders.* New York: International Universities Press.

Buunk, B. P., Collins, R. L., Taylor, S.E., VanYperen, N. W., & Dakof, G. A. (1990). The affective consequences of social comparison: Either direction has its ups and downs. *Journal of Personality and Social Psychology, 59,* 1238–1249.

Collins, R. L. (1996). For better or for worse: The impact of upward social comparison on self-evaluations. *Psychological Bulletin, 119,* 51–69.

Coyne, J. C. (1994). Self-reported distress: Analog or ersatz depression? *Psychological Bulletin, 116,* 29–45.

Coyne, J. C., Burchill, S. A. L., & Stiles, W. B. (1990). An interactional perspective on depression. In C. R. Snyder & D. O. Forsyth (Eds.), *Handbook of social and clinical psychology: The health perspective.* New York: Pergamon.

Davila, J., Hammen, C., Burge, D., Paley, B., & Daley, S. E. (1995). Poor interpersonal problem solving as a mechanism of stress generation in depression among adolescent women. *Journal of Abnormal Psychology, 104,* 592–600.

DeVellis, R. F., Holt, K., Renner, B. A., Blalock, S. J., Blanchard, L. W., Cook, H. L., Klotz, M. L., Mikow, V., & Harring, K. (1990). The relationship of social comparison to rheumatoid arthritis symptoms and affect. *Basic and Applied Social Psychology, 11,* 1–18.

Dixon, J. F., & Ahrens, A. H. (1992). Stress and attributional style as predictors of self-reported depression in children. *Cognitive Therapy and Research, 16,* 623–634.

Flett, G. L., Vredenburg, K., Pliner, P., & Krames, L. (1987). Depression and social comparison information-seeking. *Journal of Social Behavior and Personality, 2,* 473–484.

Freud, S. (1957). Mourning and melancholia. In J. Strachey (Ed.), *The complete psychological works of Sigmund Freud* (Vol. 14). London: Hogarth Press. (Original work published 1917)

Gibbons, F. X. (1986). Social comparison and depression: Company's effect on misery. *Journal of Personality and Social Psychology, 51,* 140–148.

Gibbons, F. X., Blanton, H., Gerrard, M., & Eggleston, T. J. (1996). *Does social comparison make a difference? The influence of comparison level on outcome.* Unpublished manuscript, Iowa State University Des Moines.

Gibbons, F. X., & Boney McCoy, S. (1991). Self-esteem, similarity, and reactions to active versus passive downward comparison. *Journal of Personality and Social Psychology, 60,* 414–424.

Golin, S., Terrell, F., & Johnson, B. (1977). Depression and the illusion of control. *Journal of Abnormal Psychology, 86,* 440–442.

Golin, S., Terrell, F., Weitz, J., & Drost, P. L. (1979). The illusion of control among depressed patients. *Journal of Abnormal Psychology, 88,* 454–457.

Haaga, D. A. F, Dyck, M. J., & Ernst, D. (1991). Empirical status of cognitive theory of depression. *Psychological Bulletin, 110,* 215–236.

Hahn-Smith, S. T., & Agostinelli, G. (1993). Effects of normative information on task persistence among depressed and nondepressed individuals. *Journal of Social Behavior and Personality, 8,* 715–728.

Heidrich, S. M., & Ryff, C. D. (1993). The role of social comparisons processes in the psychological adaptation of elderly adults. *Journal of Gerontology: Psychological Sciences,*

*48,* 127-136.
Hemphill, K. J., & Lehman, D. R. (1991). Social comparisons and their affective consequences: The importance of comparison dimension and individual difference variables. *Journal of Social and Clinical Psychology, 10,* 372-394.
Joiner, T. E., & Metalsky, G. I. (1995). A prospective test of an integrative interpersonal theory of depression: A naturalistic study of college roommates. *Journal of Personality and Social Psychology, 69,* 778-788.
Kernis, M. H. (1993). The roles of stability and level of self-esteem in psychological functioning. In R. Baumeister (Ed.), *Self-esteem: The puzzle of low self-regard* (pp. 167-182). New York: Plenum.
Kuiper, N. A., & McCabe, S. B. (1985). The appropriateness of social topics: Effects of depression and cognitive vulnerability on self and other judgments. *Cognitive Therapy and Research, 9,* 371-380.
Major, B. Sciacchitano, A. M., & Crocker, J. (1993). In-group versus out-group comparisons and self-esteem. *Personality and Social Psychology Bulletin, 19,* 711-721.
Martin, D. J., Abramson, L. Y., & Alloy, L. B. (1984). The illusion of control for self and others in depressed and nondepressed college students. *Journal of Personality and Social Psychology, 46,* 125-136.
McArthur, L. Z. (1972). The how and what of why: Some determinants and consequences of causal attribution. *Journal of Personality and Social Psychology, 22,* 171-193.
McFarland, C. & Miller, D. T. (1994). The framing of relative performance feedback: Seeing the glass as half empty or half full. *Journal of Personality and Social Psychology, 66,* 1061-1073.
Metalsky, G. I., Halberstadt, L. J., & Abramson, L. Y. (1987). Vulnerability to depressive mood reactions: Toward a more powerful test of the diathesis-stress and causal mediation components of the reformulated theory of depression. *Journal of Personality and Social Psychology, 52,* 386-393.
Meyer, N. E., Dyck, D. G., & Petrinack, R. J. (1989). Cognitive appraisal and attributional correlates of depressive symptoms in children, *Journal of Abnormal Child Psychology, 17,* 325-336.
Miller, D. T., Turnbull, W., & McFarland, C. (1988). Particularistic and universalistic evaluation in the social comparison process. *Journal of Personality and Social Psychology, 55,* 908-917.
Morrow, J. & Nolen-Hoeksema, S. (1990). Effects of responses to depression on the remediation of depressive affect. *Journal of Personality and Social Psychology, 58,* 519-527.
Needles, D. J., & Abramson, L. Y. (1990). Positive life events, attributional style, and hopefulness: Testing a model of recovery from depression. *Journal of Abnormal Psychology, 99,* 156-165.
Nisbett, R. E., & Ross, L. (1980). *Human inference: Strategies and shortcomings of social judgment.* New York: Prentice-Hall.
Nolen-Hoeksema, S., Girgus, J., & Seligman, M. E. P. (1986). Learned helplessness in children: A longitudinal study of depression, achievement and explanatory style. *Journal of Personality and Social Psychology, 51,* 435-442.
Pelham, B. W. (1991). On the benefits of misery: Self-serving biases in the depressive self-concept. *Journal of Personality and Social Psychology, 61,* 670-681.
Radloff, L. (1977). The CES-D Scale: A self-report depression scale for research in the general population. *Applied Psychological Measurement, 1,* 385-401.
Roberts, J. E., & Monroe, S. M. (1994). A multidimensional model of self-esteem in depression. *Clinical Psychology Review, 14,* 161-181.
Robins, C. J., Hayes, A. M., Block, P., Kramer, R. J., & Villena, M. (1995). Interpersonal

and achievement concerns and the depressive vulnerability and symptom specificity hypotheses: A prospective study. *Cognitive Therapy and Research, 19,* 1–20.

Robinson, N. S., Garber, J., & Hilsman, R. (1995). Cognitions and stress: Direct and moderating effects on depressive versus externalizing symptoms during the junior high school transition. *Journal of Abnormal Psychology, 104,* 453–463.

Rogers, C. R. (1961). *On becoming a person.* Boston: Houghton Mifflin.

Rosenblatt, A., & Greenberg, J. (1991). Examining the world of the depressed: Do depressed people prefer others who are depressed? *Journal of Personality and Social Psychology, 60,* 620–629.

Sacco, W. P., & Graves, D. J. (1984). Childhood depression, interpersonal problem-solving, and self-ratings of performance. *Journal of Child Clinical Psychology, 13,* 10–15.

Schulz, R., & Decker, S. (1985). Long-term adjustment to physical disability: The role of social support, perceived control, and self- blame. *Journal of Personality and Social Psychology, 48,* 1162–1172.

Swallow, S. R., & Kuiper, N. A. (1988). Social comparison and negative self-evaluations: An application to depression. *Clinical Psychology Review, 8,* 55–76.

Swallow, S. R., & Kuiper, N. A. (1990). Mild depression, dysfunctional cognitions, and interest in social comparison information. *Journal of Social and Clinical Psychology, 9,* 289–302.

Swallow, S. R., & Kuiper, N. A. (1992). Mild depression and frequency of social comparison behavior. *Journal of Social and Clinical Psychology, 11,* 167–180.

Swallow, S. R., & Kuiper, N. A. (1993). Social comparison in dysphoria and nondysphoria: Differences in target similarity and specificity. *Cognitive Therapy and Research, 17,* 103–122.

Sweeney, P. D., Anderson, K., & Bailey, S. (1986). Attributional style in depression: A meta-analytic review. *Journal of Personality and Social Psychology, 50,* 974–991.

Taylor, S. E., & Lobel, M. (1989). Social comparison activity under threat: Downward evaluation and upward contacts. *Psychological Review, 96,* 569–575.

Vredenburg, K., Flett, G. L., & Krames, L. (1993). Analogue versus clinical depression: A critical reappraisal. *Psychological Bulletin, 113,* 327–344.

Weary, G., Elbin, S., & Hill, M. G. (1987). Attributional and social comparison processes in depression. *Journal of Personality and Social Psychology, 52,* 605–610.

Weary, G., Marsh, K. L, & McCormick, L. (1994). Depression and social comparison motives. *European Journal of Social Psychology,* 117–129.

Webster, D. M., & Kruglanski, A. W. (1994). Individual differences in need for closure. *Journal of Personality and Social Psychology, 67,* 1049–1062.

Wechsler, C. (1974). *Manual for the Wechsler Intelligence Scale for Children-Revised* (WISC-R). New York: Psychological Corporation.

Weissman, A. N., & Beck, A. T. (1978). *Development and Validation of the Dysfunctional Attitude Scale: A preliminary investigation.* Paper presented at the American Educational Research Association Annual Convention, Toronto, Canada.

Wheeler, L., & Miyake, K. (1992). Social comparison and everyday life. *Journal of Personality and Social Psychology, 62,* 760–773.

Wills, T. A. (1981). Downward comparison principles. *Psychological Bulletin, 90,* 245–271.

Wilson, T. D., & Linville, P. W. (1982). Improving the academic performance of college freshmen: Attribution therapy revisited. *Journal of Personality and Social Psychology, 42,* 367–376.

Wood, J. V. (1996). What is social comparison and how should we study it? *Personality and Social Psychology Bulletin, 22,* 520–537.

Wood, J. V., & Taylor, K. L., (1991). Serving self-relevant goals through social comparison.

In J. Suls & T. A. Wills (Eds.), *Social comparison: Contemporary theory and research* (pp. 23–49). Hillsdale, NJ: Lawrence Erlbaum Associates.

Ybema, J. F. (1994). *Up and down: Affective responses to social comparison*. Capelle and Yssel: Labyrint Publication.

Ybema, J. F., & Buunk, B. P. (1995). Affective responses to social comparison: A study among disabled individuals. *British Journal of Social Psychology, 34,* 279–292.

Ybema, J. F., Buunk, B. P., & Heesink, J. A. M. (1996). Affect and identification in social comparison after loss of work. *Basic and Applied Social Psychology, 18,* 151–169.

# CHAPTER 14

# Social Comparison and Health: A Process Model

Howard Leventhal
Shawna Hudson
Chantal Robitaille
*Rutgers University*

Social comparison theory was originally based on a fairly simple assumption: In times of uncertainty, when other means for objective evaluation are lacking, individuals compare themselves to similar others to evaluate their own opinions and abilities. Subsequent iterations of social comparison theory focused on further qualifying the conditions under which the social comparison process could be employed. These approaches answered, or attempted to answer, "when, why, what, and with whom" questions.

There appears to be much agreement about the answers to the when and why questions. Festinger (1954) and later architects of social comparison theory, like the contributors to this volume, agree that individuals tend to engage in social comparison when they are unsure about some particular outcome, such as their health, and they do so to reduce perceived uncertainty. Agreement quickly dissipates among social comparison theorists, however, when they begin to suggest what specific things individuals do when they make these comparisons. Some suggest that individuals simply evaluate their own abilities (Festinger, 1954) or feelings (Schachter, 1959). Others suggest social comparison is used primarily for self-enhancement (Gruder, 1977; Hakmiller, 1966; Taylor & Lobel, 1989; Wills, 1981, 1991; Wood, Taylor, & Lichtman, 1985). Similarly, there is disagreement about who is used as a comparison object—a similar (Festinger, 1954; Wills, 1981, 1991; Wood & Taylor, 1991) or dissimilar (Suls, Leventhal, & Martin, chapter 4, this volume) other. Although all of these qualifications to social comparison theory go a long way toward helping us conceptualize the circumstances under which social comparison occurs, they tell us little about the process of social comparison or about "how" it is done by real people in real settings.

Social comparison theory in its original presentation did not elaborate models of the situations in which comparisons occur. Its propositions were tested in laboratory settings where the operational definitions of ambiguity and the availability of comparison information were controlled by the experimenter (see Festinger, 1954; Hakmiller, 1966; Radloff, 1966; Schachter, 1959; Schachter & Singer, 1962). Since experimental control is lacking in studies where the model is applied to real world settings, it can be expected that social comparison will be but one of several procedures useful for uncertainty reduction (e.g., testing of alternatives, seeking information from experts, denial). The objective of social comparison, its manner of execution, the outcome of the comparison and the relative importance and durability of the outcome of the comparison, we argue, should vary by the question addressed (i.e., the uncertainty to be reduced) in a specific situation. This view of social comparison as one among many procedures for problem solving leads us to the conclusion that it might be better to regard subjects in such settings as "problem solvers" rather than as "social comparers."

## SOCIAL COMPARISON: TRAIT OR PROCESS

Although it seems especially useful to treat participants in real-life studies (i.e., nonlaboratory) as problem solvers, recognizing that participants are actively framing and generating solutions to problems does not fully constrain our conceptualization of social comparison. Specifically, we can consider social comparison as a tactical component that is determined by higher order factors such as the characteristics of the person and/or a situationally based problem-solving process, or we can treat social comparison as a trait (i.e., as an individual's characteristic style of problem solving). Modeling social comparison as a trait is similar to what has been done in studies of coping. Factorial studies of this type typically pool a wide variety of behavioral tactics and strategies into one, or at best two, problem-solving factors (e.g., Krohne, 1993; Lazarus & Folkman, 1984). As such, they fail to capture the substance and texture of problem-based coping. By encasing social comparison in a factorial framework, we ignore its unique properties and emphasize its commonalities with other social and nonsocial procedures for problem solving. Procedures for problem-based coping are incredibly varied and their problem-solving utility will vary in accord with the specifics of the problem setting. In short, coping procedures are not traits, nor is there a necessary or fixed relationship between any specific coping procedure and adaptation. Modeling social comparison as a trait assumes that the outcomes of social comparison, whether it enhances self-esteem and/or creates negative emotions, reflects a stable, individual difference in need for such outcomes.

In chapter 6, Wills, a proponent of the psychometric approach, discusses two points that support our argument. First, he states that his subjects were asked how frequently they employed particular coping mechanisms and admits, "[t]here was no attempt to gauge whether the coping was appropriately matched to the problem and situation." In so doing, he acknowledges the importance of situational factors, thus arguing against the trait position. Second, Wills recognizes that the same coping responses (e.g., social comparison) "have beneficial effects" over the short-term or different, presumably harmful, effects over the long-term. A coping procedure will be adaptive or maladaptive for the short or the long term depending on the function it serves in the situation for which it is brought into play. Having conceded that the same social comparison response can have different consequences at different times (i.e., have different functions for different situations) questions the utility of treating social comparison as a trait rather than as a coping procedure that is a product of situationally specific needs and motives. Social comparison can be best understood when placed in the context of a process model.

## APPROACHES TO STUDYING THE PROCESS OF SOCIAL COMPARISON

The authors of virtually all of the chapters in this volume recognize that social comparison is but one component of a problem-solving process and that it can serve multiple functions and produce diverse outcomes. Although the authors vary in how they identify and investigate these diverse functions, they favor one of three different themes in their approach: social comparison as a product of individual personality, of situational factors, and as a product of the interaction of personality and situation. In each of these approaches, the social comparison process is treated as a product of a higher order factor (i.e., of the person, the situation, or their interaction). Those favoring properties of the person emphasize the moderating effect of personality characteristics such as extroversion on the occurrence, direction, and outcome of the comparison process. Those stressing the properties of the situation as a moderator of social comparison, focus on questions such as, "Under what circumstances (i.e., conditions of uncertainty) will different types of social comparison (i.e., enhancement, evaluation, or coping) be employed?" If one believes that individuals behave similarly within parallel situations, knowledge of the situation may be sufficient for predicting and understanding social comparison as a coping procedure. Those favoring the person-by-situation approach introduce the concept of motivation as the determinant of social comparison. In this approach, specific motives emerge from interactions among the properties of the situation with the characteristics of the person. Thus, neither situation or person factors alone are sufficient to determine the occurrence, direction, intensity, and outcome of social comparison. Of these three views, the motivational view is most fully in accord with our suggestion that persons should be viewed as active "problem solvers."

**Properties of the Person**

A variety of individual difference factors have been proposed as potential moderators of the occurrence and direction of social comparison. For example, Wood and VanderZee (chapter 10, this volume) ask if optimists are more likely than pessimists to compare themselves with others. Ahrens and Alloy (chapter 13, this volume) ask if depressed individuals are more open to social comparisons than nondepressed individuals. Gibbons and Gerrard (chapter 3, this volume) ask if adolescents are more likely than adults to engage in social comparison and Diener and Fujita (chapter 11, this volume) suggest that individual personality characteristics such as neuroticism or extraversion affect the occurrence and direction of social comparison. The expectation underlying each of these proposals is that people with similar personality characteristics will experience and respond to uncertainty in similar ways regardless of the specific features of an eliciting situation.

Investigators have gathered data suggesting that different cognitive, expressive, and autonomic patterns are associated with each of the trait-like personality factors assumed to affect social comparison. For example, it has been suggested that trait anxiety leads people to direct attention prospectively and to focus cognitions on dreaded outcomes in response to health threats (Brownlee, Leventhal, & Balaban, 1992; Janis, 1958). Trait depression, on the other hand, is presumed to direct attention to past failures and to evoke self critical cognitions (Beck, 1967; Teasdale & Barnard, 1993) and thoughts of hopelessness and helplessness in the face of threat (Abramson, Seligman, & Teasdale, 1978). The expectation that these traits stimulate social comparison, and if they do, whether they do so in a downward or upward direction and lead to particular outcome appraisals, depends in part, on how one models the way in which traits influence the cognitive, emotional, and behavioral states that generate behavior (see Ahrens & Alloy, chapter 13, this volume). If the effects are direct, that is, if states are simple correlates of individuals' traits, as the properties of the person approach contends, a modest to moderate-size correlation might be expected between trait emotions and social comparison measures taken under threatening, emotionally provocative situations. But if traits generate motives in interaction with situational factors, motives will be the immediate antecedent mediators of social comparison behaviors and the zero order correlations between trait and social comparison measured across situations will be small in magnitude. Note that a possible exception, resulting in high correlations between trait and social comparison, would result if individuals were successful in seeking out and/or creating situations compatible with their dispositions.

**Properties of the Situation**

Several authors of chapters in this book attribute the variance in behavioral (social comparison) outcomes to situational properties. For example, Aspinwall (chapter 5, this volume) believes that comparison results will look quite different depending on whether social comparison is an effort to make sense of one's response to a prior threat situation—that is, whether social comparison is working retrospectively—or whether it is an attempt to make sense of a situation that is looming on the behavioral horizon. Wood and VanderZee (chapter 10, this volume), using a different approach, found that breast cancer patients "were not using social comparison solely . . . to self-evaluate. Rather, they seemed to be making comparisons that made themselves feel better about their own situations and themselves." It is important to note here that because situations are constantly evolving, the situation at a later point may be quite different from the situation at onset. This is abundantly clear with health threats.

It has been proposed that people respond to health threats in scripted or predetermined ways. The concept of behavioral "scripts" (Abelson, 1981) represents an attempt to simplify both cross-situational diversity and the diversity introduced by the temporal unfolding of specific situations. Scripts provide the text for the unfolding of a specific set of situations. Information seeking and social comparison are embedded in prototypic scripts, and information seeking and social comparison emerge during the unfolding of specific exemplars, most likely perhaps when a specific occasion deviates unexpectedly from the modal script. For example, studies of the restaurant script identify specific questions that are asked to reduce uncertainties at specific points in time (e.g., "The menu, please"; "Is the Peking Duck still available?" (see Bower, Black, & Turner, 1979). Social comparisons are part of these modal scripts (e.g., "What do you think is good here?" "Is there something you like that we can share?"), and social comparisons appear in response to unanticipated events within the modal script (e.g., "Does this taste right?"). The extent of social comparing will vary by setting and script as will the outcome of the comparison (e.g., people may feel positively or negatively about their experience for a short or long time).

Clearly it is possible to outline a general "illness script" and to identify scenes or frames for question asking and social comparison. The need for making comparisons is greater both during frames (points in the script) posing high levels of uncertainty about both the disease and the procedures for its prevention and/or control and when the more core values of the self are under threat. Uncertainty is typically high at points of entry, for example, when for the first time an individual takes a diagnostic test or enters a treatment situation. While the need to reduce uncertainty at such points may be very strong, the effect of the information can be transient or long lasting; the need for uncertainty reduction is independent of the duration of the effects of social comparison. For example, Kulik and Mahler's (chapter 8, this volume) coronary by-pass patients are highly motivated to compare a postoperative patient's experience with their own to reassure themselves that they will recover properly. As valuable and anxiety-reducing as the comparison may be, its impact on behavior may not extend beyond the few preoperative and postoperative hours. On the other hand, a woman feeling uncertain about her physical attractiveness, sexual function, and ability to sustain important social roles following a mastectomy may benefit over very long periods of time from satisfactory social comparisons with women who have successfully managed this very same situation.

There is every reason to expect that scripts for different diseases will differ in the frequency, location, and content (e.g., upward or downward comparisons) of their social comparison frames. Diseases with consequences that threaten core values of the physical and social self, such as cancer, AIDS, and coronary disease, will stimulate social comparisons that focus on core issues of self, whereas head colds and stomach flu—except under very special circumstances—will not. Stigmatizing diseases such as AIDS that pose a "potential loss of self-esteem, status and prestige" are likely to stimulate social comparisons for self enhancement (Buunk & Ybema, chapter 12, this volume).

Though informative, the approach of examining social comparison based on properties of the situation alone lacks the flexibility to account for the different responses and needs of different individuals. It is clear that these responses and needs play a role in determining the type of social comparison used. We therefore turn to a more integrative approach: examining the interactive effects of the person and the situation on social comparison.

## Person–Situation Interaction

A person–situation interaction model permits a more complete analysis of the conditions generating the diverse motives that drive the information gathering (i.e., social comparison process). Motivation to engage in social comparison can derive from a motivation to (a) evaluate one's opinions and expectations; (b) evaluate and enhance the facets of one's self; and (c) improve cognitive and instrumental skills. If personality variables or situational factors produced consistent main effects, the study of coping and social comparison would best proceed by the identification of the factors in each of these areas that moderate social comparison and by using them as the framework around which to organize the occurrence, direction, and outcomes of social comparison. And a psychometric strategy, such as that advocated by Wills (chapter 6, this volume), might be very useful in identifying the coping and other outcome variables affected by this framework. On the other hand, if person–situation transactions lead to different motivations in different persons in what appears to be the "same" situation, it is necessary to identify and assess these motives as well as the variables giving rise to them in order to understand the social comparison process. For example, social comparison will be influenced by the controllability of the disease presented (a situational factor) and by the individual's beliefs about the disease and the self (a personal factor). If a person believes that a disease such as rheumatoid arthritis is controllable and believes that she should be able to maintain a high level of function, we can predict that she will engage in whatever type of coping she has available to sustain function, including upward social comparison for skill acquisition. Coping procedures (comparisons) that improve function and reduce distress will be reinforced, repeated on future occasions, and automatized. Indeed, a procedure can be strengthened even when it does not alter the underlying disease or dysfunction, as long as it reduces distress: distress is part of pain and the amelioration of the former reduces the latter. On the other hand, if a person with arthritis believes her disease is controllable but doubts her ability to perform the necessary behaviors, she may avoid upward comparisons and miss the opportunity for skill acquisition because of a fear of looking inadequate. Downward comparisons, however, may also be threatening if they imply that the person's self-doubt will bring her to the level of pain and dysfunction of the suffering other. Hence, as suggested in Buunk and Ybema's identification–contrast model (chapter 12, this volume), there is no general preference for upward or downward comparison; the direction of the comparison will vary according to the characteristics of the situation and of the individual facing it (also see Wood & VanderZee, chapter 10, this volume).

Several implications can be drawn from the arthritis scenario. First, predicting what an individual will actually do and what the outcome may be requires that we understand the nature of the problem (i.e., the situation) and the characteristics of the individual (i.e., the person) at that point in time. In other words, it is essential to understand what drives coping (i.e., motivation) at a particular point in time if we are to understand whether social comparison will occur, and if it does, what its direction and outcome will be. Second, it is important to distinguish the controllability of the problem and the attributes of the disease that are in fact manageable with available resources (one's own and those of an expert). If the best medical procedures are ineffective, expectations will be violated and the individual will be forced to adopt alternative procedures for self-regulation. These may include social comparison. Third, as emotional distress is itself an integral part of the symptoms of disease, particularly of pain (Leventhal & Everhart, 1979), efforts to alleviate distress by means of social comparing will be functional. Finally, the individual's responses are active coping efforts whether they are performed automatically or deliberately: the difference is the degree to which the procedures are accompanied by conscious processes. Note that here we disagree with Tennen and Affleck's (chapter 9, this volume) assertion that coping is a deliberate, effortful, and conscious process and cannot be an automatic reaction. Although we agree with Tennen and Affleck that response acquisition is often an effortful process, we assert that coping, and by association social comparison, need not always be effortful. Comparison processes involved in the minimization of fear induced by health threats (see, e.g., Kulik & Mahler, chapter 8, this volume) do not appear to be especially effortful, but, they are still social comparisons and no less effective in that role. The conscious conduct of a coping procedure affects its properties, such as communicability, but does not make it more of a coping response than the same response performed automatically. Of course, the greater the level of conscious involvement, the greater the possibility and ease of communicating and sharing goals, procedures, and outcome evaluations. Thus clearly the type of social comparison we can most easily study with questionnaire methods is that accompanied by conscious processes (see Tennen & Affleck, chapter 9, this volume).

In summary, the person–situation (motivational) model seems the best approach to the study of social comparison. Only when we understand how the individual represents the self, the situation, and the resources available can we understand or predict the need and uses of social comparison.

## THE MOTIVATION APPROACH: A MODEL OF THE PERSON AS PROBLEM SOLVER

The examples elaborated in the discussion of person and situational contributions to social comparison strongly suggest that these factors do not operate alone; person and situation interact, giving rise to differing motives for information acquisition and increasing the complexity of the social comparison process. We offer a framework that will capture and illuminate these interactions while addressing the theoretical concerns of each of the contributing investigators in ways that allow them to pursue their proprietary ideas and preserve the insights generated by their substantial empirical work. Specifically, the framework suggests that the occurrence of social comparison; the direction of social comparison; the cognitive, affective, and behavioral consequences of social comparison; and the duration of these consequences all depend on the motive for comparison (Kruglanski & Mayseless, 1990). Put in somewhat different terms, social comparison is functional. Its occurrence and its meaning (i.e., what it tells the individual) are functions of the questions an individual asks implicitly or explicitly, at a given point in time.

To generate hypotheses we must go beyond a general statement that social comparisons are goal driven: we must specify the nature of the motives, or the specific aims and questions addressed in making comparisons. When we attempt to understand the role of social comparison in natural settings, specifically in settings where individuals, acting as "common-sense medical scientists" (Leventhal, Meyer, & Nerenz, 1980) are confronting and adapting to disease threats, a model of the threat context is essential. It defines the domain in which action will take place, that is, the motives (goals and questions) and behavioral scripts that will unfold at various points during a disease episode.

As motives and questions are products of interactions of persons with ever changing situations, it is essential to model the problem situation, that is, the person in context. We have constructed a framework for representing the person as a problem solver both in anticipation of disease threats (i.e., engaging in preventive behavior) and in coping with an existing disease threat. The framework includes three sets of elements: the representation of the disease (perceived attributes); the representation of the self; and the procedures perceived to be available from problem solution (detection, treatments, rehabilitation, etc.) including the individual's personal and social resources for managing the threat and the criteria used for evaluating change (Leventhal, Diefenbach, & E. Leventhal, 1992; Leventhal, Meyer, & Nerenz, 1980) (see Fig. 14.1). The need for information gathering via social comparison or some other means influences each of these elements of the framework, although the likelihood and direction of these comparisons may differ by area. For example, social comparisons that aim to elaborate on various features of the representation of a disease are probably best made by comparison to similar others, although the definition of similarity may differ as a function of the specific attribute under question. On the other hand, comparisons to gain procedural skills may be most beneficial and efficient if they are directed toward others who have succeeded in managing threat, because their experience can be used to enhance a person's own performance and safety.

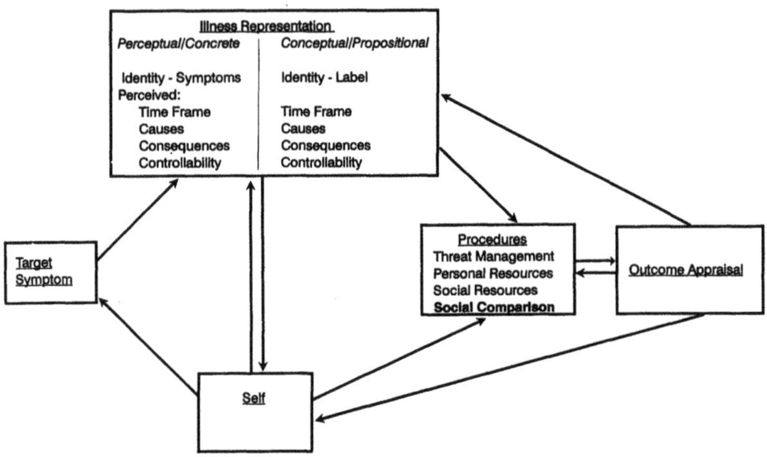


FIG. 14.1. The self-regulation (i.e., common sense) model of illness provides a framework within which the self engages in a variety of information-gathering procedures. This model regards individuals as "problem solvers" rather than "social comparers" because social comparison is but one of the procedures used by individuals in response to representations of the illness and of the self. The outcomes of these procedures are appraised and this appraisal in turn serves to modify the illness representations, the self-representations and the coping procedures. The path from self to symptoms indicates that changes in the self can change the somatic display of disease (e.g., age can blunt symptoms). The usual effect of symptoms on the self-system are indirect (i.e., through their representation). The bi-directional path from illness representation to the self creates the feeling that one is ill with a specific disease (e.g., self-knowledge of a family history of heart disease increases the likelihood that one will feel vulnerable to heart disease and label chest pain, a concrete symptom, as a heart attack).

**Representations of Disease**

Are there specific features of disease representations that are the source of ambiguity and need for information? Studies of disease models have identified five sets of attributes, each of which can be a source of ambiguity and can generate need: (a) the identity of the disease, or its label and its concrete indicators (somatic signs and symptoms); (b) its time frame (chronicity or acute state of disease indicators); (c) its causes (internal or external agents); (d) its consequences (physical, mental, social, economic effects on the person); and (e) its controllability (curability or manageability). Although we can think of each of these attributes in medical terms, it would be inappropriate to do so: they are features of an individual's common-sense views of disease threats.

The potential for ambiguity and susceptibility to clarification through social comparisons is high for each of these attributes. There are two reasons why this is so. First, as these attributes are part of everyday, or common-sense thinking, they are assumed to be culture wide and shared by others and hence open to social validation. Second, our data show that these attributes are bi-level: that is each can be described in conceptual–propositional terms and in perceptual–concrete terms (see Fig. 14.1). Both types of information can motivate and be influenced by social comparison. The meaning of *perceptual information* (the individual's observation of a symptom) is, however, often more poorly defined than *conceptual information* (the individual's knowledge that he or she has the flu) and hence in need of further specification by asking others, "What do you think this means?" In addition, these two levels may be discordant; for example, a person who feels perfectly fine can have a diagnosable cancer, and a person who is disease free, at least as far as medicine can determine, can feel quite ill. Discord creates ambiguity, which generates a need for information and opens the door to social comparison.

A powerful symmetry exists between the conceptual and perceptual facets comprising the *identity of a disease:* a symptom should have a label or diagnosis, and a label should have a concrete indicator or symptom (Baumann & Leventhal, 1985; Meyer, Leventhal, & Gutmann, 1985). The consequence of this symmetry is that the mind seeks a label for new symptoms and searches for new symptoms when it is given a label. Schachter's (1959) studies of affiliation under threat and Schachter and Singer's (1962) study of emotional contagion were based on the proposition that people have a need to label or attribute novel symptoms to specific causes and that this need is a powerful motive for social comparison. There is no shortage of studies showing that the occurrence of new symptoms or changes in existing ones leads to social contact

(Cameron, Leventhal, & Leventhal, 1993). The data are less clear, however, as to the purpose of this contact: is it intended to seek information about the meaning of the symptom? to obtain advice or consent that it is reasonable to seek medical care? or simply an effort to air one's concerns, based on the notion that sharing is stress reducing (Zola, 1973). We also suspect that the type of symptom will affect the objective of social comparison (see Suls et al., chapter 7, this volume). For example, it seems plausible that social comparison sought in response to highly unusual and severe symptoms will focus on confirming the need to seek professional care and that when symptoms are not painful or ambiguous in origin, questions for comparison will shift toward diagnosis or the meaning of symptoms.

The *time frame* for a condition is most readily represented conceptually. For example, Meyer et al. (1985) found that newly treated patients who believed that hypertension was an acute disease were much more likely to drop out of treatment once their symptoms cleared: they "felt" they had been in treatment long enough. Although it is most often presented conceptually, a time frame can also be presented perceptually. A good but unstudied perceptual example is the response of severely depressed individuals to antidepressant therapy: they "know" it will take 2 to 3 weeks for their tricyclic treatment to work, but they can "feel" it is not working as quickly as it should. The reason they feel this way is that they define "time for the drug to work" by the somatic effects (e.g., dry mouth) that appear within a day or two but that are unrelated to its psychological benefit. From the patient's common-sense experience, the drug is working within hours or days, not weeks, yet "feels" none of the expected benefits. As time frames are linked to every one of the attributes as well as to actions or procedures, they will be a frequent target for social comparison and other forms of information seeking.

Causal thinking also reflects both conceptual and perceptual processes. Misovich, Fisher, and Fisher (chapter 4, this volume) provide an excellent example of the role of perceptual cues in their discussion of the discounting of risk of AIDS by adolescents because they don't "look like" or have sex with persons who "look like" individuals at risk for AIDS. As these researchers suggest, comparisons that establish dissimilarities with another and reduce perceived vulnerability may be problematic for advocates of behavioral change. For example, a gay advocate presenting risk information to heterosexual adolescents may fail to influence them because he, the communicator, is very different from his target audience. In this situation the safe sex message activates the social comparison question, "Is this relevant to someone like me?", reinforcing existent beliefs of invulnerability that are anchored in the listener's social group. Little need be said and little effort need be invested in safe sex when AIDS victims simply "Don't look like us!" Indeed, the lower the percentage of adolescents with AIDS and the higher the percentage of gays with AIDS, the more persuasive the evidence for distancing the self from the threat (Smith, 1984). The more stereotypical the communicator's characteristics the easier it is for listeners to internalize the message that "I am different, hence not at risk." Both the disease (AIDS) and the comparison other (the gay advocate) fit schemata-based images (Gibbons & Gerrard, chapter 3, this volume) that generate a causal "question and answer" that determines the result of the social comparison process.

The perceptual level of the *consequences* attribute may be both the easiest to understand and perhaps the most frequently involved in social comparisons. Patients facing the threat of cancer or cardiac disease not only think about the abstract risks of disease and surgery, they generate images of themselves emaciated by cancer and lying on their death bed, or images of themselves in pain and mutilated by surgery (Janis, 1958). These images activate memory nodes that in turn mediate the mood, cognitive, expressive, and autonomic components of fear and depression (Leventhal, 1984). Images and their associated affects can drive avoidance as well as the search for information, for social support, and for social comparison. Kulik and Mahler's (1987; chapter 8, this volume) excellent studies of patients scheduled for coronary artery bypass surgery provide evidence of the powerful impact of perceptual cues in reducing the threatening consequences of anticipated surgery. Patients who share their hospital rooms with others who have survived surgery are less frightened and do better postoperatively than those in rooms with patients who are also awaiting surgery. The perceptual–concrete evidence that others are alive and looking well is a sufficient counter to images of mutilation, pain, and death that may fill the mind during this period of anticipation. In one way or another, most of the contributors to this volume give perceptual cues a role in the social comparison process. Assessing when and where perceptual, image-relevant data override conceptual or propositional knowledge may be an interesting and fruitful area for research.

Our examples so far have illustrated the way that social comparison might address a question about some aspect of a single representational attribute. More often than not, however, social comparisons may address more than one such attribute. Hypertensive patients provide an example of the way symptoms—the perceptual level of the identity attribute—affect beliefs about the controllability of hypertension. Patients who believe their medication is removing or controlling their symptoms are faithful users of their antihypertension medication and in better blood pressure control even though there is virtually no evidence that symptoms are related to baseline levels of blood pressure (Meyer et al., 1985). Although it is clear that the belief that hypertension is symptomatic is culture wide (Blumhagen, 1980) and inadvertently encouraged by medical practitioners, the role of social comparison in the creation and maintenance of the belief has not been studied.

**Representation of the Self**

Although questions about the *self* vary in salience and are not always easy to detect such questions are always present during the acquisition of information for regulation of illness threats (Hooker & Kaus, 1994; Gibbons & Gerrard, chapter 3, this volume). These self images can be generic or disease specific in relation to the representation of disease (e.g., schemata of the self as vulnerable or invulnerable to any disease or of the self as vulnerable to a particular disease) and in relation to the procedures for the management of disease threats and the emotional reactions associated with these threats (e.g., "I am [or am not] able to perform these exercises," and "I can [or cannot] control my fear in the presence of this threat"; Leventhal, 1970).

The presence of a generic image of the self, is apparent in what is usually the first and seemingly simplest step in symptom appraisal. When any unusual somatic event such as a lump, an ache, or a burning pain in the abdomen or chest is interpreted as a possible indicator of cancer, gastrointestinal, or cardiovascular problems, it is processed as a deviation from an implicit, or standard model of the somatic self. Similarly, the acceptance and rejection of the risk of AIDS is processed as the inclusion or exclusion of the (part of the) behavioral self-image within the prototype of the AIDS susceptible individual (Misovich et al., chapter 4, this volume). Frightening images of the somatic, economic, and social ravages of the disease are processed in terms of the self in its various guises and roles. Thus, the individual's models of both the self and the disease frame the questions and details of the social comparison process.

The following example illustrates the inclusion of the self in social comparisons involving the several functions (or questions) addressed by specific procedures for symptom control: I may use bicarbonate of soda or an antacid to treat stomach cramps or burning sensations in the gut because a friend reports successful use of such remedies whenever he has stomach problems. He is convinced, and therefore I am too, that these remedies are effective in curing minor ailments, work quickly, and prove, by their effectiveness, that the underlying condition is not serious, that is, not an ulcer or a cancer. In sum, social comparison provides me with an action plan (take 2 tablespoons full of Mylanta), a set of perceptual cues to validate that it is not a serious condition (if my dyspepsia goes away, I assume it is something less dangerous than a cancer), and a time frame to validate the efficacy of treatment.

Comparing oneself to another person to guide the selection of a procedure to manage burning sensations in the gut under the assumption that the borrowed procedure will control the symptoms and tell one if the condition is acid stomach or a serious condition implies two key assumptions about the self: the other's experience is relevant to me as we share physical similarities, and I believe myself vulnerable to ulcers and cancer and need to act to rule out these illnesses. The outcome of the procedure, (e.g., the antacid is or is not effective; it worked within an appropriate time frame or took longer than expected) informs us about ourselves (e.g., I do not have a serious disease; my body is weak and took too long to respond) and may tell us about our competencies both in using medication (I did not take it soon enough or in enough quantity) and self appraisal (my judgment about the condition was or was not correct). Thus, whereas the initial question regarding any coping procedure may be, "Did it work?" response feedback will raise questions about the accuracy of the definition of the goal (e.g., the condition may be chronic rather than acute and require a different treatment), self efficacy in its performance (e.g., I may not have used the treatment correctly), and the adequacy of one's selection of a comparison or support system for diagnosis and prescribing (e.g., my wife/friend/doctor, didn't know what it was; I need a second opinion; they should have given me an antibiotic). Social comparison, therefore, is involved in each of these questions. The evaluation of a procedure such as social comparison is inherently multidimensional.

As evaluating and conserving resources are central to the self management process, it is clear that the self will become increasingly salient and a target for comparison and information acquisition the more a disease threatens the existence of the self and disrupts its daily functions. Prior literature has focused on evaluations of the self (e.g., opinions about how well one is doing relative to others or bolstering of self-esteem resulting from downward comparisons with those performing less well). As we pointed out in our discussion, the self is present to varying degrees in the elaboration of every disease model; that is, the model has implications for the self (e.g., "Am I vulnerable?"; Gibbons & Gerrard, chapter 3, this volume; Hooker & Kaus, 1994; Klein & Weinstein, chapter 2, this volume). Indeed, the more procedures and outcome evaluations a person experiences the more salient the self is likely to become as a focus for evaluation and comparison, even for diseases that are not life threatening. Repeated performances and evaluations of treatments, especially when treatment outcomes are negative or ambiguous, raise questions as to whether the self is able to benefit from treatments, whether the performance of treatments was competent, and whether one made or is capable of making the right decisions to engage in treatment. Each question raises its respective image of the self at risk (e.g., the physical self as in some way unique and unable to profit from medication; the self failing to make an accurate diagnosis or to select the expert capable of making such a diagnosis; and the self at risk for an undiagnosed and untreated disease). Failures intensify questions about the self: for example, "Why didn't I ask more questions?" "How come I didn't understand what she said?" "Am I getting so forgetful?" "Was I so frightened that I didn't pay attention and remember? Because I was so frightened, do I have even more to worry about?" As questions accumulate and aspects of the self increasingly dominate a person's thinking, he will begin to consider fundamental questions concerning his ability to avoid risk and conserve resources (Leventhal, E. Leventhal, & Schaefer, 1991), eventually bringing strategies for self protection into play (E. Leventhal, Leventhal, Schaefer, & Easterling, 1993; E. Leventhal, Easterling, Leventhal, & Cameron, 1995).

The activation of the motive to protect oneself as distinct from the motive to avoid or cure a particular disease, such as cancer or a cardiovascular condition, will have important effects on a person's deployment of resources and may trigger a redefinition of major life values. Comparisons with individuals who have overcome a similar threat or learned to maximize their lives while living with it will be of special utility for the reappraisal of values, beliefs, and life skills under such difficult circumstances. While the objective of these comparisons—the maintenance of a world view necessary to sustain the self as a living and behaving system (see Taylor, 1983)—may be clear to the individual, he or she may be unconvinced of their utility because he or she is depressed and doubtful that he or she can make the needed adjustments, or is uncertain of his or her ability to bear the pain and distress to endure. These are the conditions where downward and upward comparison can be combined, the former to bolster self-esteem and garner the courage to move forward (Gruder, 1977; Hakmiller, 1966; Taylor & Lobel, 1989; Wills, 1981, 1991; Wood et al., 1985), the latter to model specific ways of coping with extremely difficult situations.

## Procedures and Appraisals

A wide variety of *coping procedures* exist for preventing, treating and recovering from disease; they are diverse both in their substance, that is, the complexity of their regimens, and in their objectives. The complexity exists because procedures are shaped and designed to answer questions and objectives specified by the various attributes of the representation.

The representation sets the problem, and coping procedures attempt to resolve or redefine it. Procedures vary from the relatively effortless tactics of watching and waiting to evaluate the seriousness of a symptom or the efficacy of a treatment intervention to the far more energy-demanding procedures involved in pain management for rheumatoid arthritis (Tennen & Affleck, chapter 9, this volume) and in initiating and adhering to an active exercise program. As Suls et al. (chapter 7, this volume) have suggested, comparisons aimed at acquiring new skills ("How do I do it?" "How can I do it better and/or more easily?") focus on ability and are likely to involve upward comparisons. Social comparison plays a key role in this process of information acquisition in the appraisal of outcome. It can clarify ambiguity in multiple areas; it often serves to clarify the identity of a disorder, and it can do so in relation to both the conceptual and concrete levels of identity. Social comparison is clearly one source of information for the use of many over-the-counter and home remedies, as seen in the antacid example.

Procedures typically have a plausible causal connection to the condition being treated. For example, I take an antacid by mouth and not by an injection because when I swallow, it goes right to my stomach, that is, the distressed area. The tight link of procedure to representation also supports the assumed time frame for treatment, that is, I expect to feel an immediate effect as the antacid goes right to the irritated area. Procedures activate expectations regarding their consequences; they are expected to have observable effects on the eliciting threat, and a variety of other effects, some good some bad, related to their impact on the body. In a factor analytic study of medication beliefs, Weinman, Petrie, Moss-Morris, and Horne (1996) have identified two such factors, one presents a positive view of medications as necessary to prevent and treat disease, the other a more negative view suggesting that medications are addictive, hence dangerous. These culture-wide beliefs develop from an interaction of social and personal experience; social information, often of the comparison type, establishes a framework for attending to and interpreting somatic experience during illness and treatment.

## SOCIAL COMPARISON, SIMILARITY, AND THE MINIMIZATION OF HEALTH THREATS

Kulik and Mahler's (1987) work on rooming with coronary artery bypass patients, Jemmott and Croyle's (1991) work on shared risk for pancreatic disorder, and Misovich et al.'s (chapter 4, this volume) work on the image of the AIDS-susceptible person, clearly imply that social comparison often reduces fear and feelings of threat. It would seem best to describe these comparisons as horizontal rather than downward or upward and as naturally occurring or more or less unavoidable perceptions of social reality rather than as comparisons made deliberately to achieve a particular mental state. The implications of these comparisons depend on whether the participants do or do not share a common fate. Although the informational environment appears "fixed" or "forced," the conclusions drawn from the comparison are not; the individual making the comparison can draw very different conclusions depending on whether he or she represents the other person's experience as relevant to him or herself.

The decision that another person's experience is or is not relevant to oneself requires that the problem solver evaluate whether he or she and potential others share attributes relevant to the threat and its management. In many cases, external reality establishes a framework that defines sharing or similarity: Kulik's comparer and other are both experiencing coronary artery bypass surgery; Wood et al.'s (1985) participants are cancer patients comparing themselves to other cancer patients; Misovich et al.'s (chapter 4, this volume) gay communicator and adolescent audience share exposure to information on a topic but do not share lifestyles. This process can serve to validate an individual's representation of a disease threat, to assist in the choice of treatment (coping) procedure, and to evaluate the efficacy of a treatment.

Examining the social comparison process in the context of self-regulation for the control of health threats shows that social comparison is a complex process. One part of its complexity is the selection of a comparison other, and the representation of the health threat is one of several factors that help define similarity, or relevance of experience. The "cheesecake experiment" provides a clear and simple example of the way a set of somatic events stimulates social comparison. The first step establishes shared experience, followed by environmental analysis to identify the cause and meaning of the symptomatology. This experiment began with the midnight awakening of a middle-aged man who had spent a pleasant day with his wife enjoying the sights, sounds, and tastes of the city. Experiencing nausea and severe stomach cramps, he went to the bathroom and vomited. The severity, rapid onset, and unusual nature of his symptoms evoked images of a worsening condition, perhaps an ulcer or cancer, something with imminent, life-threatening effects. At the same time, the man feared he might look foolish if he called for medical help and the pain signaled nothing more than a case of the flu. As the cramps and sick feeling returned a few minutes after the mighty heave, he was left in a state of suspended uncertainty, when at 12:35 AM, his wife awoke to the sounds of his not sufficiently muted groans. He asked her how she felt. She replied that she felt nauseous and uncomfortable and that she thought she suffered from indigestion. Is this the same nausea? The husband described his symptoms, their location and severity, and the wife responded that she felt similarly. The husband then said that he had also been feeling some fatigue and had a headache, which would suggest the flu. Because the wife did not have these symptoms, flu did not fit the shared set. As her nausea worsened, she vomited as well.

It is clear that the couple share a key set of somatic events, and this area of intersubjective agreement allows them to proceed to the next step–exploring the possible cause of their conditions. A review of the events of the day points to a possible culprit: the cheesecake at lunch! They each had different sandwiches, but they shared a piece of very tasty cheesecake. Because the weather was warm and because they questioned whether the cake had been stored properly they concluded they are suffering from food poisoning. Support for this hypothesis is strengthened further by the time frame: it is 12 hours, plus or minus 30 minutes, since they consumed the cheesecake, the right length of time for the development of a minor case of food poisoning. Having diagnosed the problem and identified its cause, the husband relaxes, feels less pain and distress, and returns to sleep.

Examples abound of the contribution of social comparison to the selection of self-care procedures. The elderly are famous for sharing their medication following discussion of their medical conditions and prescribed treatments. The selection of a similarity dimension for comparison often seems to focus on similarity of symptoms (i.e., if symptoms are similar the condition is assumed to be similar), similarity of condition (i.e., if the conditions are thought to be the same), and similarity of treatments (i.e., if the medication is thought to be similar). These similarities lead people to feel that it is legitimate to compare and to modify their medication schedules in order to reduce the number and intensity of their symptoms. Some may even go as far as to borrow another person's medication. Of course, if the symptoms monitored are related to an illness other than the disease under treatment, the variation in medication can be both nonproductive and dangerous.

## CONCLUSION

We suggested at the outset that it might be more useful to label the patient a problem solver than a social comparer. As social comparison theories were devised to help us understand the ways in which others influence our attitudes under conditions of uncertainty, their use in discussions of health seems reasonable. Uncertainty in the health arena is rampant with regard to the definition of health threats and the selection and evaluation of procedures for their containment. Upon closer examination, however, it is clear that social comparison is but one of the methods people use to reduce uncertainty about a health threat. Therefore, we conclude that social comparison must be examined within a larger health framework.

Based on our review of current trends we determined that social comparison should be approached as a process rather than a trait. This implies that the psychometric methods used to study social comparison will have to be revised. We also concluded that social comparison in real world settings is not merely a product of the individual or of the situation. Rather, it is the individual's motivation within each situation that determines the role of social comparison. Thus, a person–situation transactional model of threat is essential to our understanding of social comparison in health situations.

Our construction of a transactional model emphasizing person–situation interactions led us to conceive of new ways to apply a common-sense approach in modeling representations and procedures for coping with somatic events. The common-sense approach provides a framework in which to examine the process of information seeking, including that of social comparison. This framework emphasizes the need to represent the individual as a problem solver. It includes three sets of elements: (a) the individual's representation of the disease, (b) the individual's representation of the self, and (c) the perceived procedures available for problem solution, including the resources available. We argue that social comparison is involved in each of these areas and we show how its process can differ within and between these areas.

It is reasonable to ask whether the framework provides insight into social comparison processes. We believe it does by suggesting new interpretations for these processes and new avenues for research. We urge that future explorations of social comparison in disease threat situations include representations of the disease, of the situation, and of the self. All of these components must be present if we hope to gain a better understanding of the processes involved.

## REFERENCES

Abelson, R. (1981). Psychological status of the script concept. *American Psychologist, 36,* 715–729.

Abramson, L. Y., Seligman, M. E. P., & Teasdale, J. (1978). Learned helplessness in humans: Critique and reformulation. *Journal of Abnormal Psychology, 87,* 49–74.

Baumann, L. J., & Leventhal, H. (1985). "I can tell when my blood pressure is up, can't I?" *Health Psychology, 4,* 203–218.

Beck, A. T. (1967). *Depression: Clinical, experimental, and theoretical aspects.* New York:

Harper & Row.

Blumhagen, D. (1980). Hyper-tension: A folk illness with a medical name. *Culture, Medicine, and Psychiatry, 4,* 197–227.

Bower, G. H., Black, J. B., & Turner, T. J. (1979). Scripts in memory of text. *Cognitive Psychology, 11,* 177–220.

Brownlee, S., Leventhal, H., & Balaban, M. (1992). Autonomic correlates of illness imagery. *Psychophysiology, 29,* 1–13.

Cameron, L., Leventhal, E. A., & Leventhal, H. (1993). Symptom representations and affect as determinants of care seeking in a community dwelling adult sample population. *Health Psychology, 12,* 171–179.

Festinger, L. (1954). A theory of social comparison processes. *Human Relations, 7,* 117–140.

Gruder, C. (1977). Choice of comparison persons in evaluating one's self. In J. Suls & R. Miller (Eds.), *Social comparison processes: Theoretical and empirical perspectives* (pp. 21–42). Washington, DC: Hemisphere.

Hakmiller, K. L. (1966). Threat as a determinant of downward comparison. *Journal of Experimental Social Psychology Supplement, 1,* 32–39.

Hooker, K., & Kaus, C. R. (1994). Health-related possible selves in young and middle adulthood. *Psychology and Aging, 9,* 126–133.

Janis, I. L. (1958). *Psychological stress.* New York: Wiley.

Jemmott, J. B., & Croyle, R. T. (1991). Psychological reactions to risk factor testing. In J. A. Skelton & R. T. Croyle (Eds.), *Mental representation in health and illness* (pp. 1–31). New York: Springer-Verlag.

Kurglanski, A. W., & Mayseless, O. (1990). Classic and current social comparison research: Expanding the perspective. *Psychological Bulletin, 108,* 195–208.

Krohne, H. W. (1993). Vigilance and cognitive avoidance as concepts in coping research. In H. W. Krohne (Ed.), *Attention and avoidance* (pp. 19–50). Seattle, WA: Hogrefe & Huber.

Kulik, J. A., & Mahler, H. I. M. (1987). The effects of preoperative roommate assignment on preoperative anxiety and postoperative recovery from bypass surgery. *Health Psychology, 6,* 525–543.

Lazarus, R. S., & Folkman, S. (1984). *Stress, appraisal, and coping.* New York: Springer.

Leventhal, E. A., Easterling, D., Leventhal, H., & Cameron, L. (1995). Conservation of energy, uncertainty reduction and swift utilization of medical care among the elderly: Study II. *Medical Care, 33,* 988–1000.

Leventhal, E. A., Leventhal, H., Schaefer, P., & Easterling, D. (1993). Conservation of energy, uncertainty reduction and swift utilization of medical care among the elderly. *Journal of Gerontology: Psychological Sciences, 48,* 78–86.

Leventhal, H. (1970). Findings and theory in the study of fear communications. *Advances in Experimental Social Psychology, 5,* 119–186.

Leventhal, H. (1984). A perceptual motor theory of emotion. *Advances in Experimental Social Psychology, 17,* 117–182.

Leventhal, H., Diefenbach, M., & Leventhal, E. A. (1992). Illness cognition: Using common sense to understand adherence and affect cognition interactions. *Cognitive Therapy and Research, 16,* 143–163.

Leventhal, H., & Everhart, D. (1979). Emotion, pain, and physical illness. In C. E. Izard (Ed.), *Emotions and psychopathology* (pp. 263–299). New York: Plenum Press.

Leventhal, H., Leventhal, E. A., & Schaefer, P. (1991). Vigilant coping and health behavior: A life span problem. In M. Ory & R. Abeles (Eds.), *Aging, health, and behavior* (pp. 109–140). Baltimore: Johns Hopkins.

Leventhal, H., Meyer, D., & Nerenz, D. (1980). The common sense representation of illness danger. In S. Rachman (Ed.), *Contributions to medical psychology* (Vol. 2, pp. 7–30). Elmsford, NY: Pergamon.

Meyer, D., Leventhal, H., & Gutmann, M. (1985). Common-sense models of illness: The example of hypertension. *Health Psychology, 4,* 115–135.
Radloff, R. (1966). Social comparison in ability evaluation. *Journal of Experimental Social Psychology, Supplement 1,* 6–26.
Schachter, S. (1959). *The psychology of affiliation.* Stanford, CA: Stanford University Press.
Schachter, S., & Singer, J. E. (1962). Cognitive, social, and physiological determinants of emotional state. *Psychological Review, 69,* 379–399.
Smith, W. P. (1984). Judgmental goals in the social comparison of ability. *Representative Research in Social Psychology, 14,* 36–51.
Taylor, S., & Lobel, M. (1989). Social comparison activity under threat: Downward evaluation and upward contacts. *Psychology Review, 96,* 569–575.
Taylor, S. E. (1983). Adjustment to threatening events: A theory of cognitive adaptation. *American Psychologist, 11,* 1161–1173.
Teasdale, J., & Barnard, P. (1993). *Affect cognition and change: Remodelling depressive thought.* Hove, UK: Lawrence Erlbaum Associates.
Thorndike, E. L. (1913). *The psychology of learning.* (Educational psychology II). New York: Teachers College.
Weinman, J., Petrie, K. J., Moss-Morris, R., & Horne, R. (1996). The illness perception questionnaire: A new method for assessing the cognitive representation of illness. *Psychology and Health: The International Review of Health Psychology, 11*(3), 431–445.
Wills, T. A. (1981). Downward comparison principles in social psychology. *Psychological Bulletin, 90*(2), 245–271.
Wills, T. A. (1991). Similarity and self-esteem in downward comparison. In J. Suls & T. A. Wills (Eds.), *Social comparison: Contemporary theory and research* (pp. 51–78). Hillsdale, NJ: Lawrence Erlbaum Associates.
Wood, J. V., & Taylor, K. L. (1991). Serving self-relevant goals through social comparison. In J. Suls & T. A. Wills (Eds.), *Social comparison: Contemporary theory and research* (pp. 23–50). Hillsdale, NJ: Lawrence Erlbaum Associates.
Wood, J. V., Taylor, S. E., & Lichtman, R. R. (1985). Social comparison in adjustment to breast cancer. *Journal of Personality and Social Psychology, 49*(5), 1169–1183.
Zola, I. K. (1973). Pathways to the doctor: From person to patient. *Social Science and Medicine, 7*(9), 677–689.

# Author Index

## C

L



M

T

Y



Z

# Subject Index

N



O



P



R



S



T



U

For Product Safety Concerns and Information please contact our EU
representative GPSR@taylorandfrancis.com
Taylor & Francis Verlag GmbH, Kaufingerstraße 24, 80331 München, Germany

www.ingramcontent.com/pod-product-compliance
Ingram Content Group UK Ltd.
Pitfield, Milton Keynes, MK11 3LW, UK
UKHW022114190926
475702UK00013B/1429
*9781138975897*